FASCIA

Clinical Applications for Health and Human Performance

By Dr. Mark Lindsay, BSc., D.C.

and Chad Robertson, BSc (Pharm), BSc (Kin)

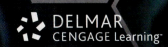

DELMAR
CENGAGE Learning™

Australia • Brazil • Japan • Korea • Mexico • Singapore • Spain • United Kingdom • United States

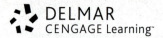

Fascia: Clinical Applications for Health and Human Performance
Dr. Mark Lindsay
Chad Robertson

Vice President, Career and Professional
  Editorial: Dave Garza

Director of Learning Solutions:
  Matthew Kane

Managing Editor: Marah Bellegarde

Acquisitions Editor: Matthew Seeley

Product Manager:
  Jadin Babin-Kavanaugh

Marketing Director: Jennifer McAvey

Senior Marketing Manager: Lynn Henn

Marketing Manager: Michele McTighe

Production Director: Carolyn Miller

Content Project Manager:
  Kenneth McGrath

Senior Art Director: Jack Pendleton

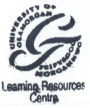
For product information and technology assistance, contact us at
Professional & Career Group Customer Support, 1-800-354-9706

For permission to use material from this text or product,
submit all requests online at **www.cengage.com/permissions**
Further permissions questions can be emailed to
permissionrequest@cengage.com

Library of Congress Control Number: 2007942498

ISBN-13: 978-1-418-05569-1

ISBN-10: 1-418-05569-7

Delmar
5 Maxwell Drive
Clifton Park, NY 12065-2919
USA

Cengage Learning is a leading provider of customized learning solutions with office locations around the globe, including Singapore, the United Kingdom, Australia, Mexico, Brazil, and Japan. Locate your local office at: **international.cengage.com/region**

Cengage Learning products are represented in Canada by Nelson Education, Ltd.

For your lifelong learning solutions, visit **delmar.cengage.com**

Visit our corporate website at **www.cengage.com**

Printed in Canada
1 2 3 4 5 6 7 11 10 09 08

CONTENTS

Foreword xv

Preface xvi

About the Authors xviii

Contributors/Reviewers xix

Chapter 1   **Histology of the Living Matrix** 1

Components of Fascia 2

Cellular Anatomy of Fascia 2

    ○ Fibroblasts 2

    ○ Mast Cells 2

    ○ Adipose Cells 3

    ○ Macrophages 4

Fascial Fibers 4

    ○ Collagen Fibers 4

    ○ Reticular Fibers 7

    ○ Elastic Fibers 7

    ○ Functions of the Collageno-elastic Complex in Fascia 8

Extracellular Matrix 8

    ○ Ground Substance 9

    ○ Proteoglycans 9

    ○ Hyaluronic Acid 9

    ○ Functions of Ground Substance 10

Summary 13

References 13

Chapter 2   **Anatomical Description of Fascia and Its Planes** 16

Anatomy and Physiology of Fascial Planes 18

Fascia Superficialis 18

Fascia Profunda (Deep) 18

Deepest Fascia 18

Cellulite 18

Variation between Sexes...18

Variations with Adiposity 19

Variations in Different Body Regions.....................................19

Zones of Adherence..19

Fascia Profunda 20

Deepest Fascia 20

Identifying Fascial Planes..20

Summary 34

References 35

Chapter 3   **Tensegrity, Thixotropy, and Somatic Recall** 36

What is Tensegrity? 38

Tensegrity at the Cellular Level 39

The Actin Filament and Cell Motility 42

Cellular Tensegrity and Mechanotransduction.....................42

Tensegrity and Myofascia 43

What is Thixotropy? 43

Thixotropy and the Musculoskeletal System 44

Sol-to-Gel Transition in Collagen 45

Somatic Recall 45

Somatic Recall and Cellular Tensegrity 46

Summary 47

References 47

Chapter 4   **Neurophysiological Basis for Fascial Plasticity** 50

**Fascial Tissue Mechanical Behavior—Biomechanical
Models** 53

Fascial Anatomy 53

Mechanical Response of Fascia to External Loading.....................53

Effect of Injury and Immobilization on Myofascial Trigger Points 55

Mechanical Effects of Fascial Manual Therapy 55

Neurophysiological Dynamics of Fascia 56

The Nervous System 56

    Central Nervous System 56

    Peripheral Nervous System 59

    Autonomic Nervous System............................60

The Reflex Arc and Reflexes 60

Fascial Sensory Receptors 60

A New Type of Receptor..61

Nociceptive Stability and Plasticity 62

Intrafascial Cells Control Contractility 63

Summary 65

References 65

Chapter 5   **Water, the Key Nutrient for Fascia** 68

Mechanical Properties of Fascia 70

Physiological Purpose of Water 70

Effects of Dehydration on the Tissue Tensegrity Matrix System 71

New Research Findings..74

Maintenance Dose of Water...................................76

Summary 77

References 77

Chapter 6   **The Role of Fascia and its Related Pathologies** 78

Mechanical Role 80

    Movement...80

    Adaptation and Protection 81

    Transmission of Force 83

Physiological Role...83

    Metabolic Role 83

    Hemodynamic Role 84

    Lymphatic Role 84

Fascia-Related Pathologies 85

    Insulin Resistance 85

Aging..85

Scar Formation 87

Compartment Syndrome 88

Infections 88

Plantar Fasciitis..88

Summary 89

References 89

Chapter 7   **Comprehensive Evaluation of Myofascial Injuries** 92

Clinical Assessment for Myofascial Injuries...........................94

Physical 94

Causes 94

Differentials..94

○ Fibromyalgia...95

○ Articular Dysfunction Requiring Manual
Mobilization 95

○ Nonmyofascial TrPs 95

○ Radiculopathy 95

Workup and Lab Studies...95

Imaging Studies..95

○ Why Image Myofascial Injuries?......................95

Normal Skeletal Muscle Anatomy and
MRI Characteristics 96

○ Characteristics of Normal Muscle Imaging 96

○ Characteristics of Injured Muscle Imaging........96

○ MRI Findings in Muscle Strain 97

Common Sports-Related Myofascial Injuries............................99

Upper Extremity..99

Pectoralis Major 99

Lower Extremity 100

Hamstring 101

Quadriceps...102

Adductors 102

Medial Gastrocnemius...102

Magnetic Resonance Imaging 103

Ultrasound 103

    Imaging Characteristics of Normal Muscle 104

    Imaging Characteristics of Injured Muscle 104

        ○ Grade I Strain 104

        ○ Grade II Strain 105

        ○ Grade III Strain 105

    Ultrasound-Guided Musculoskeletal Intervention 105

Summary 108

References 108

Chapter 8

**Manual and Rehabilitative Techniques Used
for Soft Tissue Injuries** 112

Movement Dysfunction 114

Principles of Rehabilitation 114

    Rest, Ice, Compression, and Elevation (RICE) 116

        ○ Rest 116

        ○ Ice 116

        ○ Compression 116

        ○ Elevation 116

**Rehabilitation Strategy for Restoring Dynamic Stability
and Muscular Strength** 117

    Local Stability System—Control of the Neutral Joint Position 117

    Global Stability System—Control the Direction
    of Stability Dysfunction 117

    Global Stability System—Control of Imbalance 117

Manual Therapy 118

    Stretching 118

    Articular Pumping 118

    Active Release Technique® (ART) 118

    Manual Resistance Technique (MRT) 119

    Proprioception 119

    Isometric Exercise 119

    Isotonic Exercise 120

    Plyometrics 120

Summary 120

References 120

Chapter 9   **Consevative Rehabilitation Protocols
for Fascia Injuries**..122

**Treatment and Rehabilitation of Adhesive Capsulitis:
Multiphase Approach** 124

**Phase I — Acute Trauma, Inflammation and
Phagocytosis** 124

Phase II — Initiate and Establish Healing 125

Myofascial Mobility and Articular Pumping 126

Active Release Technique® and/or Sound-Assisted Soft Tissue
Mobilization (SASTM) 133

Articular Range of Motion: Muscle Activation Technique (MAT)......133

Shoulder Stretch (posterior capsule)............................133

○ Perform Range of Motion Exercises (passive, active-assisted,
active) at a Pain-free Level 134

○ Increase Range of Motion and Restoration of Function 134

Proprioceptive Neuromuscular Facilitation (PNF) 135

Neuromuscular Control: Proprioceptive
and Kinesthetic Awareness.....................................135

○ Dynamic Joint Stability 136

○ Weight-Bearing Shift Exercises 136

○ Preparatory and Muscle Reactivation 137

○ Rhythmic Stabilization against Perturbation.....................137

○ Functional Motor Patterns......................................138

○ Active Isometric Strengthening Exercises Shoulder
Internal Rotation, Standing 138

○ Shoulder External Rotation.......................................139

○ Standing Three-Way Stretch 139

○ Dynamic Blackburn 139

○ Seated Scapular Pinches...141

○ Supine Cervical Retractions 141

Phase III — Intermediate Phase 141

Rehabilitation Protocol 142

○ PNF Exercises...142

○ Scapular Stabilization Exercises 142

○ Shoulder Plyometric Exercises..143

Phase IV — Advanced Strengthening Phase and Return to Prior Activity Level..144

Rehabilitation Protocol...145

○ Interval Throwing Program..146

○ Preparation for Returning to the Prior Activity Level (work, recreational, or sport)...146

ACL Rehabilitation Program Following ACL Reconstruction 146

Rehabilitation 148

Reconditioning 148

○ Strength and Conditioning around the Knee....................................148

Pool Training..149

○ Program Outline 149

○ Workouts..150

Cardiovascular and Strength Endurance Training Series..150

Elliptical Cross-Trainer: Hill Running 152

○ Definitions...152

○ Workout 152

Treadmill Retrograde Hill Walk 152

○ Definitions...152

○ Workout 153

Bike Conditioning Programs 154

○ Definitions...154

○ Workouts..154

ACL Rehabilitative Case Study—January 2007 155

Phase I Protocol 156

Phase II Protocol 159

Phase III Protocol 161

Phase IV Protocol 162

Summary 162

References 162

Chapter 10 **The Role of Energy Medicine in the Therapeutic Treatment of Fascia** 166

Electromagnetic Healing of Fractured Bone 168

Complementary Medicine 168

    Frequency-Specific Microcurrent Therapy 169

    Low-Level Laser Therapy...171

    Clinical Application of Low-Level Laser..172

    Acupuncture Therapy 175

        ○ Role of Connective Tissue Winding..176

        ○ Mechanical Signal Transduction..177

        ○ Potential Downstream Effects of Needle Grasp 177

    Myofascial/Active Release Therapy 179

    What Is Earthing™? 181

        ○ The Physiological Effects of Earthing™ (Grounding) in the Body...182

        ○ Clinical Applications 182

        ○ Athletic Recovery 182

    The Physiological Effects of Free Radicals in the Body....................182

        ○ Physiological Aspects of Redox Regulation 183

        ○ Molecular Aspects of Redox Regulation: Gain or Loss of Function, or Outright Destruction 183

        ○ Regulated Versus Uncontrolled Free Radical Production: Increased ROS Levels in Old Age and Disease 183

        ○ Chances for Therapeutic Intervention—Earthing™ 183

        ○ Treatment of Pathophysiological Disease and Stress.........................184

Summary 184

References 184

Chapter 11 **Nutrition and Fascial Health** 189

Nutritional Intake and Its Effects on Connective Tissue Healing 190

    Caloric Intake..190

    Protein..190

    Carbohydrates 194

    Fats...194

Specific Nutrients 195

    Arginine 195

Carnosine 196

Glutamine 196

Copper 196

Zinc 196

Orthosilicic Acid 196

EPA 196

Aloe Vera 197

Bromelain 197

Curcumin 197

Centella (Gotu Kola) 198

Superoxide Dismutase (SOD) 198

Vitamin A 198

Vitamin C (Oral) 198

Vitamin C Intravenous 199

Cetylated Monounsaturated Fatty Acid 200

Vitamin B_5 200

Summary 200

References 202

Chapter 12   **Nutritional Support for Ischemic Conditions** 204

Effects of Ischemia on Energy Production 206

Reperfusion Injury 206

**Cell Injury Due to Ischemia and
Reperfusion** 207

Reactive Oxygen Species 207

Coagulative and Fibrinolytic Pathways 208

Changes in the Microcirculation in Ischemia 210

**Ischemic Effects on Heart and
Skeletal Muscle** 210

Nutritional Treatment of Ischemia 211

Minerals 211

Enzymes 212

  ○ Bromelain 212

  ○ Nattokinase 213

  ○ Removal of Immune Complexes 213

○ Removal of Fibrin 213

○ Inhibition of Pro-inflammatory Compounds 214

Chapter 13   **Nutritional Support for Inflammatory Conditions**.................218

Acute inflammation 220

Chronic inflammation 220

The Role of Flavonoids 220

Quercetin 221

Boswellia 221

Turmeric 221

Resveratrol 222

Ginger 222

Cat's Claw 223

Other Nutrients and Inflammation...224

Vitamin B_6...224

Lactoferrin...224

Superoxide Dismutase 225

Fish Oil 225

Cetylated Monounsaturated Fatty Acid 225

Summary 225

References 225

Chapter 14   **Pharmacological Management of Fascial Pathologies** 228

Growth Factors and Immune Response 230

Epidermal Growth Factor (EGF) 230

Insulin-like Growth Factor (IGF-1 and their IGFs) 230

Human Growth Hormone (HGH) 230

Fibroblast Growth Factor-10 (FGF-10) 231

Vascular Endothelial Growth Factor (VEGF).................................231

Modulating the Immune Response During Healing...231

Antifibrotics 231

Nonsteroidal Anti-inflammatory Drugs (NSAIDs) 233

Problems with NSAIDs...234

Specific COX-2 inhibitors...234

Topical NSAIDs 235

Local Injection Therapy...235

Local Anesthetic Injections and Dry Needling 235

Local Administration of Actovegin 236

Summary 237

References 237

Chapter 15   **Management of Myofascial Injuries
in the Athlete—Case Studies**....................................240

Treating at a Global Level 243

Treatment of Fascia 243

**Case Study 1: Treatment of Proximal Hamstring Pain
Using Active Release Technique® Applied to the
Myofascial Meridians** 243

Background 244

Case History 244

Discussion...247

Conclusion..249

**Case Study 2: Global Treatment of a Surgically
Repaired Torn Supraspinatus in an
Overhand-Throwing Pitcher**......................................249

**Case Study 3: Global Treatment of a Surgically
Repaired Left Anterior Cruciate Ligament
in a Soccer Player** 251

**Case Study 4: Global Treatment of Surgically
Repaired Achilles Tendon in a Volleyball Player**.........252

Discussion...253

Conclusion..253

**Case Study 5: Quantifying Pre-Functional and
Functional Rehabilitation in an
Injured Soccer Player**...253

Case History 255

Physical Examination..255

Imaging 255

Blood Testing for the Athlete 256
    ○ Genetics and Blood Testing Interpretation 257

Diagnosis 260

Treatment..260

Abbreviations..260

Functional Rehabilitation 265

Return to Play Following Muscle Strains 266
    ○ Strength and Flexibility Testing..266
    ○ Imaging 267
    ○ Functional Field Testing..267
    ○ Risk Management Strategies 267
    ○ Results 267

Discussion..268

Summary 268

References 269

Index 273

Advances in the field of sports medicine have been evolving rapidly over the past 10 years. Athletes as well as the population in general are putting more demand on their bodies, which can result in musculoskeletal injuries. Muscle and fascial injuries are still an enigma in the hands of many physicians when it comes to appropriate treatment. Dr. Mark Lindsay has to be commended for his work on this topic. His participation in treating patients with musculoskeletal injuries in six Olympic games, and his exclusive innovation in treating elite athletes makes him a unique authority in this important part of sports medicine. This book is more than just a textbook on fascia; it is a complete multidisciplinary approach to the topic with hundreds of references. This is a well-balanced and inclusive textbook with innovative techniques and understanding of all aspects of the fascia brought by experience. This book will benefit all who are involved in the circle of sports medicine including orthopaedics surgeons and related disciplines. Dr. Mark Lindsay drew on his outstanding experience in the field and has provided us with a text that deals with all of the important points on this topic, most importantly the assessment of problems and planning in the management of patient rehabilitation. This book is a substantial achievement, and the authors and contributors should be commended for this "state of the art" advancement of the topic of fascial injuries and treatment. The field of sports medicine stands to gain from a better understanding of the clinical application and treatment of fascial injuries to improve human performance. This will allow us all to better serve our patients and clients on the sports field or in the operating room.

Marc J. Philippon, M.D.
Steadman Hawkins Clinic
Vale, Colorado

Fascia: Clinical Applications for Human Health and Performance is written for both students and practitioners in health-related disciplines who need to be firmly grounded in their understanding of the significance of fascia, the role of nutrition in fascial health, how injuries and disease impact fascia, and rehabilitative techniques to restore functional capacity of the affected tissue. For too long, therapists and health professionals have used antiquated methods in treating fascial injuries, largely because there was no knowledge base to support new treatment applications and techniques. This text offers a remedy to this situation and will serve as a unique and valuable reference, bringing together the latest trends and treatments in fascia. It is my hope that with this new guide, the fields of sports medicine, athletic training, physical therapy, massage therapy, and chiropractic will embrace these new and less invasive methods for treatment.

CONCEPTUAL APPROACH

The impetus for this book came about as a result of the dearth of material focusing on the importance of fascia and its role in overall health and functionality of the human body. Existing anatomy textbooks and atlases fail to fully appreciate and explore the complex and diverse role that the connective tissue fascia performs in the body. In order to be effective, clinicians and therapists must thoroughly understand that fascia is capable of affecting the whole body, not just one system. Thus, the conceptual approach to the book is that in order for a health professional and/or body worker to be effective in preventing and treating injuries to the fascia, they must first value its overarching role within the human body.

ORGANIZATION OF THE TEXT

The organization of this text prepares the reader to become firmly grounded in the essentials of fascia before tackling current advances in clinical application. The book is organized into four major parts:

1. Basic histology and physiology of the fascia system

2. Standard evaluation and manual treatment techniques

3. Focus on non-manual treatment techniques (nutrition and pharmacological)

4. Emphasis on sports injuries/ case studies

In order to make this book truly useful to the health practitioner and body worker, it often employs a quick reference format with its strong use of tables, lists, and text headings. This enables the reader to quickly access concepts without having to wade through excessive narrative. In addition, the use of figures strengthens the validity and clarity of text materials.

Contributions from leading researchers and practitioners ensure that our content is indeed the leading material available with regard to clinical applications in use today. Application chapters are enhanced with case studies utilizing recovery techniques which are goal oriented and comprehensive. An extensive bibliography (where applicable) encompasses each chapter to enable the curious reader to learn more and further strengthen their knowledge base on this critical subject of fascia.

The Online Companion

The publisher has provided a website that contains full-sized versions of many of the diagnostic images found in this book. To access, please go to www.delmarlearning.com/companions and search for this book using ISBN number 1-418-05569-7. The user id is 'LindsayOLC' and the password is 'enter.'

Acknowledgments

My most sincere thanks to my mentors Dr. David Leaf, Dr. Mike Leahy, Dr. Guy Voyer, and colleague Dan Pfaff whose encouragement and input provided me with a comprehensive educational and training background which challenged me to become an innovator in patient care and research. Also, my deepest appreciation to my loving wife Kate for her continuous encouragement, support, and personal sacrifices which enabled me to achieve this personal goal.

ABOUT THE AUTHORS

DR. MARK LINDSAY, BSc., D.C.

Dr. Mark Lindsay is one of the most sought after chiropractors and soft tissue specialists by professional, world, and Olympic athletes, and by organizations such as the NHL, NFL, NBA, and MLB. He is a graduate of Palmer Chiropractic College and Guelph University, where he earned a Bachelor of Science and Kinesiology. In 1996, Lindsay was named "Outstanding Field Doctor" by the Canadian Chiropractic Sports Fellowship through his intensive work with Olympic Champion Donovan Bailey.

Lindsay's work benefits from the personal understanding that he gained as a former athlete. Like his clients, he strove to push physical boundaries and had to overcome serious injury from time to time. Throughout his years in the field, Lindsay has developed a strong network of clients and professionals, each working at the top of their fields. Readers are offered the opportunity to take advantage of this network of knowledge and experience through this cutting-edge text that explores the exciting and significant field of fascia.

Dr. Lindsay has consulted for the Oakland Raiders, Denver Broncos, Toronto Maple Leafs, and the Columbus Blue Jackets. He was named a Canadian Olympic Committee Team Doctor at five Olympic Games. Dr. Lindsay is currently the President of Lindsay Sports Therapy Inc., and runs a private practice and consulting business in Toronto, Ontario.

CHAD ROBERTSON, BSc (PHARM), BSc (KIN)

Chad Robertson obtained his Bachelor of Science (Kinesiology) degree at Simon Fraser University in British Columbia in addition to a Bachelor of Pharmacy and Pharmaceutical Sciences degree at the University of Alberta. He has been formally recognized for his numerous scholastic achievements. He has broad research experience in fields ranging from cerebral autoregulation dynamics during space flight to soft tissue injuries and related pathologies. He has served as a consultant in the areas of dietary strategies and nutritional supplementation for numerous professional and Olympic athletes. In addition he has co-authored a peer-reviewed paper—"Compressive Ulnar Neuropathy at the Elbow" published in the indexed Journal of Manipulative and Physiological Therapeutics. His most recent endeavors include working as a full-time pharmacist in addition to formulating and manufacturing natural health products.

CONTRIBUTORS/ REVIEWERS

CONTRIBUTORS

Steve Haltiwanger, MD, CCN
Health and Science Director of Life Wave
www.lifewave.com
El Paso, Texas

Bill Knowles, ATC, CSCS
Director of iSPORT Training
Killington Medical Clinic
Killington, Vermont

Anthony T. Mascia, MD, FRCPC, DABR
Director of Musculoskeletal Imaging
Humber River Regional Hospital
Toronto, Ontario

Ron Otsu BSc, BSc (Pharm)
Langley, British Columbia

Dr. Jason Pajaczkowski, BSc, BS, CSCS, DC, FCCSS(C),
    DACRB, D. Ac, ART
Director, Sports Performance Centres, Ltd.
Mississauga, Ontario

Dr. John Saratsiotis, BSc, BA, DC, CSCS
Athens, Greece

Chad Robertson, BSc (Pharm), BSc (Kin)
Zanagen Limited

Dr. Andreo A. Spina, B. Kin, DC, D. Ac, ART, CCSS(C)
Director, Sports Performance Centres, Ltd.
Vaughan, Ontario

Ben Velasquez, CSCS
Somato Therapist (Performance Rehabilitation)
Certified Advanced Posturologist
New York, New York
http://www.benvelazquez.com

REVIEWERS

Lori Dewald, EdD, ATC, CHES
Associate Professor of Exercise Science
Salisbury University
Salisbury, Maryland

William Leland Elliott, MS, FT, CPT, CNMT, LMT
Exercise Physiologist and Neuromuscular
Therapist/Instructor
Colorado Institute of Massage Theraphy
Colorado Springs, Colorado

Gil Hedley, PhD
Director, Integral Anatomy Productions, LLC
Westwood, New Jersey

Taras V. Kochno, MD
Medical Director
Sports Medicine & Rehabilitation International
Bradenton, Florida

Sara Panarello
Lincoln Family Chiropractic
Lincoln, Massachusetts

Donna Redman-Bentley, PT, PhD
Professor and Associate Dean for Research
Western University of Health Sciences
Pomona, California

Pete Whitridge, BA, LMT
Instructor and Accreditation Program Manager
Florida School of Massage
Gainesville, Florida

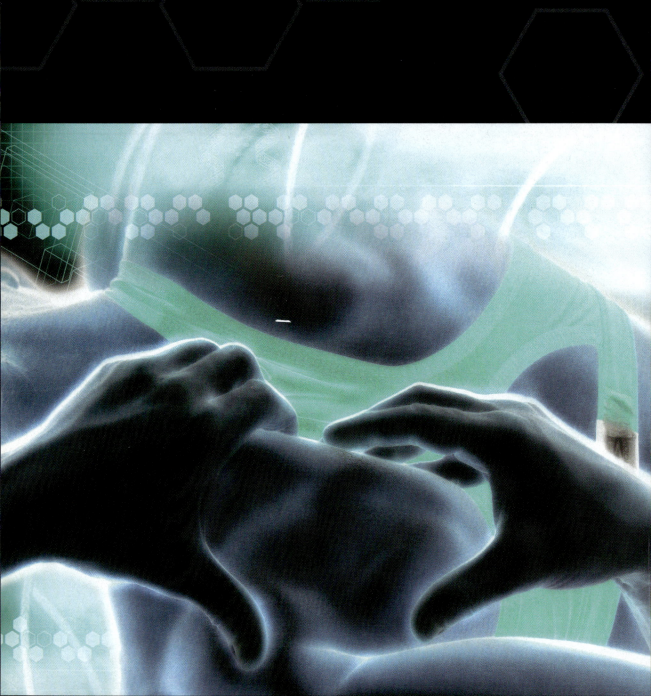

HISTOLOGY OF THE LIVING MATRIX

Connective tissue consists of a number of cells enclosed in an extracellular matrix (ECM) that contains a major portion of proteoglycans and collagen fibrils in addition to ground substance, tissue fluid, and noncollagen glycoprotein (a protein carbohydrate macromolecule (Kjaer, 2004). Connective tissue provides structural support to organs and other tissues in the body in addition to being specialized structures of blood vessels, bone, and cartilage. Together with the ECM, connective tissue forms a vast and continuous compartment throughout the body, bounded by the basal lamina of the various epithelia and by the basal or external lamina of muscle, nerve, or vascular endothelium.

Fascia is a part of the connective tissue that researchers have paid relatively little attention to in the past. Any discussion of soft tissue conditions or disorders would be incomplete and limited in scope of practice if it did not include consideration of the fascial system. Fascia and all of its components provide a contiguous connection from muscle to bone, bone to bone, and organs to their supporting structures. Together they form an independent system of strength, support, elasticity, and cushion.

COMPONENTS OF FASCIA

The cellular components of fascia consist of fibroblasts, mast cells, adipose cells, macrophages, plasma cells, and leukocytes. The fibrous components of fascia include collagen, reticular, and elastic fibers. The ground substance, a noncollagen component of the ECM, is made up of macromolecules such as proteoglycans and glycoproteins, exogenous substances, and extracellular fluid. Basically, the ECM surrounds the cell and gives support and structure to the tissue.

Hence, the fascia of the human body is comprised of three basic elements: collagen, elastic fibers, and ground substance. Each of these elements contributes to important pathological and physiological functions.

Cellular Anatomy of Fascia

As mentioned, a number of cells are found within the fascial system. All other cells—including plasma cells, monocytes, lymphocytes, multinuclear eosinophils, and basophils—can migrate within the fascia tissue.

Fibroblasts

The fibroblast is found specifically within fabrics of fascia and is the principal cell of connective tissue. It possesses unique morphological features such as a fusiform or a discoid shape with long cellular extensions. Fibroblasts are capable of a relatively high rate of synthesis of complex carbohydrates, collagen, elastic, and reticular fibers and other macromolecules of the ground substance.

Stretching and applying pressure or tension to fascia stimulates fibroblasts, as noted by Gehlsen, Ganion, and Helfst (1999). Fibroblast proliferation in response to changes in applied pressure may provide the initial stimulus for the healing cascade (Gehlsen et al., 1999). This is due to the cell's cytoskeleton functioning like a micro-tensegrity structure to transmit forces upon the cell into the interior of the cell (Ingber, 1993). Such studies have shown increased production of fibroblasts and ground matrix macromolecules, as well as orientation of newly formed fibroblasts along lines of force. Hence, mechanical force can influence fibroblasts to modify their physical and chemical properties as a result of light perturbations to the human body. This will result in changes in the fascia composition at any one time, depending on the stresses placed upon it throughout an individual's lifetime.

Helen Langevin et al. (2004) performed a study examining the dynamic response of a fibroblast's cytoskeletal response to subcutaneous tissue stretch under both ex vivo and in vivo conditions (Langevin, Cornbrooks, & Taatjes, 2004). Intra-cytoskeletal and extra-cytoskeletal applied tension forces affected the shape and consequently the function of fibroblasts. Langevin, Cornbrooks, et al. (2004) showed that shortened tissue (both in vivo and ex vivo) possessed small, globular fibroblasts with long, branching "dendritic" processes; in contrast, the fibroblasts in stretched tissue appeared wider, flatter, and possessed larger cross-sectional areas (Figure 1-1). Changes to intracellular microtubules and microfilaments are responsible for changes in fibroblast shape (Langevin, Bouffard, Badger, Iatridis, & Howe, 2004).

Cytoskeleton-dependent changes in fibroblast shape due to tissue stretch may play an important role in intracellular signaling, cell-to-cell signaling within connective tissue, and many other cellular functions (Langevin, Bouffard, et al., 2004). The implications of the Langevin, Bouffard, et al. (2004) study broaden our understanding of how connective tissue responds to changes in posture, normal movement, and exercises. Additionally, the study helps in comprehending therapeutic mechanisms of a wide variety of treatments including myofascial release, physical therapy, massage, and chiropractic.

Mast Cells

Mast cells are large and ovoid. They have a spherical nucleus and a cytoplasm filled with numerous granules. These cells are involved in immune system activity and contribute to a variety of inflammatory conditions in the brain, joints, skin, and other bodily organs (Theoharides & Cochrane, 2004). There are two types of mast cells, each containing variable amounts of proteolytic enzymes and cytokines.

Tissue Shortening

Tissue Elongation

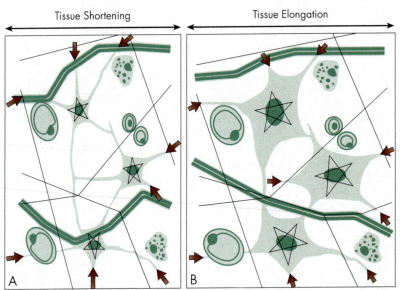

A   B

Figure 1-1 Proposed Model for Fibroblast Dynamic Cytoskeletal Response to Tissue Shortening and Elongation with Resultant Cellular and Tissue Forces. The shortened tissue (A) shows fibroblasts having a "dendritic" morphology as a result of microfilament tension, causing disassembly of the microtubule. When the force between microfilament tension and microtubule assembly is balanced, fibroblasts in elongated tissue (B) have a "sheetlike" morphology. Arrows inside fibroblasts represent tension inside the cell. Arrows outside fibroblasts represent the "pull" exerted by the cells onto the ECM.

Source: Langevin et al. (2004).

Mucosal mast cells contain tryptase enzyme (T mast cells), and connective tissue mast cells contain tryptase and chymase (TC mast cells). These mast cell types differ in the kind of stimulus required for degranulation and in the amount and type of granules they produce. Another distinguishing property is that T mast cells contain a greater proportion of chondroitin sulfate, whereas TC mast cells contain more heparin (Theoharides & Conti, 2004).

Mast cells are involved in synthesizing and secreting chemical mediators such as histamine, heparin (an anticoagulant), slow-reacting substance of anaphylaxis (SRS-A), platelet-activating factor (PAF), tumor necrosis factor-alpha (TNF-alpha), and various leukotrienes (Henz, Maurer, Lippert, Worm, & Babina, 2001). Mast cells contain receptors that bind immunoglobulin E (IgE), and when an allergen binds to IgE, this causes a disruption in the cell wall and release of chemical mediators from mast cells.

IgE has a defensive role in responding to parasitic infections and immediate hypersensitivity reactions (Luger, Crameri, Lamers, Achatz-Straussberg, & Achatz, 2006).

Adipose Cells

Adipose cells differentiate from fibroblasts and from undifferentiated mesenchymal cells. There are two types of adipose tissue: white adipose tissue (WAT) and brown adipose tissue (BAT). WAT cells accumulate and store large quantities of lipids (triglycerides, free fatty acids) in their central vacuoles, and BAT cells use the stored lipid to generate heat in a process known as thermogenesis (A. Avram, M. Avram, & James, 2005).

Physiologically, adipose tissue plays key roles in thermogenesis, lipid storage, and breakdown into free fatty acid. It also protects underlying deep fascia against physical trauma and provides thermal insulation.

Macrophages

Two types of macrophages are derived from mono-cytes: normal and inflammatory. Normal macrophage is associated with skin, connective tissue (histiocytes), lymph nodes, spleen, liver, lung, and bone marrow. Inflammatory macrophage is found in various exudates associated with wound healing, or autoimmune inflammation (Duffield, 2003).

Macrophages possess different shapes according to whether they are motile or fixed to fibers of the matrix (Livingstone, 1995). Some organs, such as the lymph nodes and spleen, consist of both free and fixed macrophages; connective tissue is comprised of fixed macrophages, found isolated in sheets of fascia accumulating within collagen and elastin fibers. These fixed macrophages are able to phagocytize and scavenge cellular debris. Free, or motile, macrophages also possess phagocytic action; but they migrate to areas of inflammation and infection where they present an antigenic peptide to activate lymphocytes which in turn secrete interferon molecules that hinder viral multiplication (Lloberas & Celada, 2002). Mechanical disruption placed on a fascial sheet due to either chronic or acute trauma leads to an activation of the macrophages, leading to secretion of enzymes (collagenase and elastase) that degrade collagen and elastic fibers to contribute

to the remodeling process as well as to initiate an inflammatory reaction (Nénan, Boichot, Lagente, & Bertrand, 2005; Werb & Gordon, 2005).

Fascial Fibers

Three types of fibers are normally found in fascia—collagen fibers, reticular fibers, and elastic fibers.

Collagen Fibers

Collagen fibers are a product of the superfamily of closely related genes that produce highly characteristic fibrous proteins found in all multicellular animals. Currently, 25 distinct collagen alpha chains have been found, each encoded by a separate gene. From these 25 collagen chains, 15 types of collagen molecules have been identified (I–XV). The main types of collagen found in connective tissue are I, II, III, V, and XI (with type I collagen being the most abundant; Vuokko, 2002). Tendons are made up of predominantly type I collagen, while all types of collagen are found in the skin (see Table 1-1). The epimysium of muscle contains mostly type I fibers; the perimysium is composed mainly of type I and III collagen; and the endomysium incorporates collagen fibers I, III, IV, and V (Light & Champion, 1984).

The basic unit of collagen is made up of three closely intertwined polypeptide chains forming a triple-helical structure 300 nm long and 1.5 nm in diameter. This triple-helical structure, also known as procollagen, is produced in the endoplasmic reticulum of the

Collagen Type	Structure	Tissue Location/Distribution	Function
I	Fibril Forming	Connective tissue of skin, bone, tendon, ligaments, dentin, sclera, fascia, and organ capsules (accounts for 90% of body collagen)	Provides resistance to force, tension, and stretch
II	Fibril Forming	Cartilage (hyaline and elastic), notochord, intervertebral disc, vitreous humor of the eye	Provides resistance to pressure

Table 1-1 Collagen Types in the Human Body

(continued)

Table 1-1 Collagen Types in the Human Body (continued)

Collagen Type	Structure	Tissue Location/Distribution	Function
III	Fibril Forming	Connective tissue of organs (uterus, liver, spleen, kidney, lungs, etc.), smooth muscle, endoneurium, blood vessels, and fetal skin	Provides structural support and elasticity
IV	Sheet-like Network	Basal laminae of epithelial and endothelial cells, kidney glomeruli, and lens capsule	Provides support and filtration barrier
V	Fibril Forming (with Type I)	Distributed uniformly throughout connective tissue stroma; may be related to reticular network	Provides support (other roles not yet defined)
VI	Network Forming	Appears to originate from a microfibrillar component of connective tissues similar to those found at the interface between elastic and collagen fibrils	Not yet determined
VII	Network Forming	Isolated from human skin (beneath stratified squamous epithelia) and amniotic epithelial cells, present in anchoring fibrils	Secures basal lamina to connective tissue
VIII	Fibril Associated	Product of aortic endothelial cells (initially described as EC collagen) and a variety of normal and tumor cell lines, presumably broadly distributed	Not yet determined
IX	Fibril Associated	Obtained as synthetic product of in vitro cartilage organ culture	Contributes to stabilization of network of cartilage collagen fibers by interaction at their intersections
XI	Fibril Forming (with type II)	Cartilage (hyaline and elastic), notochord, intervertebral disc, vitreous humor of the eye	Provides resistance to pressure
XII	Fibril Associated (with type I)	Distributed throughout tendons, ligaments, and other tissues where type I fibrils are found	Assists type I in providing resistance to force, tension, and stretch

Note: Collagen types X, XIII, XIV, and XV were not discussed.

Each collagen molecule is composed of three polypeptide α chains intertwined in a helical formation. The Roman numerals in the parentheses under "molecular formula" indicate that the α chains have a distinctive structure that differs from the chains with different numerals. Thus, collagen type I has two identical α 1 chains and one α 2 chain, while collagen type II has three identical α 1 chains.

Note: From *Histology: A Text and Atlas*, 3rd rev. ed. (p. 100), by M. H. Ross, L. J. Romrell, and G. I. Kaye, 1995, Baltimore: Williams & Wilkins. Copyright 1995 by Williams and Wilkins. Reprinted with permission.

fibroblast cell by hydroxylation of lysine and proline residues (Vuokko, 2002). Ascorbic acid (vitamin C) is essential for hydroxylation to form the final collagen molecule (May & Qu, 2005). Next, the Golgi organ packages procollagen into secretory vesicles and transports them to the cell surface, where the contents are then released into the extracellular environment. Cleavage of the terminal ends of the procollagen molecule forms tropocollagen, which is then polymerized into a collagen fibril. Fibroblasts are stimulated to increase collagen precursor production as the tissue grows or is stressed. Fibrils combine and associate to form collagen fibers, which are sometimes found intertwined with elastin fibers (collageno-elastic complex; Vuokko, 2002). Collagen fibers orient themselves in two distinct planes: unidirectional (or uni-tendinous) or multidirectional (or multi-tendinous). In unidirectional orientation, the fibers lie in a single direction corresponding to the direction of force applied to the tissue (Vuokko, 2002). An example is the dense regular connective tissue found primarily in ligaments whose primary role is mechanical. Multidirectional orientation is seen where collagen fibers are arranged in several different superficial planes. Examples of body locations include aponeurosis, capsules of the kidney and liver, tendon sheaths, peritoneum, pleura and pericardium, and stroma of the cornea.

Collagen fibers are flexible and provide an extracellular framework of considerable tensile strength, thus preventing weak points that might give way under tension. In fascia, collagen contributes strength to fascial tissue and guards against overextension.

This strength is achieved through covalent bonding between the collagen molecules of adjacent rows rather than head-to-tail attachment of the molecules (Vuokko, 2002). These bonding cross-bridges provide structural support to normal connective tissue. Injury and repair may cause excessive bonding, leading to the formation of scars and adhesions that limit the movement of these usually resilient tissues. However, regenerating myofibers form new myotendinous junctions by attaching to the scars. The myofibers are then able to transmit force across the scars (Arimaa et al., 2004). The loss of the tissue's lengthening potential is not so much due to the

volume of collagen, but to the random pattern in which it is laid down and the abnormal cross-bridges that prevent normal movement. Movement encourages collagen fibers to align themselves along the lines of structural stress—an especially important characteristic when connective tissue healing follows trauma. Without movement, the patterns of deposition may be more random and lead to adhesions. In addition, studies have shown that stretching prevents the downregulation of fibrillar collagen I and III gene expression. Alternatively, immobilization of muscle showed a decrease in activity of PH4 (Vuokko, 2002). PH4 is the rate-limiting enzyme involved in collagen synthesis. Therefore, following tissue injury, activity that is introduced early in the recovery period may help to prevent maturation of the scar tissue and development of adhesive cross-links.

With advancing age of an individual, the tissue forms glycosylation cross-links. These types of cross-links are nonenzymatic in nature and lead to increased tensile strength, decreased solubility of the fibers, and an increased resistance to digestion by certain enzymes such as proteases and collagenase. A stabilizing factor renders an increasing proportion of the collagen less susceptible to rapid digestion and solubilization. Preliminary studies suggest that the stabilizing factor may be lost during collagenase digestion. This can be detrimental to tissues, resulting in an individual being more prone to injury and scar tissue buildup (Hamlin & Kohn, 1971).

Elastic fibers are also found in association with collagen, providing the necessary tension and rearrangement of these fibers after stretching (Barros et al., 2002). Loss of elasticity due to aging can contribute to deformation and injury. This is due to degenerative changes in the quantity and quality of the ECM of elastic and collagen fibers.

Collagen fibers have other properties in addition to providing tensile strength. They are resistive to traction and mechanical forces and can stretch to 5% of their original length. Furthermore, collagen fibers are insoluble in cold water but soluble in hot water, which gives them a gelatinous property. Collagen can also affect cells in the surrounding environment. Collagen fibers have been shown to neutralize electric charges along the surface of other cells (Meyers, Armstrong, & Mow, 1988). In addition, collagen fibers are mechanically connected to the endothelial cells that make up lymphatic capillaries. As a result, collagen fiber movement produces movement in the endothelial cells, which causes opening of the capillaries and thus allows for passage of various molecules (water, proteins).

A significant trait of collagen is its piezoelectrical property (Hastings & Mahmud, 1988; Silva et al., 2001). During the organization of tropocollagen molecules into collagen fibrils, the molecules are arranged due to their polarity. Since tropocollagen has an asymmetrical structure, it has different polar ends. Therefore, it is obvious how collagen fibers possess longitudinal piezoelectric activity. However, electrical activity also takes place at right angles to the fibers. This can be explained by the hexagonal packaging of the fibers and by the ultrastructure of the collagen molecule itself. Where these concepts come into play is during repair processes. Structures are able to communicate through this electrical potential pattern and regulate the reconstruction of the supporting structures accordingly.

Reticular Fibers

Reticular fibers are closely related to collagenous fibers; both of them consist of collagen fibrils. The individual fibrils that constitute reticular fibers are uniform and thin in diameter, and they typically do not bundle to form thicker fibers (Ushiki, 2002). Under an electron microscope, reticular fibers appear as either individual collagen fibrils or small fibril bundles. In loose connective tissue, networks of reticular fibers are found at the boundary of connective tissue with epithelium. In addition, reticular fibers can be found around adipose cells, nerves, muscle cells (skeletal and smooth), and blood vessels. In most locations (except peripheral nerve endoneurium and lymphatic or hemopoietic tissue) the reticular fiber is produced by fibroblasts but is much thinner than a collagen fiber. Another structural difference is that type I fibers comprise collagen fibers, whereas type III fibers are the main constituents of reticular fibers.

The meshlike structure of reticular fibers provides strength, support, and a framework for many viscera.

These fibers also function as a selective filter, provide elastic support to known and underlying tissues, and serve as a skeleton for healing and restoration of soft tissue.

Elastic Fibers

Elastic fibers are produced as proelastin subunits by the same cells that produce collagen and reticular fibers—namely, fibroblasts. In contrast to collagen, elastic fibers are comprised of two structural components: elastin and microfibrils.

Microfibrils form the scaffolding structure to which elastic fibers are formed during the early stages of development (Kozel, Ciliberto, & Mecham, 2004). Microfibrils are thin (10 to 15 nm diameter) and relatively straight. They are formed through the process of oligomerization (conversion of monomers into oligomers) of fibrillin molecules with other proteins (TGF-B binding protein, fibrulin, and microfibril-associated glycoproteins). Abnormal elastic tissue can result from a defect in the fibrillin gene expression, as in Marfan's syndrome.

Elastin is a protein rich in glycine (33%) and is similar to collagen. But unlike collagen, it has more hydrophobic amino acids such as valine and alanine, is poor in both proline and hydroxyproline, and lacks hydroxylysine. Due to its hydrophobic nature, elastin is not glycosylated and does not form a triple helix. The basic unit of elastin is tropoelastin (similar to tropocollagen), which is secreted by elastin-producing cells. To be functional, tropoelastin must be properly aligned so that cross-linking can occur in a sequential manner (Kozel, Rongish, et al., 2006). Like collagen, elastic fibers provide strength; but unlike collagen, whose fibers are uniform in size, the elastic fiber's size and shape varies during its formation and location within organs and different tissues (Ushiki, 2002). For example, in the aorta, elastic fibers have a sheetlike appearance, whereas in loose connective tissue they are organized as a loose network of fibers. In addition, elastic fibers can be stretched up to 150% (20–30 times that of collagen) of their relaxed length without breaking. Elastic fibers are found predominantly in the skin, blood vessels, and lungs, where they form three-dimensional networks that are not affected by heat, acids, or alkalines and have a poor solubility. Like collagen, elastin has its highest functional capacity (rubbery and flexible) at 37°C but takes on a glasslike consistency at 20°C and becomes brittle.

While collagen provides stability and a limit to connective tissue movement, elastin provides an elastic-like stretch to the limit of the collagen fiber's length while absorbing tensile force. Continuous overstretching of elastic fibers may cause it to lose its ability to recoil. An example of this effect is enormous weight loss or following pregnancy; in both cases, the stretched skin sags and is difficult to return to normal.

Heavy pressure or excessive tension applied to the connective tissue may cause it to respond in a brittle manner and result in tearing. However, stress applied more slowly results in tissue that can be stretched to the limit of the collagen fiber length. The degree of flexibility will depend upon elastic quality, quantity, and the extent of cross-bridging that has occurred between the collagen fibers. The quantity of elastic fibers found in tissue varies depending on the type of fascia considered.

Elastic fibers are characterized as being long and rectilinear. They anastomose to one another and sometimes attach to collagen fibers. However, the interlacing elastic fibers of the superficial fascia do not anastomose, but instead are arranged in multiple layers to form a network (Braverman, 1988). Cross sections of loose connective tissue show that each elastic layer is associated with undulating collagen bundles and fibroblasts, and the layers are separated from each other by an intercalated empty zone. The superficial fascia, as a unit of loose connective tissue, allows the skin and muscle to move relatively independently of each other. The layers of differently oriented elastic fibers provide for some of the integrity of this fascia in addition to balancing the elastic and tensile stresses generated during the movement of skin and muscle.

The relationships between elastin and collagen determine the mechanical capacity of connective tissue. Elastin fibers are laid down in parallel with an excess length of collagen fibers in places where elasticity is required, such as skin or arteries. The collagen and elastic fibers are organized in different but complementary ways in fascia.

Functions of the Collageno-elastic Complex in Fascia

In tissue, including fascia, elastic fibers are interwoven with collagen fibers. This property—as well as the ratio of elastic to collagen fibers—is crucial in determining not only the mechanical properties of fascia but also the way fascia responds to inner and outer forces. Usually, the collagen fibers are wrapped around the elastic fibers and have common attachment sites. The connection between the two fibers is transverse, which seemingly allows the collagen to return to its initial length following any type of pressure, or tension, being applied to the fascia (Upledger, 1995).

Studies have shown that this collageno-elastic complex responds to forces differently depending on how extensive the deformation of the tissue is following application of force to that tissue. Consequently, if the fascia is stretched to approximately 30% of its original length, the elastic fibers stretch, followed by the collagen fibers. When the mechanical force stops, the collageno-elastic fibers enable the tissue to return to its original length—except for any inelastic collagen fibers. These fibers will remain stretched until the area of deformation is identified and addressed by a trained health professional. Another situation arises when tissues are stretched to more than 30% of their original length, in which case both collagen and elastic fibers stretch simultaneously. If the tissues remain stretched for only a short time, the fascia will return to its original length. If, however, the fibers remain stretched for an extended period of time, not only will the fibers not return to initial length, but the surrounding fascial matrix will be affected. The goal of the trained professional is to return the fibers to their original length while depolymerizing the matrix to restore increased tissue fluidity.

Extracellular Matrix

The extracellular matrix (ECM) occupies the intercellular space within a given tissue and is composed of collagenous and noncollagenous proteins. It is a complex structural network that includes the fibrous proteins, proteoglycans, and several glycoproteins. These macromolecular structures are classically known to provide mechanical support, physical strength, and elasticity to tissues.

The current view of the extracellular components of connective tissue and their functional role reveals a dynamic system in which fibers, proteoglycans (some associated with ground substance and with surfaces), and specific glycoproteins such as fibronectin and laminin interact with other components. This section details the various components of ECM.

Ground Substance

Ground substance is a viscous, clear substance with a slippery feel. It possesses high water content and a structureless nature that makes its morphology not very distinct or consistent. Ground substance is often referred to as the "polysaccharide gel complex" that fills the space between the fibers and the cells (fibroblasts) of fascia. Ground substance provides the immediate environment for every cell in the body. The physical properties of ground substance, from its viscous nature in loose connective tissue to its more turgid character in cartilage, function to permit diffusion of oxygen and nutrients between the microvasculature and adjacent tissues. This is due to the macromolecules (collagens and proteoglycans) it contains. The proteoglycan component is hydrophilic, attracting water into the area and producing a cushion effect as well as maintaining space between the collagen fibers. The other main component of ground substance is hyaluronic acid (HA).

Proteoglycans

Proteoglycans are peptide chains that form the gel of the ground substance. They have a brushlike structure with a protein backbone approximately 300 nm in length; and due to their mutually electronegative repulsion, the oligosaccharide chains form the long, stretched (60 nm to 100 nm) bristles. The molecular weight of proteoglycans lies between 10^6 and 10^9 daltons. These large macromolecules are comprised of a core protein to which many glycosaminoglycan

molecules are covalently bound. Glycosaminoglycans (GAGs) are long-chain polysaccharides made up of repeating disaccharide units. One of the two sugars in this disaccharide is a hexosamine (D-glucosamine or D-galactosamine), while the other saccharide is uronic acid (D-glucuronic acid, L-iduronic acid). GAGs are highly negatively charged due to sulfate and carboxyl groups located on many of the sugar groups. This results in attraction of water molecules to form a hydrated gel. This physical property permits easy diffusion of water-soluble molecules but inhibits the movement of larger molecules and bacteria. In addition, its high water content makes this substance very shock-absorbent so that it is able to absorb compressive forces placed upon it. Besides their mechanical properties, proteoglycans are involved in cell adhesion, differentiation, and development. Other processes in the body such as metastasis and angiogenesis involve interactions between cells or between cells and the ECM where proteoglycans are involved. (Garcia-Manyes et al., 2005).

Depending on the degree of sulfation, specific sugar group attachments, and types of linkages, there are approximately seven types of GAGs (Table 1-2).

GAGs account for 1 to 5% of the ECM. Through mutual charge loss, these long polymers are stretched; this action determines their biological characteristics and reciprocal effects with other molecules.

Hyaluronic Acid

The second component of ground substance is hyaluronic acid, which is one of the seven GAGs currently recognized. However, it differs from the other GAGs in several aspects. Firstly, it is much longer, being thousands of residues in length (molecular weight of about 100,000 to several million daltons). Secondly, hyaluronic acid is not bound to a protein in order to form a proteoglycan; instead linker proteins bind proteoglycans indirectly to hyaluronic acid. This structure results in the formation of giant macromolecules, which are fundamental to tissue such as cartilage. These large hyaluronic acid molecules attract larger quantities of water molecules to form a viscous gel that makes joints able to withstand large amounts of compression (Price, Myers,

Table 1-2 Seven Types of Glycosaminoglycans (GAGs)

Name	Approximate Molecular Weight (in daltons)	Disaccharide Composition
Hyaluronic acid	1,000,000	D-glucuronic acid + N-acetylglucosamine
Chondroitin 4-sulfate	25,000	D-glucuronic acid + N-acetylgalactosamine 4-sulfate
Chondroitin 6-sulfate	25,000	D-glucuronic acid + N-acetylgalactosamine 6-sulfate
Dermatan sulfate	35,000	L-Iduronic acid + N-acetylgalactosamine 4-sulfate
Keratan sulfate	10,000	Galactose (or galactose 6-sulfate) + N-acetylglucosamine 6-sulfate
Heparan sulfate	15,000	Glucuronic acid or L-iduronic acid 2-sulfate + N-sulfamylglucosamine or N-acetylglucosamine
Heparin	40,000	Glucuronic acid or L-iduronic acid 2-sulfate + N-sulfamylglucosamine or N-acetylglucosamine 6-sulfate

Note: From *Histology: A Text and Atlas*, 3rd rev. ed. (p. 107), by M. H. Ross, L. J. Romrell, and G. I. Kaye, 1995, Baltimore: Williams & Wilkins. Copyright 1995 by Williams and Wilkins. Reprinted with permission.

Leigh, & Navsaria, 2005). The movement of water is made possible by a polymerizing/depolymerizing action of the enzyme hyaloronidase (also known as diffusion factor). Polymerization forms large hyaluronic acid molecules, while depolymerization breaks down hyaluronic acid into smaller molecules. These actions of hyaloronidase cause fascia to fluctuate between a fluid state and a more gel-like state.

Due to its highly viscous nature, hyaluronic acid lubricates collagen, elastin, and muscle fibers, allowing them to slide over each other with minimal friction. This lubrication is vital in preventing collagen fibers from forming cross-links and adhering to one another.

Functions of Ground Substance

Ground substance has several primary functions besides structural support. Due to its high proportion of water content, a primary function of ground substance involves diffusion of nutrients and other substances including gases, hormones, white blood cells (leukocytes), antibodies, and cellular waste.

This property is important to the cells in the surrounding area since it provides a means of exchanging substances between blood and cells. Proper diffusion rates will help keep the cells healthy and functioning effectively and efficiently. The high water content of ground substance also enables it to absorb and disperse shock throughout the body. If the ground substance of fascia has inadequate water content at the time of injury or trauma, the body cannot efficiently absorb and disperse the impact of forces acting on it.

While ground substance is an effective exchange medium, it also functions as an important barrier against any invading bacteria or other microorganisms. Since connective tissue cells are part of the reticulo-endothelial system, they provide the first line of defense against invading organisms.

Ground substance also functions to keep the connective tissue fibers lubricated to allow easier sliding over one another, although this is more a function of hyaluronic acid. Collagen fibers that approximate one another can potentially adhere together if a certain distance, known as critical interfiber distance, is not maintained between them. The ground substance, which provides some of the tissue volume, can effectively maintain the distance between fibers to prevent microadhesions and maintain extensibility.

With increasing age, the ground substance content in connective tissue decreases. Decreased ground substance can lead to the formation of numerous microadhesions, and possibly contribute to a decrease in flexibility. Decrease in flexibility and movement will result in the ground substance changing from a fluid to a more solid form. When it is left immobile and undisturbed, ground substance has a tendency to further solidify. This in turn results in solidification of synovium and connective tissue, leaving an individual much more vulnerable to injury. Unless irreversible fibrotic changes have occurred or other underlying pathologies exist, the state of an individual's connective tissue can be changed from a gel-like substance (which limits movement) to a more watery and flexible solute through therapeutic intervention applied by a trained practitioner. Interventions might include introduction of energy through muscular activity, soft tissue manipulation, heat, and vibration.

Water

Water accounts for 70% of the ECM (25% of the fascia) and flows freely, carrying oxygen, electrolytes, and salts between spaces created by the fibers. Water movement through fascia is affected by several factors such as the presence of macromolecules and the attachment of their chemical groups (side chains) and polymerization of hyaluronic acid (discussed earlier).

The dipolar nature of water (electrically charged) attracts the large macromolecules found in the ground substance and ECM. The number of macromolecules present definitely affects the hydration, viscosity, and permeability of the matrix.

Glycoproteins

Glycoproteins are short chains formed by sugars bound to a polypeptide chain. Unlike proteoglycans, glycoproteins have a hydrophobic property that plays a role in the formation of intermolecular

bridges and orientation of fibrous proteins. The ECM has a number of noncollagenous adhesive proteins. Typically, these proteins have multiple domains, each with specific binding sites for other matrix macromolecules and for receptors on the surface of cells. Fibronectin and laminin are two characteristic glycoproteins. Both of these high molecular glycoproteins mediate between cell surfaces and the ECM due to their collagen-binding capacity, and they are easily degraded by proteases.

Fibronectin

Fibronectin is a large glycoprotein found in all vertebrates, where it exists as a monomeric, dimeric, and polymeric molecule. It appears in vertebrate blood as a dimer composed of two very large subunits joined by a pair of disulfide bonds near the carboxyl terminus. In addition to blood plasma, fibronectin has been found in amniotic fluid and cerebrospinal fluid (CSF). Fibronectin has multiple binding domains; it binds to collagen, heparin, cell surface, heparin sulfate, hyaluronic acid, proteoglycans, and actin. The actin-binding site is of interest since it indicates that fibronectin can very likely connect with the actin filaments of the cellular cytoskeleton.

Fibronectin is important for normal growth and adhesion of cells, cell migration, and tissue growth (Mao & Schwarzbauer, 2005). It promotes cell migration by helping cells attach to the matrix, and it interconnects the macromolecules of the ECM with each another and with the glycocalyxes of cell surfaces. This process is exact so that migrating cells attach to the matrix without becoming stuck to it. Due to the high proteolytic sensitivity of fibronectin, a nonphysiological increase in proteases can disrupt the information coupling between the cells and the ECM. Increases in protease content can be due to autoimmune diseases and/or inflammation. As a protective measure, the sugar content of fibronectin prevents both proteolytic splitting and turnover of the polypeptide chains from occurring too rapidly.

Laminin

Laminin is one of the first ECM proteins synthesized in a developing embryo. During early development, the basal lamina contains little or no type IV collagen;

instead, it consists mainly of a laminin network. This glycoprotein is found in the basement membrane as a large molecule consisting of three long, flexible polypeptide chains interconnected via disulfide bonds.

Laminin is involved in the adhesion of epithelia to type IV collagen; both of these molecules are ubiquitous and integral parts of the basal lamina. The fundamental role of laminin is to maintain cell polarity, organizing cells into tissues through extracellular signaling for completion and assembly of the basement membrane (Kao, Huang, Hedgecock, Hall, & Wadsworth, 2006).

Like many other extracellular proteins, laminin contains a number of binding domains. These binding sites include one for type IV collagen, one for heparin sulfate, one for entactin, and two or more for laminin receptor proteins found on cell surfaces. A single dumbbell-shaped entactin molecule binds tightly to each laminin molecule, and since entactin also has an affinity for type IV collagen, it can act as an extra connection between type IV collagen and laminin in basal membranes.

Severe progressive muscle-wasting diseases, such as congenital muscular dystrophies, are a result of mutations in the laminin alpha-2 chain, which is the most prominent alpha chain in muscle and peripheral nerve.

Fibroblasts and the ECM

One question that scientists were concerned with for some time was whether fibroblasts rest passively within the ECM, or whether in fact some type of mechanical attachment was connecting the two. Of course, as explained earlier, the fibroblast is important in producing and maintaining the ECM. Nonetheless, research has shown that the two are indeed connected mechanically and that these attachments are critical in cell movement. Two types of attachments deserve special attention. First is a class of surface receptors (the *glycocalyx*) for proteins found in collagen fibrils and glycoproteins (such as fibronectin and laminin, discussed earlier). The second type of attachment involves a specific

integral plasma membrane protein (*integrin*) that covalently has an affinity for GAGs.

The Glycocalyx: Sugars of the Cell Surface

On the extracellular surface of the plasma membrane, carbohydrates are attached either to protein molecules (glycoproteins) or lipids of the bilayer (glycolipids). These complex carbohydrates, consisting of branched oligosaccharides with terminal N-acetylneuraminic acid, extend into the proteins and lipids of the cell membrane. These polysaccharide-rich components constitute a layer at the surface of all cells and are referred to as glycocalyxes (Basivireddy, Jacob, Ramamoorthy, & Balasubramanian, 2005).

The glycocalyx usually contains both glycoproteins and glycosaminoglycans that have been secreted into the ECM, and they then migrate onto the cell surface. Many of these absorbed macromolecules are components of the extracellular matrix, which makes the division between the plasma membrane and the ECM almost indistinguishable. In this way, the glycocalyx mediates functionally between the cell interior and the extracellular space.

The function of the glycocalyx depends on its location in the body. In the intestines, it has multiple functions: protects the underlying villi from infectious bacteria and stomach acids, serves as a platform for normal bacterial flora, and allows transport of nutrients across the microvilli (Horiuchi et al., 2005). The endothelial glycocalyx protects blood vessels from ischemia/reperfusion injury and formation of atherogenic plaque (Nieuwdorp et al., 2005).

Integrins

The principal receptors on the cell surface for binding most ECM proteins—including collagen, fibronectin, and laminin—are the integrins. They are a large family of homologous, transmembrane linker proteins composed of two noncovalently bound transmembrane glycoprotein subunits (a heterodimer), both of which contribute to the binding of the matrix protein. Most integrins bind to one specific molecule; however, integrins found in fibroblasts bind to collagen, fibronectin, and laminin. Laminin deposition into the ECM is controlled by integrins (Li, Rao, Burkin, Kaufman, & Wu, 2003). Integrins differ from other cell surface receptors in that they bind their ligand with relatively low affinity and are usually present at about 10- to 100-fold higher concentration on the cell surface. This weak binding to many of the matrix molecules allows cells to move with some ease. However, if the binding to the ligand was tighter, then the cells would not be able to move freely.

Integrins mediate extracellular membrane signaling and thus play an important role in differentiation, migration, and proliferation of cells (Tarone et al., 2000). Mutated fibroblasts have been shown to produce less fibronectin than normal cells, while not adhering properly to the substratum and failing to develop organized actin filament bundles (Turner & Burridge, 1991). The interactions of actin filaments and fibronectin are mediated mainly by integrins. Thus, integrins are fundamental to the interactions of cells and the matrix around them.

Intracellular Components are Indirectly Attached to the ECM Cytoskeleton

The ability of cells to adopt various shapes and carry out coordinated and directed movements depends on a complex network of protein filaments that extends throughout the cytoplasm. This network is called the cytoskeleton. The cytoskeleton is directly responsible for movements such as the crawling of cells on the substratum, muscle contraction, and the many changes in shape of the developing vertebrate embryo. The ECM provides biochemical information governing cell differentiation, adhesion, intracellular movements such as transport of organelles from one place to another in the cytoplasm, and segregation of chromosomes during the process of mitosis (Oschmann, 1998).

These multiple activities of the cytoskeleton depend on three major classes of filamentous polymers: actin filaments, microtubules, and intermediate filaments. As mentioned earlier, it is these structures for which cell surface molecules, like the glycocalyx and integrins, act as a bridge connecting the ECM components (Khatiwala, Peyton, & Putnam, 2006).

Summary

The living matrix is a complex structure with diverse functions in the body. Evidence accumulates in support of the thesis that nuclear matrices, cytoskeletons, and extracellular matrices are mechanically, chemomechanically, electromechanically, and functionally interconnected throughout the organism (Oschmann, 1998). The entire molecular continuum has been called a tissue tensegrity matrix system, or simply the living matrix. More research is required to foster an understanding of the importance of individual living matrix components in relation to their synergistic and complementary action on the fascial system. Research is also required to comprehend the changes in cellular components of fascia that occur during the aging process and learn how these age-related changes can be mitigated to preserve the overall functioning of the fascia.

References

Arimaa, V. A., Kääriäinen, M., Vaittinen, S., Tanner, J., Järvinen, T., Best, T., et al. (2004). Restoration of myofiber continuity after transection injury in the rat soleus. *Neuromuscular Disorders, 14,* 421–428.

Avram, A. S., Avram, M. M., & James, W. D. (2005). Subcutaneous fat in normal and diseased states: Anatomy and physiology of white and brown adipose tissue. *Journal of the American Academy of Dermatology, 53,* 671–683.

Barros, E. M. K. P., Rodrigues, C. J., Rodrigues, N. R., Oliveir, R. P., Barros, T. E. P., & Rodrigues, A. J., Jr. (2002). Aging of the elastic and collagen fibers in the human cervical interspinous ligaments. *Spine Journal, 2,* 57–62.

Basivireddy, J., Jacob, M., Ramamoorthy, P., & Balasubramanian, K. A. (2005). Alterations in the intestinal glycocalyx and bacterial flora in response to oral indomethacin. *International Journal of Biochemistry & Cell Biology, 37,* 2321–2332.

Duffield, J. S. (2003). The inflammatory macrophage: A story of Jekyll and Hyde. *Clinical Science, 104,* 27–38.

Garcia-Manyes, S., Bucior, I., Ros, R., Anselmetti, D., Sanz, F., Burger, M. M., et al. (2005). Proteoglycan mechanics studied by single-molecule force spectroscopy of allotypic cell adhesion glycans. *Journal of Biological Chemistry,* Vol. 281, Issue 9, 5992–5999.

Gehlsen, G. M., Ganion, L. R., & Helfst, R. (1999). Fibroblast responses to variation in soft tissue mobilization pressure. *Medicine & Science in Sports & Exercise, 31,* 531–535.

Gray, H. (1995). *Gray's Anatomy,* 38th ed., Sydney, Churchill Livingstone, New York.

Hamlin, C. R., & Kohn, R. R. (1971). Evidence for progressive, age-related structural changes in post-mature human collagen. *Biochimica et Biophysica Acta, 236,* 458–467.

Hastings. G. W., & Mahmud, F. A. (1988). Electrical effects in bone. *Journal of Biomedical Engineering, 10,* 515–521.

Henz, B. M., Maurer, M., Lippert, U., Worm, M., & Babina, M. (2001). Mast cells as initiators of immunity and host defense. *Experimental Dermatology, 10,* 1–10.

Horiuchi, K., Naito, I., Nakano, K., Nakatani, S., Nishida, K., Taguchi, T., et al. (2005). Three-dimensional ultrastructure of the brush border glycocalyx in the mouse small intestine: A high-resolution scanning electron microscopic study. *Archives of Histology & Cytology, 68,* 51–56.

Imayama, S., & Braverman, I. M. (1988). Scanning electron microscope study of elastic fibers of the loose connective tissue (superficial fascia) in the rat. *Anatomical Record, 222,* 115–120.

Ingber, D. E. (1993). Cellular tensegrity: Defining new rules of biological design that govern the cytoskeleton. *Journal of Cell Science, 104,* 613–627.

Kao, G., Huang, C. C., Hedgecock, E. M., Hall, D. H., & Wadsworth, W. G. (2005). The role of the laminin h subunit in laminin heterotrimer assembly and basement membrane function and development in *C. elegans. Developmental Biology, 290,* 211–219.

Khatiwala, C. B., Peyton, S. R., & Putnam, A. J. (2006). The intrinsic mechanical properties of the extracellular matrix affect the behavior of preosteoblastic MC3T3-E1 cells. *American Journal of Physiology Cell Physiology, 290(6),* C1640–50.

Kjaer, M. (2004). Role of extracellular matrix in adaptation of tendon and skeletal muscle to mechanical loading. *Physiological Review, 84,* 649–698.

Kozel, B. A., Ciliberto, C. H., & Mecham, R. P. (2004). Deposition of tropoelastin into the extracellular matrix requires a competent elastic fiber scaffold but not live cells. *Matrix Biology, 23,* 23–34.

Kozel, B. A., Rongish, B. J., Czirok, A., Zach, J., Little, C. D., Davis, E. C., et al. (2006). Elastic fiber formation: A dynamic view of extracellular matrix assembly using timer reporters. *Journal of Cellular Physiology, 207,* 87–96.

Langevin, H. M., Bouffard, N. A., Badger, G. J., Iatridis, J. C., & Howe, A. K. (2004). Dynamics fibroblast cytoskeletal response to subcutaneous tissue stretch ex vivo and in vivo. *American Journal of Physiology Cell Physiology, 288,* C747–C756.

Langevin, H. M., Cornbrooks, C. J., & Taatjes, D. J. (2004). Fibroblasts form a body-wide cellular network. *Histochemical Cell Biology, 122,* 7–15.

Li, J., Rao, H., Burkin, D., Kaufman, S. J., & Wu, C. (2003). The muscle integrin binding protein (MIBP) interacts with $a7\beta1$ integrin and regulates cell adhesion and laminin matrix deposition. *Developmental Biology, 261,* 209–219.

Light, N., & Champion, A. E. (1984). Characterization of muscle epimysium, perimysium, and endomysium collagens. *Biochemical Journal, 219,* 1017–1026.

Lloberas, J., & Celada, A. (2002). Effect of aging on macrophage function. *Experimental Gerontology, 37,* 1323–1329.

Luger, E., Crameri, R., Lamers, R., Achatz-Straussberger, G., & Achatz, G. (2006). Regulation of the IgE response at the molecular level: Impact on the development of systemic anti IgE therapeutic strategies. *Chemical Immunology & Allergy, 91,* 204–217.

Mao, Y., & Schwarzbauer, J. E. (2005). Fibronectin fibrillogenesis: A cell-mediated matrix assembly process. *Matrix Biology, 24,* 389–399.

May, J. M., & Qu, Z.-c. (2005). Transport and intracellular accumulation of vitamin C in endothelial cells: Relevance to collagen synthesis. *Archives of Biochemistry and Biophysics, 434,* 178–186.

Myers E. R., Armstrong C. G., Mow V. C. (1986). Swelling pressure and collagen tension. In: Hukins D. W. L., editor. *Connective tissue matrix.* London: Macmillan.

Nénan, S., Boichot, E. Lagente, V. & Bertrand, C. P. (2005). Macrophage elastase (MMP-12): A pro-inflammatory mediator. In *Memorias do Instituto Oswaldo Cruz, 100*(Suppl. I), 167–172.

Nieuwdorp, M., Meuwese, M. C., Vink, H., Hoekstra, J. B., Kastelein, J. J., & Stroes, E. S. (2005). The endothelial glycocalyx: A potential barrier between health and vascular disease. *Current Opinion in Lipidology, 16,* 507–511.

Oschmann, J. L. (1998). The cytoskeleton: Mechanical, physical, and biological interactions. *Biological Bulletin, 194,* 321–418.

Price, R. D., Myers, S., Leigh, I. M., Navsaria, H. A. (2005). The role of hyaluronic acid in wound healing assessment of clinical evidence. *American Journal of Clinical Dermatology, 6,* 393–402.

Silva, C. C., Thomazini, D., Pinheiro, A.G., Aranha, N., Figueiró, S. D., Góes, J. C., et al. (2001). Collagen–hydroxyapatite films: Piezoelectric properties. *Materials Science & Engineering, B86,* 210–218.

Tarone, G., Hirsch, E., Brancaccio, M., De Acetis, M., Barberis, L., Balzac, F., et al. (2000). Integrin function and regulation in development. *International Journal of Developmental Biology, 44,* 725–731.

Theoharides, T. C., & Cochrane, D. E. (2004). Critical role of mast cells in inflammatory diseases and the effect of acute stress. *Journal of Neuroimmunology, 146,* 1–12.

Theoharides, T. C., & Conti, P. (2004). Mast cells: The Jekyll and Hyde of tumor growth. *Trends in Immunology, 25,* 235–241

Turner, C. E., & Burridge, K. (1991). Transmembrane molecular assemblies in cell–extracellular matrix interactions. *Current Opinion in Cell Biology, 5,* 849–853.

Upledger, J. E. (1995). Craniosacral therapy. *Physical Therapy, 75,* 328–330.

Ushiki, T. (2002). Collagen fibers, reticular fibers and elastic fibers: A comprehensive understanding from a morphological viewpoint. *Archives of Histology & Cytology, 65,* 109–126.

Vuokko, K. (2002). Intramuscular extracellular matrix: Complex environment of muscle cells. *Exercise & Sport Science Reviews, 30*(1): 20–25.

Werb, Z., & Gordon, S. (2005). Secretion of a specific collagenase by stimulated macrophages. *Journal of Experimental Medicine, 142,* 346–360.

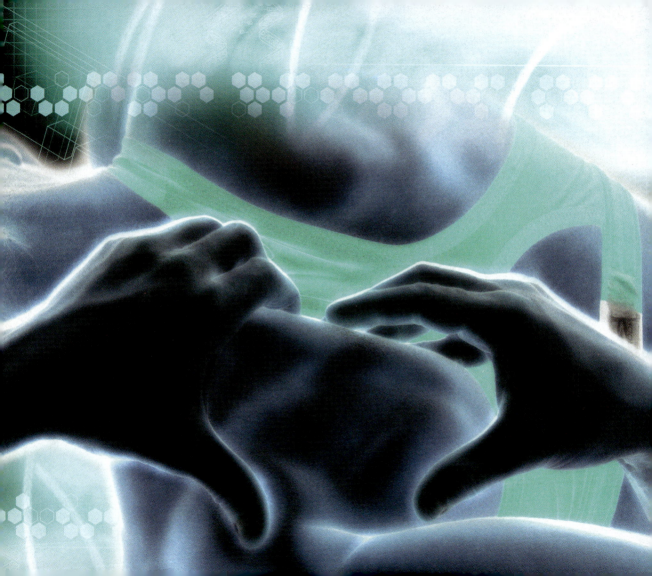

CHAPTER 2

ANATOMICAL DESCRIPTION OF FASCIA AND ITS PLANES

This chapter deals with the anatomy and physiology of fascia based on work by Myers. The anatomical description of the various types of fascia and their fascial anatomy planes throughout the body is presented. Fascial chains and trains, which are uninterrupted "tracks" of connective tissue running up and down the body, will be described.

ANATOMY AND PHYSIOLOGY OF FASCIAL PLANES

Fascia is a tough connective tissue that spreads throughout the body in a three-dimensional web from head to foot without interruption. The fascia surrounds every muscle, bone, nerve, blood vessel, and organ of the body, down to the cellular level. Fascia can be categorized into three divisions: fascia superficialis, fascia profunda, and deepest fascia.

Fascia Superficialis

A layer of loose connective tissue located beneath the dermis of the skin, and sometimes referred to as the subcutaneous tissue, is called the fascia superficialis. It serves as a passageway for nerves and blood vessels, and in some areas of the body it houses skeletal muscles and various quantities of adipose tissue.

The superficial fascia layer is more prominent in the posterior half of the body than in the anterior half. The main functions of this layer are protective and supportive. It anchors the skin onto the underlying myofascia while providing (along with the skin and superficial fat) a cushion for protection. Because of the variety in the physiology of this layer, only two fasciae are identified in the fascia superficialis: Scarpa's fascia (anterior trunk) and Colles' fascia (perineum). Furthermore, in the extremities (both upper and lower), it is much more difficult to separate the type of fascia superficialis.

Fascia Profunda (Deep)

The fascia profunda is a fibrous layer of connective tissue found beneath the superficial fascia. It is also involved in passageways for nerves and blood vessels. Fascia profunda invests muscles and other internal structures.

Deepest Fascia

The deepest fascia is also known as the dural tube. This fascia surrounds and protects the brain and spinal cord.

Cellulite

Fascia superficialis consists of one to several horizontal layers containing various amounts of superficial fat deposits, which change the physiology of this layer. For example, an increased number of fat cells give rise to cellulite. This is primarily seen in women or obese individuals. Cellulite due to hypertrophy of adipose (fat) cells is known as primary cellulite. Its presence is noticeable when the patient is in the erect or supine position. Primary cellulite is normally seen in younger women and is not generally improved with surgery, although it can be corrected through weight loss. Secondary cellulite usually appears after 35 years of age and may be combined with primary cellulite. It is associated with aging, sun damage, dramatic weight loss, and liposuction. Secondary cellulite results in skin laxity compounded by gravitational forces along the vertical or oblique fibrous septum that extends from the dermis to the superficial fascial layers. Because of the damage done to this layer, weight loss is not very effective in reducing secondary cellulite. Surgical correction (plastic surgery) might be more effective in decreasing the effects of cellulite.

Variation between Sexes

The superficial fascia varies between sexes in the breast and pelvic areas. In the female breast, fascia superficialis splits into an anterior and a posterior division. The anterior division attaches to the dermis while the posterior division connects to the pectoralis musculature. This allows female breasts to increase in size; but as they do, the connections become looser as a result of gravitational forces and the retromammary space is formed.

A sexual difference is also noted in the pelvic region. In females, the fascia superficialis is not as closely adhered to the pelvic musculature (gluteals, etc.), which allows for easier and larger fat deposition in this area. The fascia superficialis in males is tightly attached to the pelvic musculature a few centimeters below the iliac crest and forms the roof of the localized fat deposit that overlies the crest. This explains the differences in lateral truncal contour seen between the two sexes. The superficial fascial layer forms peaks and valleys along our bodies (zones of adherence). Areas where the superficial fascial system is most adherent to underlying muscle fascia or periosteum are the creases of the skin and certain plateaus, such as those found on the bridge of the nose, whereas areas of least adherence are the bulges where the superficial fascial system forms the roof over localized deep fat deposits, as seen in the abdominal area or hips.

Variations with Adiposity

As the degree of adiposity changes, the superficial fascial system anatomy varies significantly. There is a significant amount of fat separating the layers of the superficial fascial system, even in nonobese individuals. Obesity further separates the fascial layers until they become indistinct and are not easily recognizable. The same quantity of connective tissue remains, but it is diluted by the adipose tissue.

Variations in Different Body Regions

A confusing feature of the superficial fascial system is the inconsistent anatomy from one body region to another. In areas such as the lower anterior trunk

(Scarpa's) and the perineum (Colles'), the superficial fascial system consists of a well-defined single membranous sheet. Scarpa's and Colles' are the only named superficial fasciae in the body. In most other areas of the trunk, there may be more than one superficial fascial system layer separating the superficial fat from the deep fat or muscle.

Interestingly, the superficial fascial system is more prominent on the posterior half of the trunk and thighs than on the anterior half. The appearance of the superficial fascial system can become diffuse in the extremities. This is seen in parts of the trunk (epigastrium) and in obese individuals, where it is difficult to separate superficial fat from the fat within the horizontal superficial fascial system layers. Therefore, all fat superficial to the deepest superficial fascial system layer should be termed superficial fat.

Zones of Adherence

The topographic features of the human body are largely the result of superficial fascial system anatomy and its relationships to fat and muscle fascia. Varying zones of adherence of the superficial fascial system cover the trunk and extremities. Together with the fat, these zones of adherence produce creases, folds, valleys, plateaus, and bulges of the normal body contour.

Table 2-1 Superficial Fascial System Zones of Adherence

Most Adherent	Adherent	Least Adherent
Skin creases: inframammary, groin, gluteal, joint	All areas of trunk and extremities without significant deep fat	Areas of localized fat deposits
Plateaus		
Vertical		
Posterior midline		
Anterior midline		
Horizontal: inguinal to lateral gluteal depression		

Fascia is a tissue that forms a whole-body continuous three-dimensional matrix of structural support. Fascia interpenetrates and surrounds all organs, muscles, bones and nerve fibers, creating a unique environment for body systems functioning. Fascia extends to all fibrous connective tissues, including aponeuroses, ligaments, tendons, retinaculae, joint capsules, organ and vessel tunics, the epineurium, the meninges, the periostea, and all the endomysial and intermuscular fibers of the myofasciae. This text will be adapting a more traditional presentation of fascia via its anatomical location to describe its locations in the human body.

FASCIA PROFUNDA

The fascial layer known as the fascia profunda is found just under the fascia superficialis layer, where it encapsulates individual muscles as well as groups of muscles. This is the middle of the three layers of connective tissue. The physical characteristics of this layer consist of occasional fat and a fibrous membrane of bluish-white color. It has the tendency to fuse with the periosteum of bony protuberances such as the linea nuchae superior, linea temporalis superior, arcus zygomaticus, margo inferior mandibulae, clavicula, spina scapulae, sternum, crista iliaca, linea innominata, processi spinosi of the vertebrae of the trunk, and protuberances around the joints of

the extremities. The fascia profunda also encloses the glands and forms sheaths for nerves (epineurium, perineurium, endoneurium) and vessels.

DEEPEST FASCIA

The deepest fascia layer is situated within the dura of the cranial sacral system surrounding the central nervous system. This is the deepest, and final, layer of fascia that is identified in our bodies. It surrounds and protects the brain and spinal cord from injury. Dysfunction in these tissues can have significant and widespread neurological effects.

IDENTIFYING FASCIAL PLANES

Much of the information provided in Tables 2-2 through 2-9 (see following pages) can be obtained in most anatomy books or atlases. This information was compiled using Edward Singer's work *in Fasciae of the Human Body and Their Relations to the Organs They Envelop* (Singer, 1935). This information has been taken and the following tables created in order to organize the material better. A more thorough and detailed description of fascial anatomy can be gotten by reading Singer's work.

Table 2-2 Fascia of the Head	
Fascia capitis superficialis	Fascia covering the face and cranium.
	Variable thickness throughout, depending on area; over the nose it has a spongy character; over the eyelids less fat.
	Before the external acoustic meatus, this fascia joins the fascia profunda and they continue together over the trigonum laterale colli.
Fascia capitis profunda	Envelops superficial masticatory muscles of the buccinator and salivary glands.
	(continued)

Table 2-2 Fascia of the Head (continued)

	Cannot be traced over the regions of the head that are occupied by the mimic muscles.
	Made up of four divisions (see following).
Fascia buccopharyngea (buccal aponeurosis)	Covers the buccinator muscle and the superior pharyngeal constrictors.
	Is distinct on the posterior part of the buccinator, while the anterior part is thinned out.
	Attaches onto the alveolar process of the linea mylohyoidea and the mandibular ramus.
	Forms the pterygomandibular ligament, which serves as the origins of the buccinator and superior pharyngeal constrictor muscles.
Fascia temporalis	Covers the external surface of the temporalis.
	Its external layer attaches to the zygomatic arch.
	Connects to the superficial fascia anterior to the sternocleidomastoid SCM; from it originate the superficial bundles of the temporalis.
	Its deepest layer passes over the internal surface of the masseter and attaches onto the mandible.
Fascia interpterygoidea	Covers both lateral (external) and medial (internal) pterygoids.
	Originates from pterygoid process and inserts onto mandible just above the pterygoid muscle insertion
Fascia parotideomasseterica	Forms the compartment for the parotid gland and anterior covering for the masseter.
	Thickest on the external surface of the gland, under the skin.

Table 2-3 Fascia of the Neck

Fascia colli superficialis	A continuation of the fascia superficialis capitis, while anteriorly it blends with the fascia superficialis thoracis.
	Along with fascia colli profunda, forms the fascia nuchae around the posterior margin of the platysma muscle.

(continued)

Table 2-3 Fascia of the Neck (continued)

Fascia colli profunda	Forms a complex number of compartments to account for the various movements of the muscles of the head, neck, shoulders, vertebral column, and upper intestinal tract. Forms part of fascia nuchae (along with fascia colli superficialis). Made up of three layers: lamina superficialis, lamina media, and lamina profunda (see following).
Lamina superficialis	Found underneath the platysma; extends along the linea nuchae superiorly to the mastoid process and the mandible and inferiorly onto the manubrium and outside surface of the clavicles. Very thin tissue, thicker at the superior attachment of the sternocleidomastoid (SCM). Over supraclavicular space, it forms a sheet that overlies the supraclavicular lymph nodes, the superficial cervical artery, and the external jugular vein. In its cranial part, lamina superficialis is connected with the fascia parotideomasseterica, while along its caudal portion, it blends in with the fascia pectoralis and the fascia dorsi.
Lamina media	Its superior portion (posterior margin of the SCM) is in contact with the lamina superficialis, while its inferior portion is thinner, separated from the lamina superficialis (by fat tissue). Attaches to the posterior aspect of the clavicles and surrounds the subclavius muscle; from there, it travels down into the thorax and blends with the pericardial tissue. Also forms part of the carotid sheath (lateral portion) and surrounds the omohyoid, sternohyoid, and sternothyroid muscles.
Lamina profunda (fascia paravertebralis)	Covers the deep muscles of the neck. Originates at the base of the skull, attaches to vertebral transverse processes and extends into the posterior mediastinum. In the upper part of the neck, it lies over the scalenes and levator scapulae and forms the boundary between the nape and the neck. Inferiorly, it encloses the levator scapulae, serratus anterior, and rhomboids major and minor.

(continued)

Table 2-3 Fascia of the Neck (continued)

	In the lower neck region, it surrounds the scalenes, brachial plexus, and serratus posterior superior; attaches to the scapula; and fuses with the lumbodorsal fascia.
	Forms part of the carotid sheath (with lamina media) and is attached to the thyroid gland.
	Connects with the tunica externa of the esophagus, forming part of the retropharyngeal space (lateral border).
Fascia nuchae superficialis	This is the superficial fascia of the nape.
	It is a continuation of the fascia superficialis colli.
	Continuous with skin and fascia nuchae profunda.
Fascia nuchae profunda	Continuous with the lamina superficialis and the lamina profunda.
	The continuation of the lamina superficialis portion forms the layer above the trapezius muscle, while the continuation of the lamina profunda portion forms the layer under the levator scapulae and rhomboideus muscles.

Table 2-4 Fascia of the Thorax

Fascia pectoralis superficialis	Superiorly, the fascia pectoralis superficialis is continuous with the fascia colli superficialis (see Table 2-3).
	Inferiorly, it is continuous with the fascia abdominalis, and laterally it is continuous with the fascia axillaries and fuses at this locale with the fascia pectoralis profunda.
	This fascia contains a considerable amount of fat in which the mammary glands are embedded.
	In the upper medial part of the thorax, the fascia is relatively well separated from the fascia pectoralis profunda by radiating, small tendons of platysma muscle.
Fascia pectoralis profunda	Medially, the fascia pectoralis profunda is attached to the sternum.
	Laterally, it is attached to the clavicle and is continuous with the fascia axillaries.

(continued)

Table 2-4 Fascia of the Thorax (continued)

	Inferiorly, it is connected with the fascia profunda of the abdominal wall.
	The fascia pectoralis profunda covers the surface of the pectoralis major and sends numerous septa between the bundles of this muscle.
	At the superomedial portion of the pectoralis major, this fascia is a firm layer; inferolaterally, it thins out into the fascia pectoralis superficialis.
Fascia clavipectoralis	The deeper surface of the pectoralis major is covered by a strong fascia that arises from the clavicle beneath the layer that covers the upper surface of this muscle (fascia pectoralis) and extends over the subclavius muscle. From here, the fascia clavipectoralis extends to the upper border of the pectoralis minor muscle and to the medial end of the ribs and fuses with the fascia of the intercostals (also known as fascia coracoclavicularis).
	At the upper border of the pectoralis minor, the fascia clavipectoralis divides to envelop the muscle; then it unites and runs on the undersurface of the pectoralis major, at whose lower border the fascia clavipectoralis unites with the fascia of the external surface of the pectoralis major.
Fascia coracoclavicularis	This triangular fascia lies between the pectoralis minor and the clavicle, runs medially to the ribs, and fuses with the fascia of the intercostal musculature.
	Medially it also lies over the subclavius muscle and the first rib. It thins out into the fascia of the first intercostal space with a few fibers reaching the second rib.
	Its lateral border, extending from the coroid process of the scapula to the cartilage of the first rib, becomes thickened and is known as the costocoracoid ligament.
	Structures such as the anterior thoracic artery, anterior thoracic nerve, and cephalic vein all pierce this fascia.
	This fascia forms the anterior wall of the axilla and separates the cavity of the axilla from the anterior chest wall.
Fascia endothoracica	The inner cavity of the thorax is lined by the fascia endothoracica, which is found between the serous sacs of the thorax and the intercostal muscles, ribs, and diaphragm.

(continued)

Table 2-4 Fascia of the Thorax (continued)

	The fascia is strongest where the diaphragm is uncovered by the pleura. The fascia passes along the line of the diaphragmatic reflection of the pleura costalis, which it fastens to the diaphragm and to the costal cartilages.
Fascia axillaris	The axilla is a pyramidal space bordered by the upper part of the brachium and the lateral wall of the thorax. This space is filled with a plug of fibrous tissue and fat, contains many lymph nodes, and is pierced by a great number of nerves and vessels.
	Laterally, the fascia formed by this plug passes over into the fascia superficialis and fascia profunda of the upper extremity (see Table 2-7).
	Medially, the fascia axillaris is connected with the part of the fascia profunda that envelops the serratus anterior muscle.
	Anteriorly, the fascia axillaris is connected with the fascia pectoralis superficialis and the fascia corococlavicularis.
	Posteriorly, the fascia axillaris is connected with the fascia of the latissimus dorsi.

Table 2-5 Fascia of the Abdomen (external and internal)

External Abdominal Fascia	
Fascia abdominis superficialis	This fascia is the continuation of the fascia pectoralis superficialis.
	Posteriorly, it joins into the fascia superficialis dorsi.
	Inferiorly, it connects into the fascia of the anterior surface of the thigh.
	This fascia contains fat in most individuals, but the part around the umbilicus never contains any fat.
Lamina superficialis fasciae abdominis superficialis (Camper's fascia)	This superficial fatty layer covers the subcutaneous vessels and is continued over the fascia lata as fascia superficialis femoris.
Lamina profunda fasciae abdominis superficialis (Scarpa's fascia)	This fibrous layer underlies the subcutaneous vessels; in some places, it is firmly connected to the fascia abdominis profunda (especially around the umbilicus and on the linea alba).

(continued)

Table 2-5 Fascia of the Abdomen (external and internal) (continued)

Fascia abdominis profunda (fascia abdominalis superficialis and abdominalis externa)—"the deep fascia"	At the linea alba in the regio pubica, the lamina profunda of the fascia abdominis superficialis consists mostly of elastic fibers and forms the fundiform and suspensory ligaments of the penis/clitoris. In males, this fascia continues inferiorly as the tunica dartos. Toward the perineum, it forms the lamina profunda fasciae superficialis perinea (fascia of Colles). This is a clearly distinguishable layer above the muscle fibers of the oblique abdominis externus. Over the aponeurosis of this muscle, the fascia is almost unrecognizable and is intimately connected with the aponeurosis. From the anterior superior iliac spine, it sends out fibers in the shape of a fan across the tendinous fibers of the oblique abdominis externus. Some of these fibers form an arch above the subcutaneous end of the inguinal canal. From this point on the fascia becomes very thin and fuses at the lower lateral part with the aponeurosis of the oblique abdominis externus. The upper medial part continues for a short distance, but this also soon becomes inseparable from the aponeurosis. The fusion of these two layers (fascia and aponeurosis) forms the external spermatic fascia.
Internal Abdominal Fascia	
Fascia transversalis	This is a fascial plate that covers the entire internal surface of the abdomen. It is named after the transversus abdominis muscle whose internal surface it covers; however, parts of this fascia cover other muscles lying in different regions, so they are also named accordingly: fascia diaphragmatica, fascia iliaca, and fascia levatoris ani superior. The thickness and density of this fascia vary. It often fuses with and becomes inseparable from the fascia subserosa. Under the linea semicircularis (Douglas' line), the fascia transversalis forms a part of the rectus sheath. Its lateral portion is attached to the periosteum of the iliac crest, to the inguinal ligament, and to the os pubis thus forming the dorsal wall of the inguinal ligament.

(continued)

Table 2-5 Fascia of the Abdomen (external and internal) (continued)

Fascia subserosa	The fascia leaves the abdomen with the funiculus spermaticus and becomes the fascia spermatica interna.

The fascia transversalis also leaves the abdomen with the femoral vessels to form the femoral sheath.

This fascial tissue lies between the peritoneum and the fascia transversalis and changes in character at different regions of the abdomen.

In certain areas it contains a great amount of fat, in other areas it splits into many layers, and in other areas it appears as thin fascia. The latter is true around the kidneys and in front of the bladder, where the tissue is justly named fascia subserosa (found in subserous tissue). |

Table 2-6 Fascia of the Pelvis

Fasciae pelvis	The fasciae of the pelvis have three main divisions: fascia pelvis parietalis (covering the muscles of the pelvic cavity), fascia pelvis viseralis (surrounding the pelvic intestines), and fascia perinei (lies in the urogenital trigonum).
Fascia pelvis parietalis	This fascia covers the pelvis and its muscles, and is considered by some as the continuation of the fascia transversalis.

The fascia pelvis parietalis originates anterolaterally from the linea terminalis of the os coxae, and posteriorly from the sacral promontory (sacral base), where it forms tendinous arches around the anterior sacral foramina.

Over the upper portion of the obturator internus muscle, the fascia pelvis parietalis is more strongly developed and contains a white, curved thickening—the arcus tendineus fasciae pelvis (or "white line"). This arch runs with a downward-directed curvature from the symphysis to the ischial spine. In the male it passes along the sides of the prostate gland and is called the puboprostatic ligament. In the female, it passes along the side of the bladder and is called the pubovesical ligament.

The fascia pelvis parietalis passes over the upper or intrapelvic surface of the levator ani and is called the superior pelvic diaphragmatic fascia (also known as the rectovesical fascia); along the lower or perineal surface of the levator ani, it is known as the lower pelvic diaphragmatic fascia. |

(continued)

Table 2-6 Fascia of the Pelvis (continued)

Fascia pelvis visceralis	The fascia pelvis visceralis is the visceral part of the fascia pelvis, which originates from the arcus tendineus fasciae pelvis (see fascia pelvis parietalis). It covers the prostate gland in the male and the base of the bladder in the female. The medial and inferior continuation of this fascia covers the muscles that form the pelvic diaphragm. This part of the fascia was described as superior pelvic diaphragmatic fascia.
Fascia perinea	The fascia perinea is composed of two layers of tissue: the fascia perinea superficialis and the fascia perinea profunda.
Fascia *perinea superficialis*	1. *Lamina superficialis (Scarpa's fascia):* This superficial layer of the fascia perinei superficialis is a loose, thin, fat-containing fascia; but at the posterior border of the trigonum urogenitale, it fuses with the lamina profunda, rapidly becomes very thick, and contains a coarse, fibrous septa that connects it with the lamina profunda at numerous points.
Fascia *perinea profunda*	2. *Lamina profunda (Colles' fascia):* The lamina profunda comes from the same layer of fibrous membrane that forms the tunica dartos of the scrotum and continues from there into the fascia penis. At the posterior border of the trigonum urogenitale, it is firmly attached to the fascia perinea profunda. As this layer is firmly attached to the fascia profunda in the rear and along its lateral boundary but has no attachments anteriorly, it forms a wedge-shaped fascial compartment, the spatium superficiale perinea (spatium subcutaneum), which is open toward the lower part of the abdomen. This fascia is composed of two layers: (a) fascia diaphragmatis urogenitalis inferior (superficial layer of the triangular ligament) and (b) fascia diaphragmatis urogenitalis superior (deep layer of the triangular ligament). a. The fascia diaphragmatis urogenitalis inferior is a membranous structure spreading across the triangular area formed by the arcus pubis, to which the fascia is attached. By the attachment to the periosteum of this bone, the fascia assists in completing the anterior pelvic wall. The fascia diaphragmatic urogenitalis inferior is entirely hidden in the male by the crura of the penis and the bulbus of the urethra and sends fine enveloping sheaths to the muscles of these structures. b. The fascia diaphragmatis urogenitalis superior, which is thinner than the inferior, has the same attachments. It continues with the pelvis visceralis.

Table 2-7 Fascia of the Back (Dorsi)

Fascia dorsi superficialis (superficial fascia)	The fascia dorsi superficialis is the continuation of the superficial nuchal fascia, the scapulae, and the abdomen. It contains a considerable amount of fat.
Fascia dorsi profunda (deep fascia)	The fascia dorsi profunda forms the continuation of the fascia profunda nuchae, scapulae, and abdominis; most parts of this fascia have already been described along with those fasciae (see Tables 2-3 through 2-5).
Fascia lumbodorsalis	The fascia lumbodorsalis consists of three layers: 1. The posterior, or external, layer extends from the spinous processes of the thoracic and lumbal vertebrae to the angles of the ribs and iliac crests. It is only partly a fascia because it is partly the aponeurosis of the latissimus dorsi muscles in the lower aspect of the back. 2. The middle, or second, layer originates from the transverse processes of the lumbar vertebrae. It forms a partition between the sacrospinal muscles and the quadratus lumborum musculature. 3. The anterior, or third, layer stretches from the base of the transverse processes of the lumbar vertebrae in front of the quadratus lumborum to its lateral border and continues with the fascia transversalis. Of note is that the three layers of the fascia lumbodorsalis serve as the origin for the oblique muscles of the abdomen.

Table 2-8 Fascia of the Upper Extremity (superioris extremitatis)

Fascia superficialis superioris extremitatis (superficial fascia)	The fascia superficialis of the arm and forearm is a fat-containing connective tissue layer (in a female it contains a larger amount of fat than in a male). The fascia superficialis of the dorsum of the hand is thin and loose, but in the palm it is thick and has many fibrous septa that connect it with the aponeurosis pulmaris and with the skin.
Fascia profunda superioris extremitatis (deep fascia)	This description of the fascia profunda of the upper extremity is divided according to the regions it covers: the scapula, upper arm (brachii), lower arm (antebrachii), and hand.

(continued)

Table 2-8 Fascia of the Upper Extremity (superioris extremitatis) (continued)

Fascia scapulae profunda	This fascia covers the muscles of the scapula and is divided into the fascia supraspinata, infraspinata, teres major, and subscapularis.
Fascia brachii	This strong fascia forms a tubular investment around all the muscles of the arm. By sending a lateral and medial septum to the humerus, it separates the muscles of the extensor and flexor compartments.
	The two septa of the fascia brachii separate the lower two-thirds of the arm into two compartments posteriorly (extensors) and anteriorly (flexors). In the upper third of the arm, another compartment is found between these two—the compartment for the adductor group (represented by the coracobrachialis).
	The medial intermuscular septum begins proximally at the insertion of the coracobrachialis and extends distally to the medial epicondyle of the humerus. At its proximal end, it thins out into the fascia of the axilla. It is pierced by the ulnar nerve and the superior ulnar collateral artery and vein.
	The lateral intermuscular septum is much thinner. It begins proximally from the insertion of the deltoideus and extends to the lateral epicondyle of the humerus, separating the m. triceps from mm. brachialis and brachioradialis. It is pierced by the radial nerve and profunda brachii artery and vein.
Fascia antebrachii	The fascia antebrachii surrounds the forearm and continues as the fascia carpi of the hand. In the region of the elbow, it is firmly adhered to the superficial muscles.
	At the olecranon, at the posterior margin of the ulna, and at the lateral distal end of the radius, it is connected with the periosteum of the bone.
	In the fossa cubiti, it is connected with the tendon of the biceps brachii. This part of the fascia also has a number of oblique fibers and is called the lacertus fibrosus (semilunar fascia of the biceps).
	At the dorsal aspect of the wrist, the fascia is greatly strengthened by transverse fibers and forms the transverse carpal ligament and retinaculum.
Fascia volaris manus	This fascia is composed of the firm aponeurosis palmaris, the thin fascia of the thenar, and a thin fascia of the hypothenar muscles.

(continued)

Table 2-8 Fascia of the Upper Extremity (superioris extremitatis) (continued)

Aponeurosis palmaris	The aponeurosis palmaris is a triangular, fan-shaped, firm sheet of fascia with a proximally directed apex, where it is thickest and where the palmaris longus inserts.
	Laterally, and distally, it thins out into the thenar and hypothenar fasciae.
	It is connected with the fascia superficialis and sends out five terminal bundles that insert partly into the fascia superficialis of the fingers and thumb and partly into the capsules of the metacarpophalangeal joints.
	Its most distal end, which lies directly under the web of the fingers, consists of strong fibers that stretch across the interdigital spaces and form the fasciculi transversi ("natatorium ligament").
Thenar fascia	This fascia stretches from the base of the first phalynx of the thumb and from the first metacarpal to the third metacarpal, where it fuses with the deep layer of the anterior interosseous fascia.
	It covers the opponens, abductor, flexor brevis, and abductor muscles.
Fascia of hypothenar	The fascia of hypothenar originates along the ulnar margin of the fifth metacarpal, and—after enveloping the opponens, abductor, and flexor brevis digiti minimi muscles—it inserts onto the radial margin of the same metacarpal.
	In its upper end, it is also connected with the base of the first phalynx of the fifth finger; in its lower end, it is connected with the pisiform.
Fascia dorsalis manus	The dorsal fascia of the hand has three layers: lamina superficialis, lamina intertendinosa, and lamina interossea dorsalis.
Lamina superficialis dorsalis manus	This layer is under the fascia superficialis and above the tendons of the extensor muscles. It is the thin continuation of the dorsal carpal ligament. On both sides of the hand, it passes over into the fascia of the volar side.
Lamina intertendinosa dorsalis manus	Between the tendons of the extensor digitorum is a connective tissue membrane that is very thin in whites but much stronger in blacks.
Fascia interossea dorsalis manus	This fascia lies above the dorsal interossei and fuses with the periosteum of each metacarpal.

(continued)

Table 2-9 Fascia of the Lower Extremity (inferioris extrematatis)

Fascia superficialis inferioris extremitatis (superficial fascia)	This fascia is the continuation of the fascia superficialis abdominis on the anterior side of the thigh and the continuation of the fascia superficialis dorsi on the posterior side of the thigh.
	In the buttocks, it is considerably thicker and contains a large amount of fat that forms the contour of the buttocks.
	In the groin, the fascia is attached to the medial part of the inguinal ligament.
	Over the fossa ovalis, it fuses with the superficial layer of the fascia lata and forms a fat plug, the fascia cribrosa.
	On the lower part of the leg, the fascia gradually loses its fat; and on the dorsum of the foot, it becomes very thin.
	Under the calcaneal tuberosities and the balls of the toes, it becomes thickened again and contains many fibrous septa that form small compartments enclosing fat droplets and thereby forming a natural, shock-absorbing, elastic, rubber heel.
Fascia profunda inferioris extremitatis (deep fascia)	Because some of the muscles of the thigh originate in the abdominal and pelvic cavities, the fascia for these muscles has been described with the fascia transversalis and fascia pelvis profunda (see Tables 2-5 and 2-6).
	The description of this fascia is divided according to the regions that it covers and includes the fascia coxae profunda, fascia lata, fascia cruris profunda, and fascia pedis profunda.
Fascia coxae profunda	As the fascia transversalis passes over the abdominal part of the psoas muscle and iliacus, the fascia coxae profunda becomes thin.
	As fascia iliopectinea, over the brim of the pelvis it is strong; the section of this part of the fascia that goes to the eminentia iliopectinea is even described as lg. iliopectineum.
	As fascia of the m. piriformis it is thin, and as fascia obturatoria it is firm.
	As fascia glutea, it is connected with the perimysium externum and sends numerous partitions between the coarse bundles of the muscle; it is also connected with the fascia superficialis. It is on account of this connection that the skin cannot be moved over the buttocks.

(continued)

Table 2-9 Fascia of the Lower Extremity (inferioris extrematatis) (continued)

Fascia lata	As fascia of the m. gluteus medius, it has a strong subcutaneous and a thin intermuscular part; and as fascia of m. gluteus minimus, it is hardly more than a perimysium externum.
	Fascia lata is the deep fascia of the thigh. It is attached at its proximal end to the periosteum of the iliac crest, to the periosteum of the pubic arch, and to the sacrotuberous and inguinal ligaments.
	At its distal end, attachments include the periosteum of the patella, the medial and lateral condyles of the tibia, and the periosteum of the fibular head.
	The fascia lata is not as strong as usually described. Its strongest parts are on the lower third of the thigh, where it has numerous strong cross-fibers; at the patella, where it forms the patellar rectinaculum (collateral ligaments of the patella); and on its lateral side, where the iliotibial band is situated. The iliotibial band is, however, partly a tendon and serves as an insertion point for the fibers of gluteus maximus and tensor fascia lata.
	The fascia lata sends septa between muscles having widely different actions. Muscles of similar action are closed in the same compartment. There are three septa. The extensor muscles are separated from the flexor muscles by the lateral intermuscular septum. The adductors and the extensors are separated by the medial intermuscular septum. The adductors and flexors are separated by the posterior intermuscular septum.
	Besides the compartments for the muscle groups, there are strong sheaths for some single muscles: sartorius, tensor fascia lata, iliopsoas, pectineus, and gracilis; the lower two-thirds of the sheath of sartorius lies over the femoral artery, vein, and saphenous nerve, thereby forming the roof of the adductor canal.
Fascia cruris profunda	The fascia cruris profunda is a continuation of the fascia lata and is a much stronger sheet.
	It envelops the muscles of the leg and the medial surface of the tibia. It is connected with the periosteum of the protruding edges of the tibia and fibula as well as with the extensor muscles at their origin.
	The fascia cruris profunda has a number of bands that are strengthened by fibers running in an oblique direction. These bands or ligaments hold the tendons of the muscles in their proper places.

(continued)

Table 2-9 Fascia of the Lower Extremity (inferioris extrematatis) (continued)

	The fascia cruris profunda divides the leg into lateral, anterior, and posterior compartments by sending two partitions—the anterior intermuscular septum and posterior intermuscular septum.
Fascia pedis profunda	The fascia pedis profunda is composed of three subdivisions: the fascia dorsalis pedis, the fascia plantaris pedis, and the spatial interaponeurotica pedis.
Fascia dorsalis pedis	1. *Fascia dorsalis pedis:* The fascia dorsalis pedis is the thin continuation of the cruciate ligaments. It covers the tendons of the long extensor muscles. Similar to the dorsum of the hand, the foot also has a fascia interossea dorsalis pedis, covering the short extensor and interossei muscles.
Fascia plantaris pedis or aponeurosis plantaris (plantar aponeurosis)	2. *Fascia plantaris pedis or aponeurosis plantaris (plantar aponeurosis):* The fascia plantaris consists of a medial long, triangular band that extends from the calcaneal tuberosity to the heads of the metatarsal bones (1–4), where it becomes connected to the capsules of the metatarsophalangeal joints, and a lateral band that extends from the same place to the tuberosity of the fifth metatarsal. The two parts are separated by the lateral plantar sulcus. Both the medial and lateral bands are connected by fibrous bands to the skin of the sole of the foot and to the long plantar ligament.
Spatia interaponeurotica pedis	3. *Spatia interaponeurotica pedis:* The fascial partitions divide the foot into a dorsal and three plantar compartments. The spatium interaponeuroticum pedis is the continuation of the extensor compartment and contains their tendons, the dorsalis pedis artery, and the deep peroneal nerve. The medial spatium interaponeuroticum plantare contains the muscles for the great toe; the middle spatium aponeuroticum plantare is the continuation of the deep flexor compartment and contains their tendons, the flexor digitorum brevis, and quadratus plantae. The lateral spatium interaponeuroticum contains the muscles for the fifth toe.

It is important to note that individual muscles do normally have a connective tissue layer surrounding themselves (epimysium), and it would be redundant to mention each and every individual muscle.

Summary

Fascia is a widespread and complex structure. It is comprised of various planes, with some notable differences of the superficial fascia, depending on body region and between sexes. Singer, through his work, has laid the foundation in describing the various components of the fascial planes according to body region. More research will be required to fully understand the physiologic and anatomic role fascia plays in the body, so that various injuries can be diagnosed and treated more effectively.

References

Myers, Thomas W. (2001). *Anatomy Trains: Myofascial Meridians for Manual and Movement Therapists, Medical.* pp. 280. Elsevier Health Sciences, Churchill Livingstone.

Singer, E. (1935). *Fasciae of the human body and their relations to the organs they envelop.* Baltimore, MD: Williams & Wilkins.

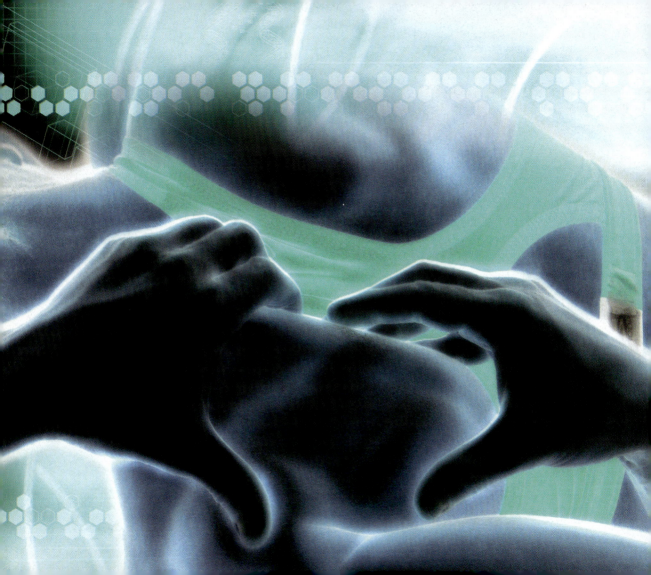

TENSEGRITY, THIXOTROPY, AND SOMATIC RECALL

This chapter takes a closer look at three concepts that are critical in understanding and treating the human fascial system; tensegrity, thixotropy, and somatic recall.

WHAT IS TENSEGRITY?

The concept of tensegrity was first introduced in 1961 by the architect Buckminster Fuller. *Tensegrity* is the union of two words: *tension* and *integrity*. Tensegrity is the property certain structures possess of maintaining their integrity as a result of continuous tensile integrity, rather than continuous compressive integrity (Pienta & Coffey, 1991). This concept is used to explain how various cells and tissues are built and to explain how fascia is structured. The ideas presented in this chapter lay the foundation for some of the discussions found later in this book.

Tensegrity-based structures are composed of a continuous series of tension-resistant components and a series of discontinuous compression-resistant (struts) elements. This is the only requirement of the tensegrity model: tension must be continuous, and compression must be localized. The tensegrity structure was visualized by Kenneth Snelson through his sculpture of stainless steel bars held in place by tension cables (Figure 3-1A).

Even though it is clear that both components can support either tensile or compressive forces simultaneously, individual elements need only support either tensile or compressive forces at a local level. Components of tensegrity structures are positioned effectively and offer a great deal of strength to withstand any stresses placed upon them. Tensegrity-based structures are independent of gravity; gravity-dependent structures would not be able to withstand applied tensile forces. Tensegrity structures are pre-stressed in that they require continuous transmission of internal tension to maintain stability. They are composed of tension-resistant structures that pull inward and compressive structures that tend to push outward. These are intermediate filaments and cytoskeletal microfilaments that produce tensional force and are balanced by the extracellular matrix (ECM), adhesions, and internal microtubule struts (Figure 3-1B). This balancing of forces stabilizes the overall structure.

Cells are built, based on a tensegrity model, so as to resist or accommodate for the various external

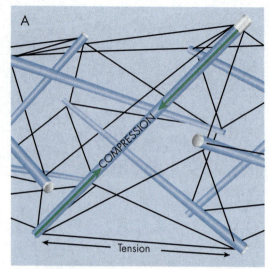

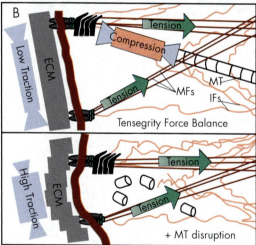

Figure 3-1 Compression and Tension Forces (A) A magnified view of a Snelson Model, displaying compression and tension forces to help visualize how tensegrity forces remain balanced. (B) A schematic representation of tensegrity force balance and disruption of microtubules by compressive forces affecting the ECM adhesions by transferring of forces from microtubules to ECM. (MF = microfilament, IF = intermediate filaments, MT = microtubules.)

Source: Ingber, (2003).

and internal forces acting upon them. So before discussing fascia, this section first takes a few steps back and looks at tensegrity at a molecular level.

Tensegrity at the Cellular Level

Chapter 1 revealed microscopic components of fascia and how these components are interconnected to form an uninterrupted system of connections from the inner parts of the cell to the outer ECM and ground substance. The connections are continuous enough that some studies have shown that applying mechanical stress to integrins (adhesion receptors located on the cell surface that link the ECM on the outside of a cell to the cytoskeleton on the inside of the cell) can affect cellular function, stimulate signal transduction, and affect gene expression (Ingber, 2003).

As mentioned earlier, tensegrity structures are not dependent on gravity. Applying this knowledge at a microscopic level, it is safe to say that cells do not have a gravity-dependent ultrastructure. At a cellular level, gravity is almost nonexistent when compared to local force interactions (Ingber, 1993).

The cellular cytoskeleton responds to stresses placed upon it by rearranging itself in a way that does not disrupt the internal cellular structures. Zaner and Valberg's (1989) study showed that laboratory-constructed, noncontinuous actin filaments that were not prestressed (i.e., not tensegrity based) did not exhibit a stiffening response to applied force (Zaner & Valberg, 1989). On the other hand, in living cells, the cytoskeletal and nucleus shapes change in an integrated manner (Emerman & Pitelka, 1977). Cellular components such as intermediate filaments are able to couple between integrins and the nucleus. In addition, they stabilize the microtubules and microfilament networks and thus prevent tearing of the cytoplasm. Local and distant changes occur when mechanical stress is placed on integrin cell receptors. These changes of cytoplasmic realignment and molecular repositioning were observed experimentally (Figure 3-2). Such studies further support the hypothesis that the cellular cytoskeleton is built on the idea of tensegrity, and they give evidence of the importance of molecular components of the framework interconnecting the cell surface and cytoplasm.

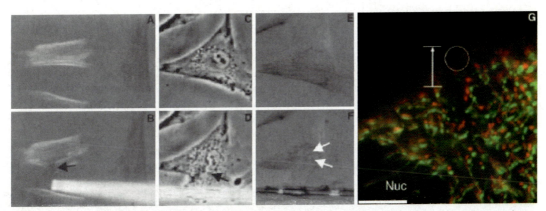

Figure 3-2 How Force Is Transferred via Molecular Networks in Cells. Different views are used: polarization (A, B, E, F), phase contrast (C, D), and fluorescence (G) to observe the cell's integrin receptors being stressed by micropipettes coated with fibronectin (A–F) or uncoated with ECM-coated microbeads (G). In photo (A), double refraction shows cytoskeletal bundles as white (positive) and black (negative), aligned vertically and horizontally in the cytoplasm. When integrins were pulled laterally, this tensional force caused the cytoskeletal bundles to realign vertically along the axis of the applied force and change from white to black (see black arrow in b). Photos (c) and (e) show an adherent cell just before tensional force was applied to integrin receptors bounded by fibronectin-coated micropipettes and pulled laterally (down) by micromanipulators (D, F). With applied tension, nuclear elongation occurs along the lines of tensional force (black arrow in D). When mechanical stress was applied to integrins (microns away) on the cell surface, molecular realignment was induced within the nucleoli of the nucleus (F), seen as white arrows on white double-refraction spots. Tension applied to a cell (G) using a surface-bound RGD microbead depicts a mitochondrion (labeled EYFP) displaced in the direction of the white arrow as a result of integrins. Green is the position before stress application, and red after stress was applied. (Nuc = cell nucleus.)

The three components of the cell cytoskeleton include microfilaments, microtubules, and intermediate filaments, as briefly mentioned earlier. What is known is that contractile microfilaments produce forces that create and propagate tension through the cytoskeleton of a cell. On the other hand, microtubules are more representative of the compression-resistant struts that oppose tension as already discussed (Lamoureux et al., 1990). Intermediate filaments are usually described as the "mechanical integrators" since they are positioned between microfilaments and microtubules. In cells found in the epidermis, intermediate filaments have been known to resist mechanical stress; but in any other cell, these filaments are not associated with cell shape control. Looking more closely at the components of the cytoskeleton under microscopy, microtubules appear curved in nature, particularly near the distal ends (Figure 3-3A).

This provides some evidence that these are indeed more compression-resistant structures. Microfilaments are straight and appear to intersect at 90° and 120° angles, which are the same angles that are seen in tensegrity-based models (Figure 3-3B). On the other hand, intermediate filaments resemble a network radiating from the cell nucleus (Figure 3-3C).

There have been numerous theories explaining how exactly cells spread and move under stressful conditions (Ingber, 1993). Using experimental data obtained from studies, along with examination of some of these cell motility theories, certain similarities are revealed. First, a cell attaches to the ECM through transmembrane linker glycoproteins, known as integrins. These connections form what are known as focal adhesion complexes (FACs). Interestingly, FACs formed between fibroblasts and the ECM are the most studied. In these studies, fibroblasts appear to be positioned a certain distance from the substratum; but at certain points, this distance is reduced by approximately one-fifth. At these points, the integrin molecule is attached to the ECM components on one side and to actin filaments on the cytoplasmic side of the cell. Thus, FACs act as a bridge connecting the outer ECM environment to the inner cytoskeletal fibers of the cell (Figure 3-4).

However, FACs are not only structural connections. They also act as an information highway, relaying messages from the ECM into the cytoplasm. Phosphorylation of various molecules by kinase proteins, found at the FAC sites, are to some degree controlled by the type of substratum the cell is attached to. In fact, cell spreading is controlled by the type of substratum it is attached to. If attached to a flat/planar surface, a cell tends to spread; however, if a cell is not attached or is attached to a malleable substratum, then it becomes spherical in shape (Volokh, 2003; Volokh, Vilnay, & Belsky, 2000). This latter phenomenon occurs because tensegrity models (such as fibroblasts) always try to be in a structure of minimal stress. Phosphorylation reactions are important in cell growth, movement, and differentiation. Therefore, the ECM environment of a cell is important in regulating cell activity. Consequently, any abnormalities in ECM composition can affect fibroblast activity and, in the end, can alter connective tissue and fascia properties and function.

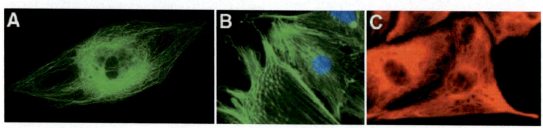

Figure 3-3 Shapes of Microfilaments and Intermediate filaments. (A) Microtubules (curved shape) in the cytoplasm of endothelial cell. (B) Microfilaments are linear shaped "within long stress fibers and triangulated actin "geodomes." Blue stains are nuclei. (C) Intermediate filaments in red form a network pattern within a spread cell.
Source: Ingber (2003).

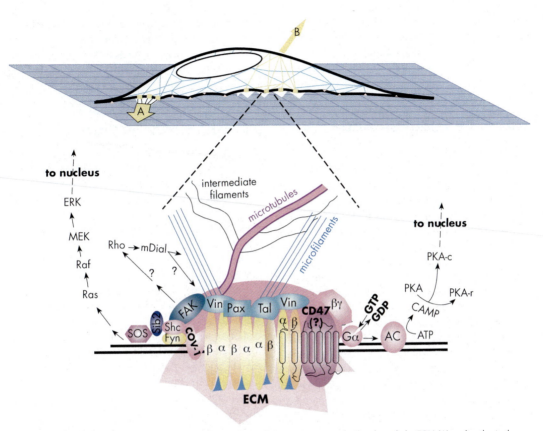

Figure 3-4 A Magnified View of How Applied Force Is Transmitted. Force is transmitted either through the ECM (A) or directly via the cell surface (B) to integrin focal adhesions below. Forces that build up within focal adhesion can stimulate a and b, integrin receptors to bring about engagement of focal adhesion proteins (Vin, Pax, and Tal). These adhesion proteins have an indirect connection to microtubules and intermediate filaments and a direct connection to microfilaments. This complex can stimulate signaling cascades such as focal adhesion kinase (FAK) and extracellular signal-regulated protein kinase (ERK) among others.

Source: Ingber (2003).

Once the FAC is attached to the ECM, Lotz, Burdsal, Erikson, and McClay (1989) discovered that tension is exerted by the cells onto the FACs within 20 minutes of FAC creation. If tension is continuous (the basis of tensegrity models), microfilaments restructure themselves into linear bundles, better known as "stress fibers," and the cells flatten out (Kreis & Birchmeiser, 1980). Stress fibers are prominent components of the cytoskeleton of fibroblasts and are an example of a temporary contractile bundle of actin filaments and myosin II type fibers. At one end they insert onto the FAC; at the other, they are either attached to another FAC or to intermediate filaments that surround the nucleus. Stress fibers are created as a

result of tensional forces and are dissolved if this tension is eliminated (this occurs either when the cell detaches from the substratum or by breaking the connection of the stress fiber with the FAC).

This situation is true for microfilaments directly attached to the FAC. Microfilaments within the same cell that are far removed from the FAC also undergo structural modifications. These filaments instead form triangular structures referred to as "actin geodomes" (Heuser & Kirschner, 1980).

Actin geodomes appear to be important to cellular motility. Obviously, cellular motility and cellular spreading are not the same thing. The vertices of these actin geodomes function as sites of actin polymerization during lamellipodia organization. What are lamellipodia? Let us look at cell motility much more closely.

The Actin Filament and Cell Motility

As mentioned earlier in this chapter, actin filaments are the tension-resistant structures of the cell. It is these molecules that give cells their tensegrity properties, so that they can change their shape in response to stress or movement. In a fibroblast, half the actin molecules are arranged in filaments; the other half exist as monomers. Several proteins associated with the plasma membrane are bound to monomer actin molecules, thus preventing them from binding to actin filaments. One such monomer-binding protein, profilin, is known to accelerate ATP exchange and to play a part in stimulating actin polymerization during cellular movement. When a cell moves, its leading edge produces flat distensions or processes known as lamellipodia. The actin filaments in a lamellipodium are well organized and project outward, forming the actin geodomes already mentioned.

At this leading edge of the cell, it appears the actin is continuously polymerized; near the core of the cell, however, the actin continuously depolymerizes. The rapid assembly of actin filaments within the lamellipodium requires release of monomer-binding proteins from actin monomers. Actin polymerization appears to be regulated by extracellular signals binding to cell surface receptors that act through G proteins. It is clear that actin forms the basis of cell motility.

In general terms, three stages have been identified in the movement of a cell: protrusion, attachment, and traction. Protrusion is a function of the leading edge of the cell. This stage involves the actin polymerization just described. Next, the actin filaments attach to the substratum through FAC creation. These focal complexes are temporary; as the cell moves, its FACs repeatedly are broken and made again. Finally, traction is the movement of the back

of the cell forward. The mechanism for this action is still not completely understood. One theory is that movement generated at the leading edge of the cell drags the rear end of the cell with it.

Cellular Tensegrity and Mechanotransduction

Mechanotransduction is the cell's ability to convert a mechanical signal into a biochemical one. First, cells contain mechanosensitive ion channels that are activated, or deactivated, by mechanical stimulation of the cell membrane. In addition, G-protein activation, release of chemical second messengers (cyclic AMP), protein phosphorylation, secretion of growth factors, remodeling of cell–ECM adhesions, and changes in gene expression also occur within seconds to minutes following mechanical perturbation (Ingber, 1993). However, it is interesting to note that many of these reactions can take place without stimulation of mechanosensitive ion channels. Therefore, mechanotransduction must be explained using the internal structural framework that exists within cells (Ingber, 1993). This internal structural organization is of course based on the tensegrity model, as discussed already.

The chemical reactions mediating protein synthesis, RNA transport, glycolysis, and DNA synthesis all appear to involve channeling of sequestered substrates and products from along the cytoskeletal filaments and nuclear matrix scaffolds (Ingber, 1993). Signal transduction may be similarly regulated since it has been demonstrated that multiple signaling molecules that are activated by integrins and growth factors become physically associated with the cellular framework of the FAC (Ingber, 1993). Because these signaling molecules lie in the main path for mechanical force transfer, the FAC represents a potential site for translating the mechanical stresses into a biochemical response. This is supported by the finding that mechanical stretch increases phosphorylation of the focal adhesion protein, tyrosine kinase (Ingber, 1993).

Thus, mechanical disturbances in cell shape definitely affect cellular biochemistry and behavior.

Changing the tension placed on a cell will change cellular and—on a higher level—tissue tone. Stiffening of the cell can potentially alter not only cellular mechanics but also vibrational frequencies, which in turn affect reaction rates. Obviously, cellular changes produce a cumulative effect that will be expressed at the tissue level. For example, look at how bone responds to stress. If an area of an osseous structure is stressed, more bone will be deposited in that area. This theory is better known as Wolff's law.

Tensegrity and Myofascia

Organs and tissues are dynamic structures that change in response to variations in pressure or stress. The restructuring obviously occurs at the cellular level and is grossly seen at a tissue level. Individual cells change shape and orientation, and they move to adapt to changing environments and forces placed upon them. The changes occurring within each cell, as well as through the ECM and into the next cell, are seen and felt by a trained practitioner when examining connective tissue and fascia integrity. Ingber (1993) stated that "only tensegrity can explain how every time that you move your arm, your skin stretches, your ECM extends, your cells distort, and the interconnected molecules that constitute the internal framework of the cell feel the pull—all without any breakage or discontinuity."

Thus, we can extrapolate this tensegrity model as seen at the cellular level to a more macroscopic level. The musculoskeletal system as a whole demonstrates components of tensegrity. The skeletal system (bones) can be envisioned as the compressive struts described earlier, while myofascia (muscles, ligaments, tendons) represents the tension components of the model. As explained, tensegrity models depend on a balance between these two components: tension structures and compression struts. If there is balance between the two, then the body can function effectively and without injury.

Applying a force to one area of a tensegrity structure will result in restructuring of the whole in order to accommodate. Again, quoting Donald Ingber (1993), "An increase in tension of one of the members results in increased tension in members throughout the structure, even ones on the opposite side." This situation can be compared to that of the spider web. If something gets caught within one end of the spider web, the whole web shifts, or is pulled, to that side. Tension occurs even in areas far removed from the snag in the web.

All this research points to a holistic role for the mechanical distribution of strain in the body that goes far beyond dealing with localized tissue pain. Creating an even tone across the myofascial meridians, and further across the entire fascial net, could have profound implications for health—both cellular and general. Very simply, transmission of tension through a tensegrity array provides a means to distribute forces to all interconnected elements, and at the same time to couple or *tune* the whole system mechanically as one. This role for manual and movement therapy of tuning the entire fascial system could have long-term effects in immunological health, as well as in an individual's sense of self integrity.

WHAT IS THIXOTROPY?

Thixotropy is derived form the Greek words *thixis* (touch) and *tropos* (transformation); it refers to the state of stiffness of a substance, particularly fluids. In 1927, Peterfi was the first to introduce the idea after he witnessed a reduction in cytoplasm viscosity of sea urchin eggs following their disturbance with a needle. Furthermore, thixotropy describes variations in the physical characteristics of a substance as a result of movement. For example, if a thixotropic substance is mechanically disturbed, then it will become more fluid. On the other hand, if the same substance is allowed to stand, or if the force applied is below a certain level, then the substance will have stiffer physical properties (Proske, Morgan, & Gregory, 1993). In other words, "an increase in viscosity in a state of rest, and a decrease in viscosity when exposed to shear stress" (Proske et al., 1993). When dealing with muscle tissue, thixotropy refers to the "dry friction-like behavior of passive muscle to movement, as distinct from its elastic (length dependent) and/or viscous (velocity dependent) behavior" (Proske et al., 1993).

However, this is only one theory. In fact, there are several theories explaining the hypothetical mechanisms of thixotropy observed in muscle.

Thixotropy and the Musculoskeletal System

One of the most popular theories for thixotropy mechanisms and muscle tissue involves the early work of D. K. Hill. In 1968, Hill described the short-range elastic component (SREC) of muscle tissue and attributed the thixotropic properties to myofibril cross-bridging. During his experimentation, Hill (1968) discovered that tension of the tissue did not vary with either length or velocity. Instead, tension increased until approximately 0.2% of tissue length and then surprisingly remained constant. According to the definition of thixotropy borrowed from Proske et al. (1993), the SREC could account for the thixotropic properties of muscle since it does not vary directly with changes in length or velocity (except for the initial elastic portion). Due to the SREC phenomenon, Hill (1968) hypothesized that this occurred because a number of "slower" cross-bridges are present in resting muscle tissue (between myosin and actin) that do not exist in active muscle.

Subsequent work has supported some of the ideas presented by Hill. Lakie and Robson (1988) discovered that stiffness of muscle tissue, in this case frog tissue, depends on prior movement of the tissue as well as on the amount of force used. Small forces applied to the frog muscle produce greater stiffness within the SREC range (0.2% of muscle length). Along the same lines, when the force applied was small, stirring the muscle (i.e., movement) decreased stiffness of the tissue for a period of time after which the original stiffness level returned (Lakie & Robson, 1968). This finding supported the theory that cross-bridging and the SREC are related to thixotropy in muscle. In the same experiment, Lakie and Robson discovered that applying larger forces produced a larger stretch, thus rupturing the SREC and producing decreased stiffness and a smaller thixotropic effect. Therefore, passive motion decreases stiffness. In a follow-up experiment, the same authors discovered that stiffness is also

temporarily decreased by prior titanic electrical stimulation under isometric conditions (Lakie & Robson, 1968). Finally, changes in temperature do not significantly affect the thixotropic properties of the tissue (Walsh & Wright, 1988).

In an extensive review of thixotropy, Proske et al. (1993) concluded that thixotropy depends on whether "stirring" will break the SREC complex. If the SREC complex is broken, stable cross-bridges will take less than two seconds to reform and, depending on the length at which the muscle is held during this reformation period, slack might or might not develop (Proske et al., 1993). According to Proske et al. (1993), slack forms at a muscle length longer than that at which the muscle is held subsequently, and its purpose is to raise muscle compliance and increase the delay time for onset of tension during a muscle contraction. However, since thixotropy is controlled by several variables, the onset of tension during muscle contraction can be unpredictable (Proske et al., 1993). Proske et al. (1993) extrapolate from these findings and suggest that warming up prior to exercise will theoretically improve performance due to more predictable muscle contractions. In addition, pre-activity warm-ups can provide slack not only to the agonists, but to the antagonists as well. Stretched antagonistic muscles will have more slack; consequently, they will not be as stiff during passive resistance (Proske et al., 1993).

However, it is important to remember that myofascial structures are anchored to the skeletal system. In determining the SREC of a specific muscle, the joint that muscle crosses—or is attached to—does affect the SREC value. Consequently, the joints affect the thixotropy of the tissues. Research in this area has shown that if joint movement occurs within a small amplitude, then muscle stiffness in the surrounding tissues increases (Walsh & Wright, 1988). At the same time, further research has indicated that joints themselves, and tendinous structures, do not exhibit the thixotropic properties of muscles (Gandevia & McCloskey, 1976), although the ground substance in skin displays thixotropic behavior (Finlay, 1978).

The information gained from the studies just described can be valuable in designing a treatment plan for myofascial injuries. By taking into consideration some of the evidence provided, therapists are in a position to design a more effective treatment. However, in a study by Vattanasil, Ada, and Crosbie (2000), it was found that the thixotropic response was not higher in neurologically normal subjects versus patients impaired after stroke. According to the authors, this finding suggests that although thixotropy may produce enough immediate resistance to impede movement in those who are weak, it does not contribute significantly to long-term muscle stiffness. Contracture did, however, contribute to muscle stiffness (Vattanasil et al., 2000). Hence, while thixotropy is important to consider when providing treatment, long-term stiffness has to be accounted for by some other property.

Sol-to-Gel Transition in Collagen

As pointed out earlier, thixotropy is a property of numerous tissues (muscles, fascia, connective and vascular tissues). Since the main focus of this book is the fascial system, it is time to take a closer look at what affects the thixotropic properties of connective tissue. More specifically, this section examines the idea that the thixotropy seen in connective tissue is a direct result of what is occurring at a molecular level: the collagen fiber.

In attempting to understand how connective tissue stiffening occurs, many researchers have used gelatin as the substance of choice for studying the properties of such tissue. The reason for this choice is that gelatin gel is composed of cross-linked polypeptide chains (similar to collagen triple helices). One substance that seems to be critical in understanding the molecular mechanism of gelation (transformation from sol to gel) is water. Water is an important stabilizing factor in the organization of connective tissue. Macromolecules have a tendency to unfold and dissociate in high-pressure environments (Fukamizu & Grinnel, 1990; Heremans, 1982). One study suggested that the pressure stabilization of gelatin gels could be attributed mainly to the specific hydration structures formed between water molecules and the polypeptide chains. In fact, it was shown that under high pressures (the result of dehydration and random association of polypeptide chains), gelation is suppressed. In similar studies, it was shown that under high pressure, the melting temperature of gelatin is increased, collagen triple helices are stabilized, and fibril formation is decreased (Gandevia & McCloskey, 1976). The importance of water in maintaining organization and tissue integrity is once again seen.

SOMATIC RECALL

"Most of us have had similar experiences, in which a glimpse of some long-forgotten place or object, or a particular odor, taste, sound, or even a movement, elicits the recall of a scene from our distant past" (J. Oschman & N. Oschman, 1994). These are the experiences that James Oschman finds analogous to what health-care practitioners, particularly hands-on practitioners, feel during treatment—and describe as transient sensations that something has happened before. Oschman, who has done extensive work in this area of recurrent "flashbacks," coined the term *somatic recall* to describe these experiences.

Thus, somatic recall is the body's way of storing somatic experiences that can resurface by means of touch. In fact, manual therapists feel these somatic experiences are indeed stored by the body's myofascial system. Furthermore, these experiences, according to practitioners, are simultaneously felt by both the client and the therapist. On the one hand, when the therapist touches areas of the patient's body, there may be a sudden recall of past somatic experiences from the client's perspective. On the other hand, these flashbacks are felt, and erased, by the soft tissue practitioner as the ground substance, extracellular, and intracellular components depolymerize and become more flexible and fluid (J. Oschman & N. Oschman, 1994).

Research in this area is new and sparse, so there is not much support for some of the ideas introduced in this section. Nevertheless, Oschman claims that these experiences occur on a regular basis and that they can help shed some light on the areas of memory, learning, consciousness, and the effects of touch (J. Oschman & N. Oschman, 1994).

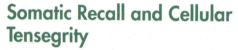

Somatic Recall and Cellular Tensegrity

This chapter began by discussing the importance of tensegrity in both maintaining cellular structure as well as accommodating for changes in tension and pull. It further discussed how the tensegrity model, observed at a cellular level, is a microcosm of what is happening at the system, or organ, level. It was shown how there are interconnections that start at the cellular/nuclear level and extend through the ECM (through FACs), on to the next cell, and consequently throughout the entire connective tissue system. In fact, Chapter 1 referred to several studies supporting

the theory that the fascial system is indeed one continuous, interconnecting system (Brodland & Gordon, 1987; Thiery, Duband, Rocher, & Yamada, 1986) and that mechanical stimulation of fascia at a global level can have noteworthy effects on processes such as neurulation, granulation, and DNA replication.

Because of this continuity, the fascial system acts as an "information highway" through the process of mechanotransduction. Oschman theorizes that signal production and distribution are the result of six fascial characteristics: semiconduction, piezoelectricity, crystallinity, coherence, hydration, and continuity (see Table 3-1). Oschman refers to this

Table 3-1 Continuum Communication: Fascial Properties Responsible for Signal Production and Distribution	
Semiconduction	All fascial components are semiconductors. They can both conduct and process vibrational information, much like an integrated circuit or microprocessor in a computer. They also convert energy from one form to another.
Piezoelectricity	Waves of mechanical vibration moving through the living matrix produce electrical fields, and vice versa.
Crystallinity	Much of the living matrix consists of molecules that are regularly arrayed in a crystalline lattice. This includes lipids in cell membranes, collagen molecules of connective tissue, actin and myosin molecules of muscle, and components of the cytoskeleton.
Coherence	The highly regular macromolecular structures found within connective tissue produce giant coherent or laserlike oscillations that move rapidly throughout the living matrix and are radiated into the environment. These vibrations, referred to as Frohlich oscillations, occur at particular frequencies in the microwave and visible portions of the electromagnetic spectrum of light. A number of scientists have detected these signals.
Hydration	On average, 15,000 water molecules are associated with each matrix protein. Since many of the proteins are highly ordered, the associated water molecules are also highly ordered. Water molecules are also polarized (dipoles). The living matrix organizes the dipolar water molecules in a way that constrains or restricts their ability to vibrate or rotate or wiggle about in a different spatial plane. Water molecules are free to vibrate or spin only in particular directions.
Continuity	While individual organs, tissues, cells, and molecules might be examined separately, connective tissue is a continuous and unbroken whole.

process as "continuum communication" (J. Oschman & N. Oschman, 1994).

According to Oschman, all six of these characteristics help assist in transfer of information between two distant locations. When information passage is obstructed or hindered due to trauma, infection, or stress, then disease and/or pain are the result (J. Oschman & N. Oschman, 1994).

So how does somatic recall fit into all this? When mechanical stimulation excites the tissue, the signal can be altered or obstructed by previously stored memories and information (J. Oschman & N. Oschman, 1994). The goal of manual practitioners is to return the tissue to its original integrity, free of any obstructions (scar tissue, pain, etc.). By manipulating the tissues, the practitioner attempts to bring fluidity back to the tissues. This is where the concept of thixotropy comes into play. As discussed, application of pressure, in addition to increases in temperature, can bring back a tissue's fluid physical properties and decrease stiffness. In addition to restoring tissue integrity, manipulation of soft tissue structures has the ability to release toxic substances trapped within these tissues (J. Oschman & N. Oschman, 1994). Once released, these toxins are absorbed by the lymphatic and vascular systems and, finally, excreted by the body. This is why practitioners often recommend that patients consume moderate amounts of water following soft tissue work. The purpose is to assist the body in excreting these "free-floating toxins" (J. Oschman & N. Oschman, 1994).

Thus, soft tissue therapy is critical in stimulating and releasing old somatic experiences—referred to as somatic recall. The result is to remove obstacles, restore tissue integrity, and allow for free passage of signals throughout the connective tissue system.

Summary

Although the tensegrity model cannot explain all of the biochemical functions that allow cells to adapt and survive in a particular environment, it does provide a model that represents organization and stability of the cytoskeletal system of cells. This model increases understanding of how the bones, tendons, muscles, fascial system, and other organs of the body are structured to provide stability, support, and shape. In addition, based on the tensegrity principle, it can be seen that mechanical stress placed upon the body induces molecular changes at the cellular levels.

Muscles possess thixotropic properties that are largely based on the individual's immediate prior history of movements and contractions. After contractions and stretches, the mechanical tension of muscle changes by reducing stiffness and improving the range of joint motion.

The idea that memory is stored in the tissues of the myofascial system has given rise to research on how the living matrix is able to communicate via various signals known as the continuum communication model. This model suggests that every action in the body produces vibrations throughout the living matrix to distribute regulatory information; and any disruptions in the flow and processing of information lead to disease and disorder. Message therapists have taken advantage of this concept and turned it into practical methods of healing the body.

References

Brodland, G. W., & Gordon, R. (1987). The cytoskeletal mechanics of brain morphogenesis: Cell state splitters cause neural induction. *Cell Biophysics, 11,* 177–238.

Emerman, J. T., & Pitelka, D. R. (1977). Maintenance and induction of morphological differentiation in dissociated mammary epithelium on floating collagen membranes. *In Vitro Cellular & Developmental Biology, 5,* 316–328.

Finlay, J. B. (1978). Thixotropy in human skin. *Journal of Biomechanics, 11,* 333–342.

Fukamizu, H., & Grinnel, F. (1990). Spatial organization of extracellular matrix and fibro-blast activity: Effect of serum transforming growth beta and fibronectin. *Experimental Cell Research, 199,* 276–282.

Gandevia, S. C., & McCloskey, D. I. (1976). Joint sense, muscle sense, and their combination as position sense measured at the distal interphalangeal joint of the middle finger. *Journal of Physiology, 260,* 387–407.

Heremans, K. (1982). High-pressure effects on proteins and other biomolecules. *Annual Review of Biophysics & Bioengineering, 11,* 1–21.

Heuser, J. E., & Kirschner, M. W. (1980). Filament organization revealed in platinum replicas of freeze-dried cytoskeletons. *Journal of Cell Biology, 86,* 212–234.

Hill, D. K. (1968). Tension due to interaction between sliding filaments in resting striated muscle: The effect of stimulation. *Journal of Physiology, 199,* 637–684.

Ingber, D. E. (2003). Tensegrity I: Cell structure and hierarchical systems. *Journal of Cell Science 116,* 1157–1173.

Ingber, D. E. (1993). Cellular tensegrity: Defining new rules of biological design that govern the cytoskeleton. *Journal of Cell Science, 104,* 613–627.

Ingber, D. E. (2003). Tensegrity II: How structural networks influence cellular information processing networks. *Journal of Cell Science 116,* 1397–1408.

Kreis, T. E., & Birchmeiser, W. (1980). Stress fiber sarcomeres of fibroblasts are contractile. *Cell 22,* 555–561.

Lakie, M., & Robson, L. G. (1988). Thixotropy: The effect of stretch size in relaxed frog muscle. *Quarterly Journal of Experimental Physiology, 73,* 127–129.

Lamoureux, P., Steel, V. L., Regal, C., Adgate, L., Buxbaum, R. E., & Heldemann. S. R. (1990). Extracellular matrix allows PC12 neurite elongation in the absence of microtubules. *Journal of Cell Biology, 110,* 71–79.

Lotz, M. M., Burdsal, C. A., Erikson, H. P., & McClay, D. R. (1989). Cell adhesion to fibronectin and tenascin: Quantitative measurements of initial binding and subsequent strengthening response. *Journal of Cell Biology, 109,* 1795–1805.

Oschman, J. L., & Oschman, N. H. (1994). Somatic recall, Parts I–II: Soft tissue memory/soft tissue holography, massage therapy. *American Journal of Massage Therapy Association, 34,* 36–45, 66–67, 101–167.

Pienta, K. J., & Coffey, D. S. (1991). Cellular harmonic information transfer through a tissue tensegrity-matrix system. *Medical Hypotheses, 34,* 88–95.

Proske, U., Morgan, D. L., & Gregory, J. E. (1993). Thixotropy in skeletal muscle and in muscle spindles. *Progress in Neurobiology, 41,* 705–721.

Thiery, J. P., Duband, J. L., Rocher, S., & Yamada, K. M. (1986). Adhesion and migration of avian neural crest cells: An evaluation of the role of several extracellular matrix components. *Progress in Clinical & Biological Research, 217B,* 155–168.

Vattanasil, P. W., Ada, L., & Crosbie, J. (2000). Contribution of thixotropy, spasticity and contracture to ankle stiffness after stroke. *Journal of Neurology, Neurosurgery, & Psychiatry, 69,* 34–39.

Volokh, K. Y. (2003). Cytoskeletal architecture and mechanical behavior of living cells. *Biorheology, 40,* 213–220.

Volokh, K. Y., Vilnay, O., & Belsky, M. (2000). Tensegrity architecture explains linear stiffening

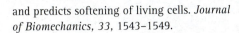

and predicts softening of living cells. *Journal of Biomechanics, 33,* 1543–1549.

Walsh, E. G., & Wright, G. W. (1988). Postural thixotropy at the human hip. *Quarterly Journal of Experimental Physiology, 73,* 369–377.

Zaner, K. S., & Valberg, P. A. (1989). Viscoelasticity of F-actin measured with magnetic microparticles. *Journal of Cell Biology, 109,* 2233–2243.

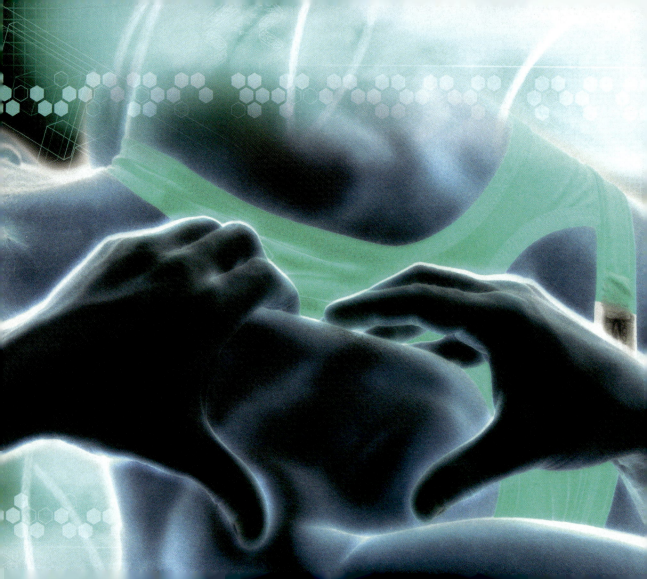

NEUROPHYSIOLOGICAL BASIS FOR FASCIAL PLASTICITY

The purpose of this chapter is to examine the known and theoretical mechanical effects of therapeutic myofascial treatment on fascia. Older models relying predominantly on mechanotransduction have failed to fully explain the observed changes in the viscoelastic property of fascia when treated using manual myofascial therapy. Recent research has shifted the focus away from a mechanical body concept and instead has moved toward a cybernetic model in which the clinician's intervention is seen as stimulation for self-regulatory processes within the patient.

The concept of tissue plasticity and ideas throughout this chapter are based on the extensive work of Schleip (2002a, 2002b). Most theories (thixotropic based) account for the changes in fascia's physical properties following treatment as resulting from the application of energy (Barnes, 1990; Cantu & Grodin, 1992; Chaitow, 1980; Paoletti, 1998; Rolf, 1977; Ward, 1993). This energy can take the form of heat (hot pack) application or mechanical compression (e.g., trigger point therapy). The result is a change in ground substance/matrix consistency from a solid gel state to a more fluid state (Zaner & Valberg, 1989). Researchers argue that thixotropy cannot explain the short-term changes occurring in fascial tissue during times of stress or treatment, but can account only for the long-term changes that fascia undergoes in adapting to stresses placed upon it. Thixotropy does not provide support for the immediate changes (less than 2–3 minutes) seen following treatment by a trained health-care practitioner. In fact, it has been demonstrated that a lengthy amount of time and a higher amount of force are required to permanently deform connective tissues, including fascia (Currier & Nelson, 1992).

Threlkeld (1992) did a study that specifically looked at "time and force dependency of connective tissue plasticity" and verified that considerable time and force were required for deformation of connective tissue fibers to occur (Threlkeld, 1992). A 1 to 1.5% percent fiber elongation for over an hour, or a forceful stretch of 3 to 8% fiber elongation over a shorter period of time, was required to deform the collagen fibers permanently with no reversibility (Threlkeld, 1992). For this latter point, it took approximately 60 kg of force to elongate the iliotibial band by 18 mm. In addition, the thixotropic effect in colloidal substances lasts only as long as energy is applied; once the energy is removed, the tissue returns to its original physiology. Thus, thixotropy cannot explain these short-term changes. Another model has to be used to explain this short-term plasticity of fascia following treatment.

Piezoelectricity has been used to explain the plasticity changes occurring following treatment. Living organisms and tissue, including fascia, usually have some type of electrical charge. Researchers have speculated that connective tissue cells, specifically fibroblasts (collagen producers), are sensitive to electrical changes within the tissue (Oschman, 2000; Athenstaedt, 1974). Mechanical pressure from treatment can either increase or decrease the electric charge, stimulating fibroblasts to produce more collagen fibers and matrix macromolecules in the area. Although this theory is currently speculative, other tissues like bone are capable of undergoing osteogenesis and remodeling following mechanical stress as a result of the piezoelectric properties of collagen (Silva et al., 2001). In addition, studies have shown that the half-life of normal collagen fibers ranges between 400 and 500 days, while the ground matrix has a half-life of approximately 2–8 days (Cantu & Grodin, 1992). Even though half-life is for normal tissue, injured fascia may be similar, although this length of time does not correlate to the sometimes immediate effects of fascial tissue treatment. Another traditional model that attempts to account for a full explanation of the viscoelastic changes occurring to tissue in a manual therapy treatment session is biomechanical and will be discussed in the following section.

FASCIAL TISSUE MECHANICAL BEHAVIOR— BIOMECHANICAL MODELS

The mechanical response of dense connective tissue that gives rise to ligaments, tendons, and fascia is reviewed here. The purpose is to provide a framework for discussion of the clinical effects of myofascial therapy on connective tissue like fascia.

Fascial Anatomy

Fascia is comprised predominantly of fibroblasts and collagen fibers. Fascia consists of collagen bundles organized into multilayered sheets or lamellae. The bundles within individual layers are roughly parallel but often have some undulations or waviness. This wave formation allows collagen fibers to stretch during compression. The amount of waviness or crimping is affected by aging (Figure 4-1). Fiber bundles in adjacent layers may not have the same direction, although fibers will often pass between adjacent layers as well as into adjacent loose connective tissue. The fibroblasts found in fascia and aponeuroses are sparse and variable in shape. Ground substance and elastin content are low in fascia.

Mechanical Response of Fascia to External Loading

The crimping of the collagen fibers in fascia accounts for a variable amount of slack. When a tensile force is applied, such as during a myofascial stretch, the superficial fascia is loaded asynchronously. Only after most of the collagen bundles that make up the superficial fascia are placed in a stretch will the superficial fascia undergo deformation. The resistance of fascia to deformation can be graphically represented using a stress-strain curve (Figure 4-2).

Periarticular connective tissue structures such as fascia are typically tested under tensile loading to

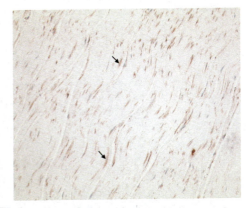

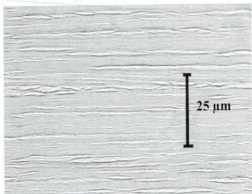

Figure 4-1 A Significantly Higher Collagen Fiber Density Is Seen in the Younger Age Group than in the Older Group. The density correlates with the crimp amplitude of the collagen fibers. (A) Sample from a 19-year-old man shows plenty of darkly stained contractile cells and extensive crimping or wave formation. (B) With the 76-year-old donor, there is neither crimp formation nor contractile cells.
Source: Robert Schleip, Werner Klingler MD, Frank Lehmann-Horn PhD (2004, November). Presentation to the Fifth Interdisciplinary World Congress on Low Back and Pelvic Pain, City, Country (slides and text of oral presentation).

determine their maximal mechanical behavior. Tensile testing of connective tissue produces a stress-strain curve that represents the load and resulting connective tissue deformation, and this curve has been divided into several functionally important regions. The clinical test region is the same as the toe region shown in Figure 4-2 and represents the level of load and deformation at which crimping is being taken out of the connective tissue structure. The

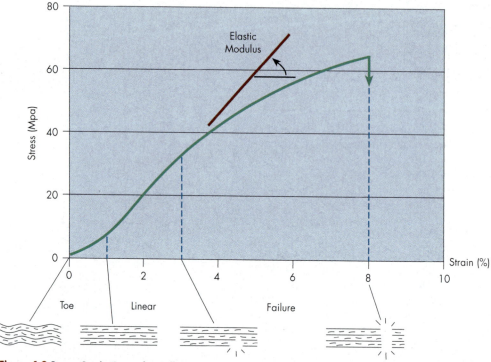

Figure 4-2 Stress-Strain Curve for Collagen. An increase in stress (tensile force) results in physical changes to collagen to the point of fiber breakage (shown as failure).

Source: Butler D. L., Grood E. S., & Noyes F. R. (1978). Biomechanics of ligaments and tendons. *Exercise and sports science reviews, 6,* 125–181.

presence and shape of the stress-strain curve in the toe region are variable and dependent on the internal structural organization of the tissue. The more regular and parallel the collagenous bundle in the superficial fascia, the shorter the toe segment. In myofascial therapy, the act of elongating connective tissue through the toe region is known as taking out the slack. The graded mobilizations that are intended primarily to relieve pain but not to elongate connective tissue are supposedly conducted in this range.

The physiological loading region of the stress-strain curve represents the range of forces that usually act on connective tissue in vivo and implies that primarily elastic deformation occurs at these loads. The region of microfailure overlaps

the end of the physiologic loading zone. Micro-failure represents the breakage of the individual collagen fibers and fiber bundles that are placed under the greatest tension during progressive deformation. The remaining intact fibers and bundles that may have not been directly aligned with the force, or those that had more intrinsic length, absorb a greater proportion of the load. The result is progressive, permanent (plastic) deformation of the connective tissue structure. If the force is released, the broken fibers will not contribute to the recoil of the tissue. A new length of the connective tissue (CT) structure is established that reflects the balance between the elastic recoil of the remaining intact collagen and the resistance of the intrinsic water and glycosaminoglycans (GAGs) to compression. Microfailure is a desired outcome of some manual stretching techniques that are intended to produce permanent elongation of the fascia. The breaking of collagen cross-links, which are responsible for the fibrotic scarring and myofascial trigger points established throughout superficial and deep fascia, will be followed by a cycle of inflammation, repair, and remodeling that should be therapeutically managed to maintain the desired fascia elongation.

Plastic deformation should not be confused with the phenomenon of creep. Creep is a time-dependent deformation that occurs over a prolonged period rather than suddenly. This deformity occurs to relieve stress, and the result is permanent. On the other hand, plastic deformation occurs following elastic deformity of tissues. Here, the change in shape is temporary under low stress and within the elastic limits of the tissue, causing the tissue to return to its original shape once the load is removed. However, if the stress load exceeds the elastic limits of the material, permanent plastic deformation results (Figure 4-3).

In biological tissues, the phenomenon of creep primarily represents the redistribution of water from the tissue to the anatomical spaces surrounding the tissue. Some elongation of tissues that results from manual stretching and massage techniques may reflect impermanent creep deformation. To detect this phenomenon, clinical research designs examining manual therapy techniques should incorporate several repeated measurements of elongation up to 24 hours after application of the myofascial stretch.

Effect of Injury and Immobilization on Myofascial Trigger Points

An acute injury to myofascial connective tissue will be followed by inflammation and subsequent fibrosis, resulting in a remodeled connective tissue with lower tensile stiffness and a lower ultimate strength than normal tissue. This weakening is caused by the more randomized collagen fiber direction, by the inability of collagen bundles to slide easily past one another (cross-linking and loss of water), and possibly by the substitution of collagen types that are not as strong as the original collagen.

Mechanical Effects of Fascial Manual Therapy

Manual soft tissue technique such as myofascial and/or active release use the examiner's hands to reestablish motion between fascial planes, thus reducing fibrous adhesions and reestablishing neural and myofascial glide between tissues. These techniques work on the presumption that they preload the fascia by taking slack out through alternating active patient muscle contraction with passive stretching. The end result should allow the collagen fiber crimping to be removed from the connective tissue and for some amount of creep deformation to occur. These are temporary lengthening phenomena demonstrating a damped elastic response, and they can easily be misinterpreted as permanent lengthening. Plastic deformation does not take place until the forces within the tissue reach a higher level.

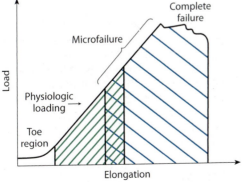

Figure 4-3 Stress-Strain Curve of Dense Connective Tissue. The physiologic loading zone represents forces that produce elastic deformation in the linear region of the curve. Microfailure and plastic deformation occurs at the greatest physiologic loads, including complete failure zone.

Source: Schleip (2003a).

All of this research leads to a simple thought experiment. In everyday life, the body is often exposed to pressure similar to the application of manual pressure in a myofascial stretch or active release therapeutic technique. While the body naturally adapts structurally to long-term furniture use, it is impossible to conceive that adaptations could occur so rapidly that any uneven load distribution in sitting would permanently alter the shape of your pelvis within a minute.

Since no theory exists as to how fascia adapts to short-term changes, many have turned to the nervous system to explain this phenomenon. Fascia is closely related to the nervous system; it is traversed by nerves, it envelops the nervous system, and fascial plasticity is reliant upon the nervous system. Studies have shown that without a proper neural connection, the tissue does not respond as well to treatment as it does under normal neuronal functioning (Schleip, 1989).

Neurophysiological Dynamics of Fascia

Studies involving the use of human cadavers and immunohistochemical technology on animal and/or human fascia have revealed some interesting findings. The chronological development of the neurophysiology of fascia has been studied as early as in prenatal ontogeny. The first neural fibers have been seen in as early as 8- to 9-week-old embryos. Cholinesterase and catecholamines are detected in nerves of the vegetative neural system in the 11th to 12th week of intrauterine life, thus demonstrating the appearance of a functioning autonomic nervous system. Mechanoreceptors have appeared in the fascia of 3- to $3\frac{1}{2}$-month-old fetuses. During prenatal ontogenesis, the neural fibers start increasing in number and become more complex with cholinergic and adrenergic nerve fibers forming plexuses in fascia.

Electron photomicrography of the fascia cruris, which encases the lower leg, has shown nerves innervating the fascia (Figure 4-4). Additional studies have shown the presence of adrenergic nerve fibers along with blood vessels penetrating the fascia at points similar to acupuncture pressure points (Figure 4-5).

Furthermore, the neural structure of the shoulder capsule of mice has revealed the ultrastructure and location of nerve endings, along with lamellated Pacini-type and Ruffini-type mechanoreceptors in the fibrous fascia sheath of the shoulder capsule. The presence of small, uniformly shaped, lamellated corpuscles of the Pacini type in qualitatively different areas of surrounding tissue implies that they are susceptible to different kinds of mechanical stimuli.

The clinical implications of discovering the presence of both mechanoreceptors and sensory receptors in fascia could possibly account for myofascial pain. If a clinician using manual therapy or any other adjunct therapy could influence the response of these fascial receptors, then therapeutic outcomes could be clinically significant. Additionally, the direct neural connection between fascia and the autonomic nervous system may be responsible for fascial tonus, which can have ramifications for biomechanics, transmission of muscular force, circulation (blood, lymph), and soft tissue pain.

THE NERVOUS SYSTEM

The nervous system consists of all the nervous tissue in the body. It can be divided into the central nervous system (CNS) and the peripheral nervous system (PNS). The CNS consists of the brain and the spinal cord; the PNS is composed of cranial and peripheral nerves, collections of nerve cells outside the CNS known as ganglia, and both motor and sensory nerve endings. Nerves consist of bundles of myelinated neuronal axons that may carry either sensory information to the CNS (afferent) or motor information from the CNS (efferent).

Central Nervous System

The entire CNS is protected by a bony encasement; the cranium, which surrounds the brain, and the vertebral column, which surrounds the spinal cord. Between the bone and the soft tissue of the CNS is a

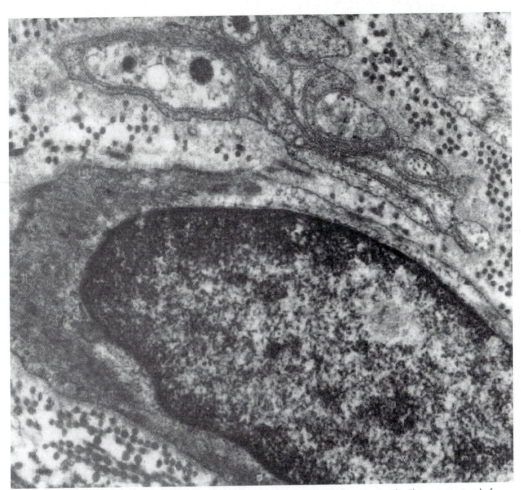

Figure 4-4 An Electron Micrograph of a Smooth Muscle Cell Within the Fascia Cruris. The uppermost end of an unmyelinated type IV sensory neuron is situated above the cell.

Source: Schleip (2003b).

protective set of membranes, the meninges. There are three layers of meninges (from the outside in): the dura mater, the arachnoid mater, and the pia mater. While the dura is thick and collagenous, the arachnoid and pia mater are both thin and transparent. The dura mater is divided into a cranial and a spinal portion to form one continuous membrane composed of a thick, dense, fibrous collagen structure with some elastic fibers. The collagen fibers are densely packed in fascicles. Although the dura mater is mainly acellular, there is evidence of fibroblasts

distributed throughout the tissue. The cranial dura mater is composed of an outer (endosteal) and an inner (meningeal) layer. The endosteal layer is continuous with the pericranium through the cranial sutures, the foramina, and the orbital periosteum through the orbital fissure; the meningeal layer envelops the 12 cranial nerves (I–XII), attaching to their respective epineuria as they pass through the various cranial foramina. The meningeal layer also forms septa that divide the brain into smaller compartments. These four septa are the falx cerebri, the

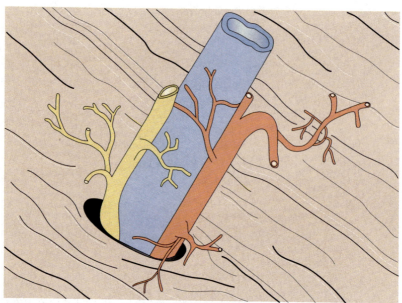

Figure 4-5 Location of Nerves and Acupuncture Points in Fascia. From left to right: a nerve, vein, and artery are shown schematically as penetrating the superficial fascia at locations similar to Chinese acupuncture pressure points.
Source: Schleip (2003b).

tentorium cerebelli, the falx cerebelli, and the diaphragma sellae.

Cerebrospinal fluid (CSF) is a clear, colorless liquid containing different electrolytes and traces of protein molecules. It bathes and circulates within the hollow ventricles of the brain, the central canal of the spinal cord, and in the subarachnoid space surrounding the entire CNS. The choroid plexus situated within the four ventricles of the brain (two lateral, third, fourth) produces the CSF and the cilia found on ependymal cells and circulates the fluid within the skull. Pulsatile movements of the various arteries, found in and around the meningeal layers, create CSF movement within the spinal cord.

As the cranial dura mater exits the foramen magnum, it forms the anterior and posterior atlanto-occipital membranes. Inferior to the foramen magnum, the spinal dura mater forms a tube that surrounds the spinal cord. The superior (upper) end is attached to the edges of the foramen magnum, to the posterior

surfaces of the second and third vertebral bodies, and to the posterior longitudinal ligament (PLL). The inferior end of the spinal dura mater merges into a conical filum terminale that is attached onto the coccygeal periosteum. Once again, more proof that connective tissues in our bodies are not limited by borders, but form an extensive network throughout the body. Within the vertebral canal and between the periosteum/ligaments and the spinal dura mater lies the extradural space, which contains loose connective tissue, adipose tissue, and venous plexi.

The middle layer of the meninges, the arachnoid mater, consists of both a cranial and spinal portion. The cranial part of this mater surrounds the brain but does not enter fissures or sulci of the brain. The space between the arachnoid and pia mater is known as the subarachnoid space; it contains the CSF as well as blood vessels and cranial nerves entering the brain. Within the arachnoid mater, particularly within fissures and sinuses, are granulations and villi that project onto a collagenous framework to move the CSF into the bloodstream by vesicular transport through the sinus endothelium. The spinal part of the arachnoid mater is continuous with the cranial portion. As nerves and vessels enter and exit the spinal cord, the arachnoid mater envelops them and adheres to the perineurium or adventitia of the vessel, once again forming a complex interconnection.

The deepest meningeal layer, the one that is closest to the brain, is the pia mater. The pia mater is a delicate, thin membrane composed of loose connective tissue only 2 to 3 cells thick; it invests the surfaces of the brain and follows all irregular contours (sulci, gyri) of the brain and spinal cord. Being highly vascular, the pia mater supports the vessels that nourish the underlying cells of the CNS. The pia mater is specialized within the walls of the ventricles, where it contributes to formation of the choroids plexus along with arachnoid mater. The spinal portion of pia mater forms lateral extensions known as ligamentum denticulatum (dentate ligaments) that separate the ventral from the dorsal roots.

These extensions attach the spinal cord to the dura mater. It has been demonstrated that dentate ligaments change in form and position during movement—particularly movement of the vertebral column.

Peripheral Nervous System

The peripheral nervous system consists only of cranial and spinal nerves that convey impulses to and from the central nervous system to the rest of the body. The 12 pairs of cranial nerves arise from the inferior surface of the brain. The cranial nerves, except for the vestibulocochlear nerve, all pass through foramina of the skull to innervate structures of the head, neck, and visceral organs of the trunk. The names of the cranial nerves are associated with their primary function or the general distribution of the fibers:

1. *Sensory (cranial) nerves:* olfactory (I), optic (II), and vestibulocochlear (VIII)

2. *Motor and sensory nerves:* trigeminal (V), glossopharyngeal (IX), and vagus (X)

3. *Motor nerves:* ophthalmic (III), trochlear (IV), abducens (VI), facial (VII), accessory (XI), and hypoglossal (XII); only the sensory fibers of these are proprioceptive

The spinal nerves consist of 31 pairs of nerves formed by the union of the anterior (ventral) and posterior (dorsal) spinal roots that emerge from the spinal cord through the intervertebral foramina. The spinal nerves are grouped according to the levels of the spinal column from which they arise, and they are numbered in sequence. Each spinal nerve consists of a posterior and anterior root of sensory fibers. The posterior root contains an enlargement called the dorsal root ganglion (sensory), where the sensory neurons are located. The axons of sensory neurons convey sensory impulses through the posterior root and into the spinal cord. The anterior root consists of axons of motor neurons that carry impulses away from the CNS.

Just beyond the intervertebral foramen, each spinal nerve divides into several branches including the meningeal branch, posterior ramus, and anterior ramus. The small meningeal branch reenters the vertebral canal to innervate the meninges, vertebrae, and vertebral ligaments. The posterior ramus innervates muscles, joints, and the skin of the back along the vertebral column. The anterior ramus innervates the muscles and skin on the lateral and anterior side of the trunk. The anterior rami of the spinal nerves (except T2–T12) combine and then split again as networks of nerves called plexuses. There are four plexuses of spinal nerves: cervical, brachial, lumbar, and sacral. Nerves that emerge from these plexuses are named according to structures they innervate or the general course they take.

Nociceptors are part of the peripheral nervous system. They are widely spread throughout the body and, depending on their location, respond to various stimuli. The stimulus of pain is transmitted by nociceptors

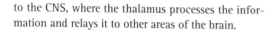

to the CNS, where the thalamus processes the information and relays it to other areas of the brain.

Autonomic Nervous System

Neurons of the peripheral nervous system that conduct impulses away from the CNS are motor or efferent neurons. There are two divisions of motor neurons: somatic and autonomic. Somatic motor neurons (cranial and spinal nerves) have their cell bodies within the CNS and send axons to skeletal muscles, which are usually under voluntary control. The autonomic nervous system is under involuntary control. The types of tissues receiving autonomic innervation include cardiac muscle, smooth muscle, and glands.

Autonomic motor control involves two neurons in the motor pathway—unlike somatic motor control, which involves only one axon from the spinal cord to the neuromuscular junction. The first of these neurons has its cell body in the brain or spinal cord, where its axon does not directly innervate the target organ but instead synapses with a second neuron within an autonomic ganglion. This neuron is known as the preganglionic neuron, and the neuron that extends from the ganglion onto the target tissue is known as the postganglionic neuron. The autonomic nervous system (ANS) is divided into a sympathetic and a parasympathetic division. The sympathetic division activates the body to "fight or flight" through adrenergic effects, while the parasympathetic division often exerts antagonistic actions ("rest and digest") through cholinergic effects.

Nerves of the peripheral system (cranial, spinal, and autonomic) branch away from the CNS and spread throughout the body, innervating a wide array of structures. These nerves pierce muscles and fascia, and they travel with various vessels (arteries, veins, lymphatics) during their course through the human body. Embryologically, the growth and migrations of the nervous system are linked to the fascial system, and fascia also plays a critical supportive role for the nervous system.

THE REFLEX ARC AND REFLEXES

Specific nerve pathways provide routes by which impulses travel through the nervous system. The simplest type of nerve pathway is the reflex arc, which involves an automatic, involuntary, quick, protective response to a potentially threatening stimulus. The conduction pathway of a reflex arc consists of the following five components:

1. Receptor
2. Sensory neuron
3. Center
4. Motor neuron
5. Target tissue/organ

The effect on the target organ is called a reflex action or a reflex. There are two types of reflexes: visceral and somatic. Visceral reflexes, also known as autonomic reflexes, cause smooth muscle to contract or glands to secrete fluids. Therefore, these reflexes help control the body's many involuntary movements such as heart rate, respiratory rate, blood flow, and digestion. Somatic reflexes involve contraction of skeletal muscles. The three main types of somatic reflexes involve the stretch reflex (monosynaptic reflex), the flexor/withdrawal reflex (polysynaptic reflex), and the crossed extensor reflex (reciprocal inhibition). Fascial plasticity is seen with somatic reflexes, particularly the stretch reflex, and they are a major component in explaining the immediate, short-term effects seen following soft tissue manipulation.

FASCIAL SENSORY RECEPTORS

A receptor is part of the conduction pathway necessary to convert a stimulus to a nerve impulse. Sensory receptors are specialized structures located at the distal tips of the peripheral processes of sensory neurons. Structurally, sensory receptors can be dendritic endings of sensory neurons that are either free (free nerve endings) or encapsulated within nonneural structures. Encapsulated receptors can be further classified into groups according to function. Extero-receptors react to stimuli from the external environment (touch, temperature, smell) and from within the body (e.g., filling or stretch of the bladder or blood vessels). Proprioceptors, on the other hand, react to stimuli from within the body (similar to enterorecep-tors) but provide sensation of body position and muscle tone/movement.

Fascia has different types of nerve endings dispersed through it, including free nerve endings, thermoreceptors (temperature stimulus), chemore-ceptors (chemical stimulus), mechanoreceptors (touch/pressure stimulus), and proprioceptors. One type of proprioceptor, Golgi receptors (type Ib), have been found to exist in dense connective tissue including ligaments, tendons, and joint capsules. Golgi tendon organs (GTO) are receptors that respond to tension (on the muscle) rather than to length (Watanabe et al., 2004). They are high-threshold receptors that exert inhibitory effects on agonist muscles and facilitative effects on antagonist muscles. When the forces of muscle contraction and those resulting from external factors reach the point where injury to the muscle tendon or bone becomes possible, the GTO inhibits agonist motor units. Due to this function of GTOs, researchers have speculated that this action causes tissue relaxation during soft tissue manipulation (Cottingham, 1985). However, evidence does suggest stimulation of Golgi tendon organs by muscle contraction and not by passive stretch of tissue. Jami (1992) showed that passive joint extension (not direct tissue pressure) did not stimulate GTO activation. Furthermore, the population of GTOs in tendons is small (10%) in comparison to the number found within muscle fibers (90%). Consequently, any relationship of GTOs to fascial plasticity is only hypothetical.

Many mechanoreceptors are found within fascia. Specifically, two types of mechanoreceptors have been identified: Pacinian corpuscles and Ruffini endings. Both these receptor types can be found in a variety of tissue, including myofascia, tendons, ligaments, and joint capsules; however, each type does have higher tendencies for certain tissues (Yahia, 1992).

Pacinian corpuscles (type II sensory fibers) are receptors that adapt rapidly to sudden changes in pressure and vibration. These receptors are located most frequently within tendons, deep layers of joint capsule, deeper spinal ligaments, and in enveloping fascia. These large, ovoid sensory organs consist of concentric layers of connective tissue surrounding a nerve ending. Examples of enveloping fascia include antebrachial, crural, abdominal, lateral compartment of the thigh, plantar, palmar, peritoneum, medial/lateral ligaments of the knee, and fascia of the masseter (Stilwell, 1957).

Ruffini endings (type II sensory fibers) are slowly adapting receptors that respond to more constant pressure, such as mechanical displacement of adjacent collagen fibers during lateral stretching (Kruger, 1987). These ovoid receptors are enclosed in a dense sheath of connective tissue within which the nerve endings end in small, circular knobs. Van den Berg and Capri (1999) also discovered that Ruffini endings might influence the sympathetic nervous system by decreasing its activity. According to Schleip (2003a), "This seems to fit the common clinical finding that slow deep tissue techniques tend to have a relaxing effect on local tissues as well as the whole organism." These receptor types are found in superficial layers of the joint capsule, dura mater, ligaments of the peripheral joints, anterior/posterior ligaments of knee, and the deeper dorsal fascia of the hand (Table 4-1; Schleip, 2003a).

A NEW TYPE OF RECEPTOR

In the study conducted by Yahia (1992), it was found that a third sensory receptor is present in fascia. Pacinian corpuscles, Ruffini endings, and Golgi tendon organs all belong in the type I and II sensory fibers. Nonetheless, research has shown that these receptors account for approximately 20% of all sensory fibers (Schleip, 2003a, b). The other 80% belong to type III (myelinated) and type IV (unmyelinated) afferent fibers, also known as interstitial receptors (Mitchell & Schmidt, 1977).

Table 4-1 Various Types of Mechanoreceptors in Fascia

	Location	Modality of Sensation	Stimulation Effects
Pacinian corpuscle (type II)	Myotendinous junctions, deep capsular layers, spinal ligaments, investing muscular tissues	Deep pressure (rapid), vibration	Used as proprioceptive feedback for movement control (kinesthesia)
Ruffini (type II)	Ligaments of peripheral joints, dura mater, outer capsular layers, and tissues associated with stretching	Sustained pressure (location and intensity), tangential forces (lateral stretch)	Inhibition of sympathetic activity
Golgi (type Ib)	Myotendinous junctions, attachment areas of aponeurosis, ligaments of peripheral joints, joint capsules	Golgi tendon organ (tension, *not* length), other Golgi receptors (strong stretch only)	Decreases tonus in related striated muscles
Interstitial (types III and IV)	Most abundant receptor type (found practically everywhere), highest density in periosteum	Pressure (both rapid *and* sustained)	Changes in vasodilation and plasma extravasation

Note: Schleip (2003a).

These interstitial receptors are slower than type I or type II fibers. They originate in free nerve endings, and they are associated with the ANS. Studies show that interstitial receptors affect blood pressure, respiration, temperature, and heart rate (Mitchell & Schmidt, 1977; Coote & Perez-Gonzales, 1970). Furthermore, they can be divided into low- and high-threshold pressure receptors, depending on their sensitivity to various amounts of pressure. Thus, although interstitial receptors can be classified as mechanoreceptors, they are also nociceptors.

As previously mentioned, nociceptors are part of the peripheral nervous system. They are widely spread throughout the body and, depending on their location, respond to various stimuli. The stimulus of pain is transmitted by nociceptors to the CNS, where the thalamus processes the information and relays it to other areas of the brain.

NOCICEPTIVE STABILITY AND PLASTICITY

Neural plasticity plays an important role in generating and perpetuating pain and hyperalgesia, including the increased efficiency of synaptic transmission and resulting in central hyperexcitability. In the past, attention to nervous system plasticity has focused on the CNS. However, it is now becoming evident that the "peripheral nociceptive system is also capable of plasticity and that this may represent a crucial process that precedes generation and maintenance of CNS plasticity" (Koltzenburg, 1995). Several lines of evidence suggest that changes in the excitability of primary nociceptive afferents in fact may be the single most important factor in generating and maintaining acute chemogenic pain or chronic neuropathic pain in humans (Koltzenburg, 1995).

Important nociceptor changes occur immediately after tissue injury, including reduced threshold. Following inflammation, the responsiveness of nociceptive receptors is doubled when exposed experimentally to a given mediator stimulus. Another important observation is that nociceptors can increase their receptive field and thereby incorporate a nearby area of tissue injury. This receptive field expansion suggests that more nociceptors can be activated by a given stimulus, resulting in spatial summation of the afferent barrage to the CNS (Koltzenburg, 1995).

Most importantly, research has found a new class of nociceptive afferent neurons—termed sleeping nociceptors, silent afferents, or mechanically insensitive afferents—that may comprise up to 25% of deep somatic tissues (Koltzenburg, 1995). According to Koltzenburg, these afferents aggressively respond to inflammatory chemicals, remaining active for prolonged periods of time after exposure and causing adverse plastic changes in the CNS. Minor tissue trauma results in temporal summation and increased responsiveness of nociceptors to a stimulus. Spatial summation, which may range from the acquisition of new receptive properties to the expansion of receptive fields, enhances the overall activity of nociceptors.

Recruitment of sleeping nociceptors requires time and tissue injury and represents a response of the peripheral nociceptive system to significant chemical tissue injury (inflammation), with implications for the development of persisting pain. While most of the changes in nociceptive function are resolved when tissue injury heals, the potential exists for permanent alteration of nociceptor activity that can result in prolonged, increased excitability of the peripheral nociceptive system and thereby exert continuous influence on central excitability (Koltzenburg, 1995).

After tissue injury, nociceptive receptors respond to released chemical mediators that promote inflammation and stimulate nociceptive pathways. When the affected area in a surrounding tissue is placed in a relaxed position, the result is improved vascular and interstitial circulation that may assist in removal of the chemical mediators reducing further release and decreasing muscle guarding. Studies have demonstrated that deep pressure exerted on soft tissue creates a reduction in muscle activity; von Euler and Soderberg (1958) discovered that light touch can affect skin temperature and reduce gamma motor neuron activity (Johansson, 1962; Folkow, Gelin, Lindell, Stenberg, & Thoren, 1962; Koizumi & Brooks, 1972; Von Euler & Soderberg, 1958). Some of these studies have discovered an increase in vagal tone during slow, deep pressure application. The increase in vagal fiber activity will lead to autonomic changes—particularly an increase in parasympathetic activity, resulting in some of the following effects: decreased heart contraction, coronary blood vessel constriction, bronchial constriction, peristalsis stimulation, and conservation of glycogen. In addition, increased vagal tone stimulates the hypothalamus and results in a generalized global reduction in muscle tone. The opposite, muscle contraction, can be seen with quick deep-pressure application (Eble, 1960). Simultaneously, Ruffini endings have been associated with sympathetic nervous system suppression (Van den Berg & Capri, 1999).

Finally, interstitial fibers (fibers III and IV) affect diffusion of blood plasma from the vascular vessels into the extracellular matrix (ECM); the result is a lower viscosity of the ECM (Cottingham, 1985). Using this fact, along with some of the other characteristics of interstitial fibers, Schleip (2003b) developed a flowchart of the processes involved in the neural dynamics of immediate tissue plasticity in myofascial manipulation (Figure 4-6).

INTRAFASCIAL CELLS CONTROL CONTRACTILITY

On closer inspection of Figure 4-6, it is evident that the flowchart includes a pathway that has not yet been discussed. Studies have shown the presence of

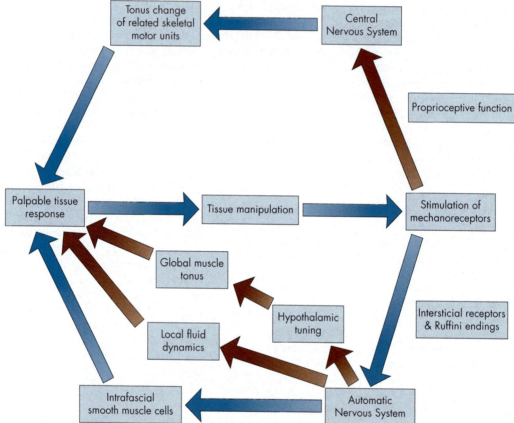

Figure 4-6 Flowchart Displaying Several Processes Involved in the Neural Dynamics of Immediate Tissue Plasticity in Myofascial Manipulation. This chart includes the four different feedback loops. The practitioner's manipulation stimulates intrafascial mechanoreceptors, which are then processed by the central nervous system (CNS) and the autonomic nervous system (ANS). The response of the CNS changes the tonus of some related striated muscle fibers. The ANS response includes an altered global muscle tonus, a change in local vasodilation and tissue viscosity, and a lowered tonus of intrafascial smooth muscle cells.

Source: Schleip (2003b).

"smooth muscle cells" (myofibroblasts) within fascial tissue (Staubesand & Li, 1996). This is how many researchers have explained the fact that fascia can actively contract, or regulate "intrafascial pre-tension."

Myofibroblasts are elongated, spindly, connective tissue cells speculated to be derivatives of fibroblasts. The reason for this speculation is that the two cells are physiologically similar. However,

myofibroblasts also have dispersed actin filaments similar to a smooth muscle cell, even though these two cells are dissimilar. While a smooth muscle cell is surrounded by an external lamina, myofibroblasts do not have such a covering.

There are theories that postulate that regulation of these intrafascial cells occurs through the sympathetic nervous system, vasoconstricting substances, and neurotransmitters (Schleip, 2003b). It is known that smooth muscle cells are usually under the regulatory control of postganglionic neurons of the ANS.

Therefore, it would make sense that in order for fascia to contract, or provide tension, the sympathetic system would be stimulated. This system is responsible for the fight-or-flight response, in which muscles need to push off their fascial surroundings to function properly. Therefore, fascia has to be tensioned, up to a point, to perform its various functions. However, heightened sympathetic system stimulation, or suppressed parasympathetics, can create prolonged tension that affects the fluidity of connective tissue. In focusing on Figure 4-6, it can be seen that stimulation of sensory fibers (Pacinian corpuscles, Ruffini endings, and interstitial fibers) can affect the ANS, which will then normalize intrafascial cell activity. This sequence of events is another plausible explanation for the immediate short-term changes seen with soft tissue manipulation.

Interestingly, evidence suggests that these intrafascial cells are also controlled by substances such as carbon dioxide (a vasoconstrictor) and a number of neurotransmitters. In one study, high levels of carbon dioxide led to immediate smooth muscle cell constriction (Staubesand & Li, 1996). Furthermore, there is evidence that serotonin and hormones released by the posterior pituitary (mainly oxytocin) have been linked to smooth muscle cell stimulation. It is stimulants like these (vasoconstrictors and neurotransmitters) that many experts in the field use to explain some of the myofascia-related conditions and injuries seen. For example, Schleip (2003b) explains how hyperventilation (increased carbon dioxide) and high levels of serotonin in the cerebrospinal fluid of fibromyalgia patients are possible causes for the generalized signs and symptoms of tension and pain felt by these patients.

Summary

This chapter attempts to explain the neurophysiology of fascial plasticity other than that based on shortcomings of thixotropy and piezoelectricity. A detailed examination of the structure of fascia and the nervous system has shown a direct connection of fascia with the autonomic nervous system (ANS) such that manipulation of the fascia affects the ANS and organs connected to it.

The network of mechanoreceptors in fascia is dense, and the degree of manual manipulation of fascia affects the involvement of different receptor types. Ruffini receptors respond to deep, slow pressure whereas Pacinian receptors react to rapid application of compression. Furthermore, the presence of smooth muscle cells embedded in fascia accounts for tissue contraction. Therapists who are familiar with the physiology and anatomy of the nervous system can improve their manual therapeutic techniques for a better tissue response.

References

Athenstaedt, H. (1974). Pyroelectric and piezoelectric properties of vertebrates. *Annals of the New York Academy of Science, 238,* 68–94.

Barnes, J. F. (1990). *Myofascial release: The search for excellence.* Paoli, PA: Rehabilitation Services, Inc.

Cantu, R. I., & Grodin, A. J. (1992). *Myofascial manipulation—Theory and clinical application.* Gaithersburg, MD: Aspen Publications.

Chaitow, L. (1980). *Soft tissue manipulations.* Wellingborough City, UK: Thorsons.

Coote, J. H., & Perez-Gonzales J. F. (1970). The response of some sympathetic neurons to volleys in various afferent nerves. *Journal of Physiology—London, 208,* 261–278.

Cottingham, J. T. (1985). *Healing through touch—A history and a quick review of the physiological evidence.* Boulder, CO: Rolf Institute Publications.

Currier, D. P., & Nelson, R. M. (1992). *Dynamics of human biologic tissues.* Philadelphia: F.A. Davis.

Eble, J. N. (1996). Patterns of response of the paravertebral musculature to visceral stimuli. *American Journal of Physiology, 198,* 429–433.

Folkow, B., Gelin, L. E., Lindell, S. E., Stenberg, K., & Thoren, O. (1962). Cardiovascular reactions during abdominal surgery. *Annals of Surgery, 156,* 905–913.

Jami, L. (1992). Golgi tendon organs in mammalian skeletal muscle: functional properties and central actions. *Physiological Reviews, 73,* 623–666.

Johansson, B. (1962). Circulatory responses to stimulation of somatic afferents with special reference to depressor effects from muscle nerves. *Acta Physiologica Scandinavica, 57* (Suppl. 198), 1–91.

Koizumi, K., & Brooks, C. M. (1972). The integration of autonomic system reactions: a discussion of autonomic reflexes, their control and their association with somatic reactions. *Ergebnisse der Physiologie, 67,* 1–68.

Koltzenburg, M. (1995). Stability and plasticity of nociceptor function. *IASP Newsletter,* January–February, 30–34.

Kruger, L. (1987). Cutaneous sensory system. In G. Adelman (Ed.), *Encyclopedia of neuroscience* (vol. 1, pp. 293–294). Birkhäuser, Boston: Elsevier Science.

Mitchell, J. H., & Schmidt, R. F. (1977). Cardiovascular reflex control by afferent fibers from skeletal muscle receptors. In J. T. Shepherd et al. (Eds.), *Handbook of Physiology* (Section. 2, no. 3). Washington, DC: American Physiological Society.

Oschman, J. L. (2000). *Energy medicine: The scientific basis.* Edinburgh: Churchill Livingstone.

Paoletti, S. (1998). Les fascias—*Rôle des tissues dans la mécanique humaine.* Vannes Cedes, France: Le Prisme.

Rolf, I. P. (1977). *Rolfing: The integration of human structures.* Santa Monica, CA: Dennis-Landman.

Schleip, R. (1989). A new explanation of the effect of rolfing. *Rolf Lines, 15*(1), 18–20.

Schleip, R. (2003a). Fascial plasticity—A new neurobiological explanation: Part 1. *Journal of Bodywork and Movement Therapies, 7*(1), 11–19.

Schleip, R. (2003b). Fascial plasticity—A new neurobiological explanation: Part 2. *Journal of Bodywork and Movement Therapies, 7*(2), 104–116.

Silva, C. C., Thomazini, D. Pinheiro, A. G., Aranha, N., Figueiró, S. D., & Góes, J. C. (2001). Collagen–hydroxyapatite films: Piezoelectric properties. *Materials Science & Engineering, B86,* 210–218.

Staubesand, J., & Li, Y. (1996). Zum feinbau der fascia cruris mit besonderer. Berucksichfingung epiund intrafascialer nerven. *Manuelle Medizin, 34,* 196–200.

Stilwell, D. (1957). Regional variations in the innervation of deep fasciae and aponeuroses. *Anatomical Record, 127,* 635–653.

Threlkeld, A. J. (1992). The effects of manual therapy on connective tissue. *Physical Therapy, 72,* 893–902.

Van den Berg, F., & Capri, E. (1999). Anjewandte physiologie—Das Bindeqewebe des bewegungs apparatus verstehen und bee influessesen. Stuttgart, Germany: Georg Thieme Verlag.

Von Euler, C., & Soderberg, U. (1958). Co-ordinated changes in temperature thresholds for thermoregulatory reflexes. *Acta Physiologica Scandinavica, 42*(4), 112–129.

Ward, R. C. (1993). Myofascial release concepts. In V. Basmajian & R. Nyberg (Eds.), *Rational manual therapies.* Baltimore: Williams & Wilkins.

Watanabe, T, Hosaka, Y., Yamamoto, E., Ueda, H., Tangkawattana, P., & Takehana, K. (2004). Morphological study of the Golgi tendon organ in equine superficial digital flexor tendon. *Okajimas Folia Anatomica Japonica, 81*(2–3), 33–37.

Yahia, L. (1992). Sensory innervation of human thoracolumbar fascia. *Acta Orthopaedica Scandinavica, 63,* 195–197.

Zaner, K. S., & Valberg, P. A. (1989). Viscoelasticity of F-actin measured with magnetic microparticles. *Journal of Cell Biology, 109,* 2233–2243.

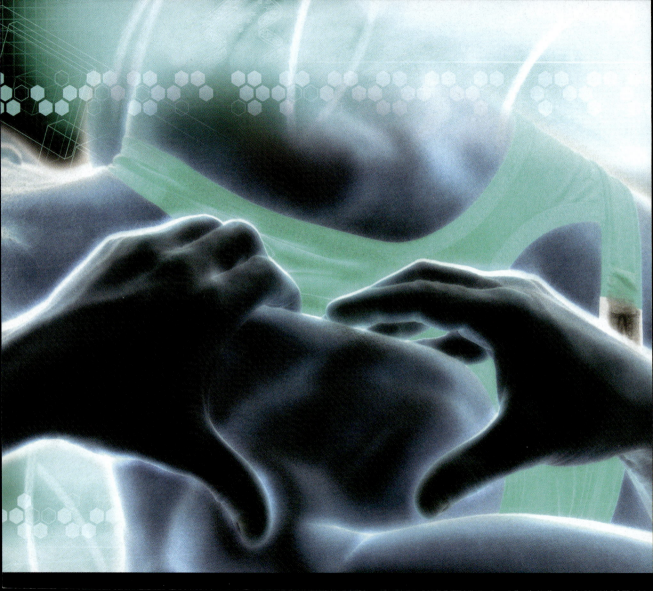

WATER, THE KEY NUTRIENT FOR FASCIA

Connective tissue consists of cells and an extracellular matrix that includes extracellular fibers, ground substance, and tissue fluid. It forms a vast and continuous compartment throughout the body, bounded by basal lamina of the various epithelia and by the basal or external lamina of muscle, nerve, or vascular endothelium.

Fascia is a part of the connective tissue system that historically has been given relatively little attention. But in fact, any discussion of soft tissue conditions or disorders is incomplete, and limited in scope of practice, if it does not include discussion of the fascial system.

The cellular components of fascia include fibroblasts, mast cells, adipose cells, macrophages, plasma cells, and leukocytes. Collagen as well as reticular and elastin fibers comprise the fibrous component of fascia; the ground matrix consists of macromolecules (proteoglycans and glycoproteins), exogenous substances, and extracellular and intracellular fluid.

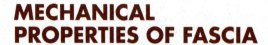
MECHANICAL PROPERTIES OF FASCIA

The water content of the tissue matrix in fascia defines tissue volume, creates space for molecular transport and for molecular dynamic organization, offers compressive resistance (as water itself is essentially incompressible), and essentially determines the mechanical properties of fascia. These properties, as seen in collagen and elastin molecules, depend on the degree of hydration (Gniadecka et al., 1998).

- ○ **Resistance** is provided by the inextensibility and organization of the collagen fibers.

- ○ **Elasticity** is determined by the presence of elastic fibers that can run in varying directions (parallel, oblique, and perpendicular) with respect to the provision of the collagen fibers and allow the fascial tissue to return to its initial length following tractional force or pressure.

- ○ **Plasticity** refers to the mechanical property of fascia to take on a certain form within certain limits provided by the presence of different fibers, adipocytes, and the colloidal state of the matrix and its relation with fibers.

- ○ **Viscosity** refers to a tissue's ability to resist or oppose forces of deformation. Regarding fascia, *viscosity* can be defined as the time-delayed modification made to fascia following the application of a force. The importance of this temporal delay and structural modification is determined by the presence of the matrix.

PHYSIOLOGICAL PURPOSE OF WATER

The human body is comprised of over 70% water, and 90% of the brain is made up of water. The effects of dehydration on the overall state of the body can be life threatening. The following are some physiological functions of water.

- ○ Water serves as the body's transportation system. It is the medium by which other nutrients and essential elements are distributed throughout the body. Without this transport of supplies, the body factory would stop. Water is also the transport system for removing waste materials, such as toxins and metabolites, from the body.

- ○ Water is a lubricant. The presence of water in and around body tissues helps defend the body against shock. The brain, eyes, and spinal cord are among the body's sensitive structures that depend on a protective water layer. Water is present in the mucus and the salivary juices of our digestive systems. It is especially important for moving food through the digestive tract. Persons who experience reduced salivary output soon will realize that foods taste different and are harder to swallow. As a lubricant, water also facilitates smooth movement of bone joints.

- ○ Water participates in the body's biochemical reactions. The digestion of protein and carbohydrates to usable and absorbable forms depends on water as part of the chemical reaction.

○ Water regulates body temperature. Our health and well-being depend on keeping body temperature within a very narrow range. The human body, which is made of 60 to 75% water, serves this function quite well. Water itself changes temperature slowly and is able to help regulate body temperature by serving as a good heat storage material.

○ Load-bearing and filtration properties of fascia result largely from the interaction of tissue components with water under the influence of various forces. At the molecular level, this function has to be interpreted in relation to the balance of osmotic and mechanical forces on the glycosaminoglycan-containing system.

○ Water is critical for collagen structure and stability. The enthalpy and the entropy of collagen melting are predominated by the effects of bound water molecules. It has been demonstrated through numerous methods of analysis that hydration forces between collagen triple helices are important for describing intermolecular interactions. Structural water, the first water adsorbed by collagenous tissue, is incorporated into the triple helix. The bound water subsequently imbibed is associated with the polar side chains, which are located in the interhelical regions within the collagen fiber. Finally, the free water along with the mucopolysaccharides makes up the interfibrillar matrix gel. The flexibility of the collagen helix is enhanced in the presence of water molecules, and water molecules probably allow rotational and translational freedom of segments of the triple helix. It is likely that, in the absence of water molecules, these water-binding sites are available to bond intermolecularly to stiffen the collagen triple helix and prevent the occurrence of slippage and translation between neighboring molecules (Kramer & Berman, 1998; Melacini, Bonvin, Goodman, Boelens, & Kaptein, 2000).

○ Water molecules in collagen play a major role in both the mechanical and electromechanical properties in bovine collagen. According to wide-angle X-ray diffraction (WAXD) and Fourier transform infrared spectroscopy (FTIR) measurements, the loss of water molecules decreases the crystallinity of collagen. The piezoelectric response observed in bovine cornea is attributed primarily to the N–H and C=O dipole polarization of the hydrogen-bonded crystal phase in the collagen (Jayasuriya, Scheinbeim, Lubkin, Bennett, & Kramer, 2003).

EFFECTS OF DEHYDRATION ON THE TISSUE TENSEGRITY MATRIX SYSTEM

Aggregation and cohesion of tropocollagen particles in collagen fibrils and fibers are further maintained by water molecules. It is especially important to realize that water molecules are influenced by the fiber lattice of collagen. When fibers align themselves with hydration, they also orient water molecules into a chain that spirals around the fiber. Those molecules that are adsorbed at low vapor pressure are tightly bound to collagen via reaction with polar functional groups. Excess water then builds up multiple layers of hydration, which force apart the fiber lattice. Liquid water then fills in and presumably moves across capillary spaces to produce a highly viscous fiber–water system at high vapor pressure. The chemical potential of these water molecules must be lower than that of extrafibrillar water, or they would not be bound. Since the quantity of water bound to collagen at saturation is 100–120% the weight of dry collagen, this represents an inactivation of a very large amount of water in mammalian systems (Elden, 1968). It is apparent that collagen–water interaction in vivo can significantly influence many biological processes, which will be discussed later in this book.

Dehydration of collagen fibers has been shown to elicit an acute inflammatory response at around 10 days, using in vitro experiments. The response consisted of an equal mixture of polymorphonuclear leukocytes and histiocytes. Many of the chemical mediators released during dehydration (e.g., histamine, heparin, dopamine, catecholamines, serotonin, etc.) contribute to maintaining tension in the fascial tissue during the early inflammatory response. Neutrophils, histiocytes, and giant cells were concentrated around areas of phagocytosis. During this early period, many of the fibers had been completely degraded while others were in various stages of resorption. The inflammatory response reached a plateau by six weeks. There were no remaining neutrophils; instead, giant cells, epithelioid cells, and fibroblasts constituted the major cell types present (Law, Parson, Silver, & Weiss, 1989). Collagen cross-linking seems to positively affect the growth and activity of the fibroblasts involved in secreting additional collagen (Law et al., 1989). The apparent advantage of having increased fibroblast activity due to collagen cross-linking is compromised by the mechanical disadvantages.

The bonding between cross-bridges provides structural support to normal connective tissue. However, injury, chronic stress by dehydration, and immobility

cause excessive bonding and lead to the formation of scars and adhesions, which limit the movement of these usually resilient tissues. With dehydration, the complexes gradually disappear from the ground substance. As a result of less water bound, the bulk of the ground substance diminishes. As this process takes place, excessive cross-linking between collagen fibers occurs. As more and more molecules crossbind, the involved connective tissue becomes less elastic. This will result in a tissue that has lost elasticity because the collagen fibers and fascial sheets have lost their ability to slide freely over one another. The loss of the tissue's lengthening potential is not due so much to the volume of collagen, but to the random pattern in which it is laid down and to the abnormal cross-bridges that prevent normal movement patterns (Wang, Pins, & Silver, 1994). Following tissue injury due to dehydration, it is essential for the human body to undergo rehydration followed by some passive activity to help prevent maturation of the scar tissue in fascia and further development of adhesive cross-links (Figure 5-1). There appears to be a rapid deterioration of mechanical strength in the collagen fibers in the wet state following hydration, and this can be attributed to a high amount of swelling instead of extensive crosslinking (Wang et al., 1994).

Collagen cross-linking on the whole does improve tensile strength of dry collagen fibers by limiting

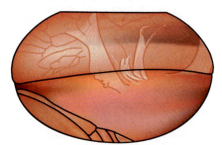

Figure 5-1 Fascial Adhesions. When the fascia is damaged, it may dehydrate to become an adhesive. Scar tissue becomes deposited around the area of injury. After being injured, a person generally becomes immobile; this results in little movement between the fascial sheaths that envelop muscle and causes the sheaths to grow into one another and form adhesions. Adhesions can also form within the fascial layers themselves when collagen fibers become intertwined and hence glued together. This type of adhesion is called cross-linkage.

interfibrillar slippage; however, in the wet state it is likely that swelling of the collagen fibers counteracts the effects of cross-linking (Wang et al., 1994). In addition, the collagen cross-links reduce the mobility of the polypeptide chains, thus augmenting the mechanical stability of the collagen fibers and in turn making it more difficult for the clinician to remove the adhesion in the fascia.

When the collagen fibers go from the dry state to the wet state, their tensile strength drops dramatically. In the dry state, collagen fibers have moduli as high as 8,000 MPa and tensile strengths up to about 600 MPa. The large decreases in these properties in the hydrated state suggest that water molecules act to break down the hydrogen and electrostatic bonds that hold collagen fibrils together. The ultimate tensile strength (UTS) of uncrosslinked collagen fibers in the wet state is less than 2 MPa, suggesting that hydrogen and electrostatic bonding between molecules plays a critical role in the load-bearing capacity of collagen. The role of cross-linking appears to be that of minimizing the distances between neighboring molecules, preventing the incorporation of excess water that would prevent hydrogen and electrostatic bond formation between molecules (Fleiss, 1992).

Dehydration of collagen can also have many other deleterious effects on the body, ranging from impairing the body's ability to communicate to initiating circulatory failure and causing a host of problems. Changes in hydration status can alter cellular activity within fascia and thereby indirectly disrupt the global communication network throughout the living matrix. When fascia becomes dehydrated, the polymerization of glycosaminoglycans reduces the fluidity and permeability of the matrix, thus reducing the ability of fascia to transfer and convey messages (in the form of hormones, neuromediators, inorganic ions, nerve potentials, growth factors, viruses, interferons, antigens, antibodies, etc.) throughout the body. As a result, the tensional integrity (tensegrity) of the organism changes, and this in turn influences enzyme activities and protein conformations involved in maintaining homeostasis (growth, wound healing, regeneration, morphogenesis, and disease resistance).

According to the continuum communication model, the living matrix creates a "symphony" of vibratory messages that travel to and fro, alerting each part of the organism about the activities taking place in each other part. Disease, disorder, and pain arise within portions of the vibratory continuum where information flows are restricted. Restrictions that occur locally can be attributed to infections, physical injury, and trauma such as dehydration that alter the properties of the fascial connective tissue. Water itself is a dynamic component of the living matrix and essentially is involved in generating and conducting vibrations that are the basis of a global communication network. When water is altered physically or chemically in any way—such as in dehydration—its ability to rotate, vibrate, or wiggle in different spatial planes is compromised, resulting in a failure in continuum communication.

Lymphatic sheets and vessels are often situated in close proximity or even attached to the fascial sheaths of blood vessels and nerves. Lymphatic capillaries are comprised of endothelial cells, to which are attached microfilaments whose movement is controlled by fascia. The structural organization of fascia controls the movement of endothelial cells, which in turn regulates the size of the openings in the walls of the lymphatic capillaries that allow for the movement of water, plasma proteins, and dissolved materials in the extracellular environment. The cleansing role and absorption of proteins and various substances in the extracellular environment by the lymphatic capillaries depends on the physical quality (mobility, fluid state) of fascia. Lymphatic congestion can result if the fascia is not properly arranged due to collagen shortening. As the collagen fibers shorten, pressure within the myofascial tissue subsequently increases, resulting in lymphatic congestion. This condition will create ischemia and induce energy-deficient contractures and fascial adhesions around organs.

Adequate perfusion and oxygenation are important for successful repair, and the speed of wound healing is limited by the oxygen supply. Molecular oxygen is essential for the hydroxylation of proline during collagen synthesis and therefore for collagen accumulation in healing wounds. Dehydration causes a reduction in oxygenation of tissues in the body.

It inevitably results in impaired collagen synthesis and hence has a deleterious effect on anastomotic healing. In addition, dehydration will reduce blood flow to some circumscribed areas and cause those tissues to become ischemic. At that point, energy-deficient contractures can form and create adhesions in the fascia. Far worse, though, is ischemia, which can cause muscle fibers to deteriorate. At the same time, fibroblasts become active and increase their synthesis and excretion of collagen, creating some degree of fascial fibrosis (Hartmann, Jonsson, & Zederfeldt, 1992). The collagen fibers of this fibrotic area are likely to form cross-links that will tighten the tissue even more.

The human body is a continuous network of tensional elements (ligaments, tendons, fascia, muscles, and cellular microfilaments) with discontinuous compressional elements (bones and cellular micro-tubules). A fascinating aspect of a tensegrity design is that an adhesion set up in the fascia is quickly conducted throughout the entire body, causing a mechanical disturbance to be set up within the fascial sheets covering the body and subsequently causing a disturbance in the body's biomechanics.

Until recently, it was thought that ground substance functioned mainly as an inert scaffolding to support tissues. Now it is clear that the ground substance is quite active in functions such as influencing tissue development, migration, proliferation, shape, and even metabolic functions. The ground substance is found within the internal environment of an organism and is closely associated with the human cardiovascular, nervous, and visceral systems. This association further explains the important role of fascia in the function of the epithelial, nervous, and muscular systems.

Hyaluronic acid and proteoglycans are two key constituents of the ground substance. They contribute to some important mechanical properties of fascia, such as cushioning and lubricating. Hyaluronic acid is a highly viscous substance that lubricates the collagen, elastin, and muscle fibers, thus allowing them to slide over each other with minimal friction. Proteoglycans are peptide chains that form the gel of the ground substance. This gel is extremely hydrophilic, allowing it to absorb compressive forces of movement (cartilage, which acts as a shock absorber, contains much water-rich gel). During dehydration, polymerization of hyaluronic acid occurs, causing loss in tissue volume; as a result, the distance between fibers decreases and cross-linking between fibers occurs. The microadhesions in fascia, as well as the reduction in water in the ground substance due to dehydration, will not disperse the forces through the body. Consequently, the body is then subjected to an intolerable impact—injury. During violent trauma, if the body is penetrated by a shock wave that reaches the interior of the body and releases a large quantity of energy, damage to internal structures and organs may occur. The role of fascia is to absorb this shock wave and disperse it in different directions to attenuate its intensity and preserve the physical integrity of the human body. If the intensity of the shock wave exceeds a certain threshold, the connective tissue will not be able to fulfill its role; lesions are the end result. Lesions most often occur to the spleen, liver, or kidneys.

Polymerization of hyaluronic acid also reduces the permeability of molecules and substances (nutrients, gases, hormones, cellular waste, antibodies, white blood cells) flowing through the fascia. The fascial membranes covering connective tissue are a site of osmotic regulation of nutrition and metabolic elimination. Abnormal pressures or tension by themselves can affect the normal osmotic exchange of fluids. Under normal conditions, there is equilibrium between normal fluid flow and tissue fluid. Tension in the tissue membranes can alter the body's hemodynamics; for instance, dehydration or drainage of fluid from the tissue will disrupt equilibrium and lead to a progressive local dysfunction and accumulation of metabolites.

NEW RESEARCH FINDINGS

Werner Klingler and colleagues recently examined the water-binding qualities of ground substance (Klingler, Schleip, & Zorn, 2004). They took strips of porcine lumbar fascia and subsequently measured the water content at various stages and at the final dry weight (after drying the strips in an oven). They reported the following observations:

○ During an isometric stretch period, water is squeezed out of the ground substance and is subsequently refilled during a rest (non-stretch) period.

○ If the applied stretch is above a threshold level and the following rest period is long enough, more water will move into the ground substance. The water content inside the ground substance will increase to a higher level than it had prior to the stretch.

A further series of tests was performed to ascertain the effect of hydration on the elastic stiffness of fascia (Klingler et al., 2004). The researchers replaced the usual physiological solution with distilled water (increases tissue hydration) or with 25% sucrose (dehydrates the tissue). The results showed that water (a hypotonic environment) increases

hydration, which increases the elastic modulus that leads to stiffness. When fascia is being stretched, water is being extruded from the ground substance and there is a subsequent change in the longitudinal arrangement of the collagen fibers (Figure 5-2). When the stretch is finished, the longitudinal relaxation of the fibers takes a few minutes to revert to the original state (provided the strain has not been too strong and there have been no microinjuries); yet the water continues to be soaked up into the tissue, to the degree that the tissue even swells and becomes stiffer than before.

It is strongly suggested that before using any connective tissue therapy directed at fascia, the clinician should first assess the patient's hydration status. As previously discussed, chronic stress by dehydration and immobility causes excessive bonding, leading to the formation of scars and adhesions and limiting the movement of these usually resilient tissues. The adhesions are relatively strong, hardened nodules in the fascia that are difficult to release due to the excessive buildup of collagen cross-linking that reinforces the adhesion structure. A patient who is dehydrated should undergo a period of hydration via oral

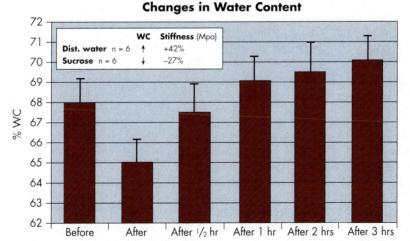

Figure 5-2 Changes in Water Content over Time. When the fascia is stretched, longitudinal relaxation changes occur in the collagen fibers and the water is squeezed out. The collagen fibers recover their original state within a few minutes. Meanwhile, water continues flooding into the tissue at an even higher percentage than before, substantially increasing the elastic stiffness. This ground substance response can be compared to the way a jellyfish shrinks and expands by changing its water content.

rehydration prior to connective tissue therapy. The clinician can use pumping and myofascial stretching to promote a more rapid uptake of water into the soft tissues. It has been suggested that to maintain optimal homeostasis in the body, the intake of water should be calculated as described in the following section.

MAINTENANCE DOSE OF WATER

The recommended daily intake of water is based on the formula:

0.6 oz. $\times$ body weight in pounds = number of ounces of water per day.

There is no scientific evidence indicating any significant benefits to fascia in consuming carbon-filtered, reverse osmosis, or distilled water.

The intake of water in the body has many benefits. Water causes collagen fibers to swell, resulting in mechanical slippage between collagen fibers so that less mechanical force is required to break the adhesion. Water removes toxins and metabolic end products (e.g., adenosine, serotonin, histamine, lactic acid, etc.) from the body, restores body temperature, and facilitates biochemical reactions. Additionally, the abundance of water resulting from rehydration will promote a greater diffusion of water molecules into the ground substance following applied manual therapy, subsequently increasing the tissues' swelling pressure and stiffness.

Fascial therapy focuses mainly on removing adhesions displaced throughout the connective tissue sheets. This approach in turn restores mobility and flexibility, opens the lines of communication throughout the body by erasing the tissue's somatic memory, clears the body of toxic substances that have been entrapped in a meshwork of fibers, and resolves soft tissue pain.

The discovery of the physiological basis of connective tissue therapy stems from the discovery of the presence of mechanoreceptors, intrafascial smooth muscle

cells, and autonomic nerves dispersed throughout the network of fascial tissue. Fascia is densely innervated by mechanoreceptors, which are responsive to manual pressure. Stimulation of these sensory receptors has been shown to lead to a lowering of sympathetic tonus as well as a change in local tissue viscosity (Schleip, 2003a). Additionally, smooth muscle cells have been discovered in fascia, which seem to be involved in active fascial contractility. Fascia and the autonomic nervous system appear to be intimately connected (Schleip, 2003b).

Fascial manipulation causes a stimulation of intrafascial mechanoreceptors, which in turn alter the proprioceptive input entering the central nervous system. This results in a change in autonomic tone via a change in gamma motor tone. Most of the fascial sensory nerve endings that are stimulated by fascial manipulation are interstitial receptors (type III and IV) that have been shown to induce a change in local vasodilation (Langevin, Bouffard, Badger, Iatridis, & Howe, 2004). The additional group of Pacinian receptors seem to be involved in high-velocity manipulation; Ruffini endings are mostly stimulated by slow deep-pressure techniques, especially if they involve tangential forces—that is, lateral stretch (Kruger, 1987). Stimulation of fascial mechanoreceptors leads to changes in muscle tonus, caused primarily by a resetting of the gamma motor system rather than the more volitional alpha motor system. Additionally, stimulation of Ruffini organs as well as many of the interstitial receptors affects the autonomic nervous system, which can result in a lowering of sympathetic tone or in changes to local vasodilation (Schleip, 2003b).

The clinician attempts to restore the fibers to their original length while also working to restore the thixotropic properties of the matrix by depolymerizing the matrix and thus increasing its fluidity. According to Kruger (1987), if the fascial interstitial fibers are strongly stimulated, there will be an extrusion of plasma from the blood vessels into the interstitial fluid matrix. Such a change in local fluid dynamics means a change in the viscosity of the extracellular matrix. Unless irreversible fibrotic changes have occurred or other pathologies exist, the state of fascia can be transformed from a gel-like substance (which limits movement) to a more watery, flexible solute state through therapeutic intervention applied by the clinician. Therapies may include introduction of energy through muscular activity (active or passive movement provided by activity or stretching), soft tissue manipulation (massage, skin rolling), heat (hydrotherapies, manual friction), vibration (manually or mechanically applied), and nutrition (rehydration).

Summary

The various components of fascia are dependent on water for maintaining proper structural integrity, protection from physical trauma, and mechanical functioning. Maintaining hydration is important. Dehydration affects the proper sliding movement of fascial sheets, interferes with biochemical messengers and intracellular signaling, and reduces healing of tissues.

References

Elden, H. R. (1968). Physical properties of collagen fibers. *International Review of Connective Tissue Research, 4*, 283–348.

Fleiss, D. J. (1992). Magnetic resonance imaging of a rupture of the medial head of the gastrocnemius muscle: A case report. *Journal of Bone & Joint Surgery American Volume, 74*, 792.

Gniadecka, M., Nielsen, O. F., Wessel, S., Heidenheim, M., Christensen, D. H., & Wulf, H.C. (1998). Water and protein structure in photo-aged and chronically aged skin. *Journal of Investigative Dermatology, 111*, 1129–1132.

Hartmann M., Jonsson K., & Zederfeldt, B. (1992). Importance of dehydration in anastomotic and subcutaneous wound healing: An experimental study in rats. *European Journal of Surgery, 158*, 79–82.

Jayasuriya, A. C., Scheinbeim, J. I., Lubkin, V., Bennett, G., & Kramer, P. (2003). Piezoelectric and mechanical properties in bovine cornea. *Journal of Biomedical Materials Research Part A, 66*(2), 260–265.

Klingler, W., Schleip, R., & Zorn, A. (2004). European fascia research report. *Structural Integration—Journal of the Rolf Institute, 32*(3).

Kramer, R. Z., & Berman, H. M. (1998). Patterns of hydration in crystalline collagen peptides. *Journal of Biomolecular Structure & Dynamics, 16*(2), 367–380.

Kruger L. (1987). Cutaneous sensory system. In G. Adelman (Ed.), *Encyclopedia of Neuroscience* (vol. 1: 293–294). Boston: Birkhäuser.

Melacini, G., Bonvin, A. M., Goodman, M., Boelens, R., & Kaptein, R. (2000). Hydration dynamics of the collagen triple helix by NMR. *Journal of Molecular Biology, 300*, 1041–1048.

Langevin, H. M., Bouffard, N. A., Badger, G. J., Iatridis, J. C., & Howe, A. K. (2004). Dynamics fibroblast cytoskeletal response to subcutaneous tissue stretch ex vivo and in vivo. *American Journal of Physiology—Cell Physiology, 288*, C747–C756.

Law, J. K., Parsons, J. R., Silver, F. H., & Weiss, A. B. (1989). An evaluation of purified reconstituted type 1 collagen fibers. *Journal of Biomedical Materials Research, 23*, 961–977.

Schleip, R. (2003a). Fascial plasticity—a new neurobiological explanation: Part 1. *Journal of Bodywork and Movement Therapies, 7*(1), 11–19.

Schleip, R. (2003b). Fascial plasticity—a new neurobiological explanation: Part 2. *Journal of Bodywork and Movement Therapies, 7*(2), 104–116.

Wang, M. C., Pins, G. D., & Silver, F. (1994). Collagen fibers with improved strength for the repair of soft tissue injuries. *Biomaterials, 15*, 507–512.

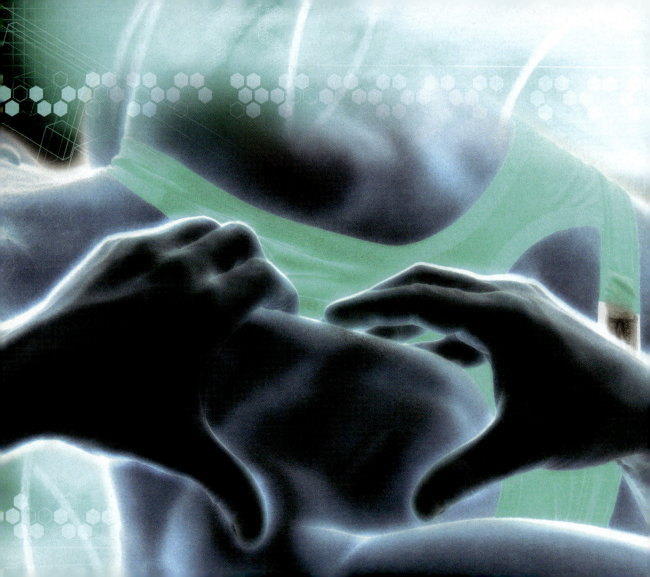

THE ROLE OF FASCIA AND ITS RELATED PATHOLOGIES

The body basically contains two types of fascia (deep and superficial). Superficial fascia is attached to the skin and is composed of connective tissue containing varying quantities of fat (adipose). This type of fascia is useful for insulation, protection from trauma, and storage, and it serves as a pathway for blood vessels and nerves. In some areas of the body it houses skeletal muscles. In contrast, deep fascia lies beneath the superficial fascia and is composed of dense collagen connective tissue that forms a sheath to hold muscles, their nerves, and blood vessels together (*Gray's Anatomy*, 1995). The deep fascia can be segregated into several investing layers: epimysium, perimysium, and endomysium. The epimysium covers the entire muscle, the perimysium covers fascicles, or bundles, of myofibers, and the endomysium surrounds individual myofibers (Huard, Li, & Fu, 2002).

Fascia has multiple functions in the body. Its mechanical roles ensure smooth transmission of muscle force and tension, support and protection for organs and vascular structures, and adaptation to tensile stress. Fascia's physiological roles involve metabolic, hemodynamic, and lymphatic functions. This chapter deals with the various properties of fascia and its related pathologies.

MECHANICAL ROLE

The mechanical roles of fascia are all interrelated. The structural components of fascia facilitate movement, which transmits force, and this role is tied into adaptation of the connective tissue to mitigate damage to underlying structure and provide protection.

Movement

Both layers of fascia (subcutaneous and deep) are capable of sliding. The initial movement of the subcutaneous connective tissue is reliant on the collagen sheets to slide, and with further sliding, the collagen fibers in each sheets alter their arrangement (parallel to the skin) to accommodate the increase in force (Kawamata, Ozawa, Hashimoto, Kurose, & Shinohara, 2003).

In the deep fascia, gliding movement over underlying muscle structures facilitates smooth and rapid motion (Wilson, Schubert, & Benjamin, 2001). In addition, physical injuries are avoided when structural layers are able to slide laterally. Despite the relatively rigid characteristic of fascia, it forms a common boundary with the underlying musculature over which it glides. Two properties demonstrate how fascia accomplishes this role: the anatomical arrangement of parallel collagen and elastic fibers (Figures 6-1 and 6-2) and the presence of hyaluronic acid.

A study by McCombe and colleagues (McCombe, Brown, Slavin, & Morrison, 2001) has revealed three distinct layers between the interface of deep fascia and the muscle: deep fascia, areolar tissue layer, and the epimysium (Figure 6-3). The deep fascia is composed of bundles of collagen fibers, most of them parallel to the underlying muscle. Also present on the deep and subcutaneous surfaces of fascia are elastic fibers. A uniform layer of mature fibroblasts represents the cellular content of fascia. Collagen strands, fat cells, and vascular components make up the areolar layer, where there is little evidence of elastin fibers. The epimysium was found to exist as a dense, thin layer of connective tissue with small amounts of elastic fibers. The presence of elastic fibers provides the necessary tension to maintain

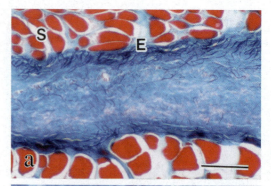
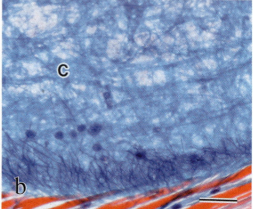
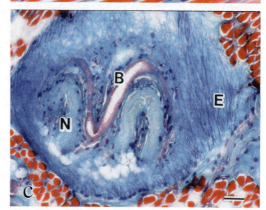

Figure 6-1 Connective Tissue without Sliding (above left). A transverse section (a) of skin-muscle flap without sliding. Collagen fibers (C) in connective tissue appear to run parallel to the skin, whereas the elastic fibers (E) branch into the connective tissue from various directions from the epimysium of skin muscle (S). The section parallel to the skin (b) shows the abundant elastic fibers and the collagen fibers (C) assuming different directions. A parallel section (c) of domed skin-muscle flap showing the nerve (N), blood vessel (B), and elastic fibers (E). Bars = 100 μm.

Source: Kawamata et al. (2003).

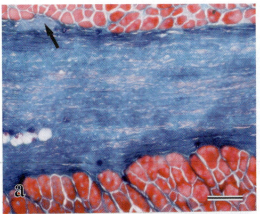

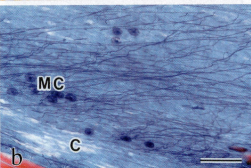

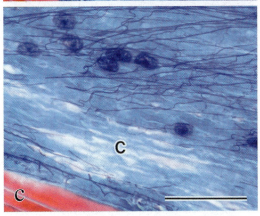

Figure 6-2 Connective Tissue with Sliding (above right). A transverse section (a) of skin-muscle flap with sliding showing the collagen and elastic fibers in parallel arrangement to skin (with 40 g load). Arrow points to a transverse section of a nerve. In the parallel section (b), collagen (C) and elastic fibers in connective tissue orient themselves in the direction of force (loaded with 30 g). MC is mast cells. A higher magnification (c) shows the parallel alignment of collagen fibers (C).

Source: Kawamata et al. (2003).

the positional balance of collagen sheets and hence results in an even distribution of stress forces.

Hyaluronic acid (HA) provides the necessary lubrication over the epimysial surface. McCombe and colleagues were also able to show its presence over the fascial-areolar plane by using HA-specific stains and thus have revealed its location in the deep surface of deep fascia and throughout the areolar section (McCombe et al., 2001). Thus, the structural components of deep fascia with the necessary lubricant properties of HA allow muscle to move freely under the relatively immobile skin covering.

Adaptation and Protection

The ability of the extracellular matrix (ECM) to adapt to local function depends on the size and organization of its type I collagen fibers and fibrils; and when force is placed on collagen fibers, their cells can change their structure (Huijing, 1999). For example, the epimysium, tendons, and aponeurosis that comprise regular, dense connective tissue have their collagen fibers organized in parallel bundles; therefore, due to their stiffness in this plane of orientation, they will mostly resist tensile force in their longitudinal direction (Schleip, Klingler, & Lehmann-Horn, 2005). The endomysium, whose collagen fibers are scattered in many directions, can resist forces in many directions (Huijing, 1999).

Work by Kawamata and colleagues has shown that the subcutaneous connective tissue layer in mammalian skin is composed of multiple thin layers of collagen sheets with elastic fibers (Kawamata et al., 2003). With shear force, the elastic fibers allowed collagen sheets to slide. With a strong shear force, the irregular arrangement of collagen fibers in each layer of sheet adapted to the local stress by assuming a more parallel alignment in the direction of the force. When the force was removed, the collagen fibers and sheets assumed their regular position and form aided by the elastic fibers. Hence, in the superficial fascial layer, collagen fibers can change their arrangement to contribute to sliding under the influence of strong shear forces and prevent damage through adjustments in tension.

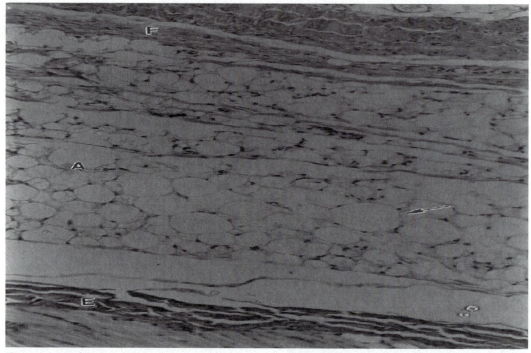

Figure 6-3 Interface (normal) between epimysium and deep fascia. (F) Deep fascia, (A) areolar layer, and (E) epimysial connective tissue layer.
Source: McCombe et al. (2001).

Elastic fibers are also capable of adapting to changes in load-bearing pressure. This is seen in the plantar aponeurosis, with its strong collagen and elastic fibers (Aquino & Payne, 1999). The elastic fibers are normally structured as a wavy, bundled network of longitudinal fibers; but with increased load, their wavy configuration changes to straight and results in increased stiffness. This adaptation to local function allows the plantar fascia to resist deformation under tremendous stress.

The nature of fascial epimysium to attach to the epitendineum (connective tissue surrounding the tendon) gives rise to the tendon's ability to transmit and absorb tensile force. Furthermore, the organization of collagen into fibrils, fibers, fiber bundles, and fascicles particularly adds high structural strength and reduces the spread of damage to the entire tendon (Kjaer, 2004). Although cross-linking and stiffness of tendons increase with age, this condition can be counteracted through low-resistance training.

Studies have shown that the total collagen content and cross-sectional area (CSA) of tendon increases with training. In elderly people, the Achilles tendon has shown a remarkable ability to adapt to an age-related decline in tensile stress by a compensatory increase in CSA. The larger the CSA of trained tendon, the less stress placed upon it during maximal isometric force compared to the tendons of untrained individuals. Moreover, a larger CSA is able to bear greater tensile loads. Correspondingly, trained muscles have larger CSA; and as the CSAs of muscle fibers increase in size, there should be a corresponding increase in the collagen content of the epimysium, perimysium, and endomysium—in direct proportion to the surface area of muscle fibers (Trotter, 2002).

The ability of fascia and associated structures to adapt to changes in shear force minimizes damage and allows varying degrees of forces to be transmitted smoothly and efficiently.

Transmission of Force

The epimysial, perimysial, and endomysial sheaths coalesce where the muscles connect to adjacent structures: tendons, aponeuroses, and fascia. The result is to give such attachments great strength since the tensile forces are distributed in the form of shear stresses, which are more easily resisted.

Fascia plays an important role in the dynamics of the musculoskeletal system, where transmission of tension across the epimysium results in muscle force. The tendon is continuous with the epimysium and perimysium, and the network of collagen fibers extends throughout the muscle from the endomysium to the tendon so that muscular contractions can be transmitted efficiently from connective tissue to bone via the myotendinous junction (Light & Champion, 1984). Force transmission also occurs laterally from neighboring fibers to fascicles (Trotter, 2002). Skeletal muscle consists of short, tapering fibers; and when contractile forces are generated, they are transmitted across the membranes of muscle cells to the basement membrane surrounding the fibers and then to the endomysium. From there, the endomysium can transmit the force across to myofibers to their basal lamina and myofilaments, which are the force-generating structures (actin and myosin).

Using low- and high-frequency stimulation conditions, Garfin and colleagues (1981) were able to show, experimentally, a 15% reduction in force at the fasciotomy site when muscle was loaded (with weight). In addition, a significant decrease in intra-compartmental pressure occurred during muscle contraction and thus a reduction in muscular strength in unconstrained fascia (Garfin et al., 1981). In contrast, (weight loaded) skin incision without including the fascia had no significant effect on these parameters. Therefore, it appears that containment by fascia drives up the interstitial pressure to result in muscle force transmission.

While fascia plays a passive role in generating mechanical tension by muscle action, there now appears to be some evidence of its role in actively contributing to "smooth-muscle-like" contractions (Schliep et al., 2005). The hypothesis centers on the

discovery that since crural fascia, ligaments, and tendons contain cells that behave like smooth muscle cells, it is reasonable to extrapolate this finding to other fascial sheets. This hypothesis was later confirmed by Schliep and colleagues in a more current study that led to the discovery of dense myofibroblasts in the perimysium that have the properties of active fascial contractions (Schliep et al., 2006).

PHYSIOLOGICAL ROLE

As noted in *Gray's Anatomy* (1995), one of the forms of fascia is evident as a constituent of loose connective tissue surrounding various components of the circulatory (blood, lymph, and the carotid and femoral arteries) and the nervous system (peripheral arteries). Anatomical studies have shown that these different systems are interconnected and linked to fascia as bands of mostly parallel fibers called neurovascular bundles. The superficial and deep fascia have distinct roles, although the physical and chemical processes involved in the functioning of the body rely directly and indirectly on the interaction between the two fascial layers.

Metabolic Role

The superficial fascia, also known as subcutaneous adipose tissue, plays a major metabolic and endocrine role. This layer is composed of both white and brown adipose tissue, which all mammals possess to some degree. White adipose tissue (WAT) is involved in lipid and glucose metabolism whereas brown adipose tissue (BAT) uses the stored fat as a source of energy to produce heat (A. Avram, M. Avram, & James, 2005).

One of the main functions of BAT is to regulate thermogenesis (heat production) to maintain normal body temperature, and obesity may be associated with an impairment in BAT in which the balance between lipolysis and storage of fat is offset (Lin & Li, 2004). The role of WAT in lipid metabolism involves the storage of fat in the form of triglycerides as a source of energy reserve. During food shortage, fat is mobilized (from storage) to meet the energy demands of metabolically active tissues. Without the subcutaneous tissue, food intake would have to be continuous. WAT contributes to glucose metabolism by regulating a transporter called glucose-4, which shuttles glucose from the circulation into cells for energy utilization. Besides the metabolic role of WAT, it also possesses autocrine and paracrine signaling functions. The hormone leptin, for example, is secreted from adipocytes and has a wide range of functions from regulating appetite to steroid hormone production in distant organs.

Hemodynamic Role

The vascular system is directly connected to the fascial system. Fascia surrounds the circulatory network of veins and arteries to aid in the dynamic regulation of blood flow and pressure. This is seen in the short saphenous vein (SSV), where two fascial connective tissues (muscular and subcutaneous fascia) encase the vein (Figure 6-4; Caggiati, 2001). The close proximity of fascia to muscle allows venous blood flow to occur. When muscle contracts, fascia develops muscular tension and pressure, which in turn compresses the vessels the fascia contain or envelope, and this serves to increase central

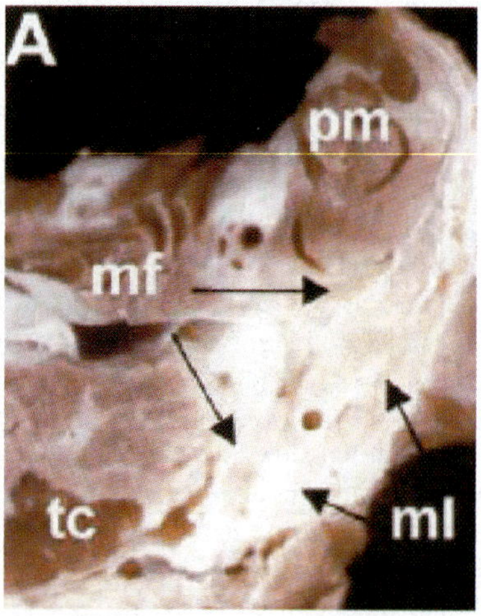

Figure 6-4 Cross Section of the SSV Encased by Two Fascial Layers. Muscular (mf) and membranous (ml) or subcutaneous layer. pm; peroneal muscles, tc; tendo calcaneus.
Source: Caggiati (2001).

venous pressure and return blood to the heart (Garfin et al., 1981).

The resistance or the ability of blood vessels to distend depends upon its two significant fibrous components, elastin and collagen (Dobrin, 1978). Elastin is an extensible fibrous protein that circumnavigates the luminal wall of arterioles in a parallel fashion; collagen is a stiff, fibrous protein with little set orientation. Therefore, movement of arteries is circumferential with little motion lengthwise. This allows fibrous components to maintain the integrity of blood vessels and permits adjustments in its hemodynamic properties to maintain normal blood pressure. When local muscular action has stopped in this region, collagen and elastic fibers in the tunica medial of veins and venules serve to compress these venous vessels and thus enhance blood return. In addition to enhancing venous circulation, the fascial connective tissues provide a structural casing to protect the vein from excessive dilation that may lead to an edematous condition or varicose veins.

Lymphatic Role

The lymphatic system functions as a drainage system to (1) transport fluid from the interstitial spaces in body tissues back into the circulating blood, where it is filtered in the lymph nodes; and (2) return plasma proteins to the blood. The lymphatics comprise a small percentage of the total tissue area compared to the muscle fibers, blood vessels in the perimysium, and interstitial space. Furthermore, their anatomical arrangement within the muscle can take on different configurations (Alitalo, Tammela, & Petrova, 2005).

Experiments by Mazzoni and colleagues have shown that in skeletal muscle with an intact fascia, the dynamic flow of lymph is influenced by external pressures and stresses on the surrounding tissue (Mazzoni, Skalak, & Schmid-Schonbein, 1990). Muscular activity increases lymph volume during the stretching phase and decreases volume during contraction. Because endothelial cells comprise the walls of lymph vessels, they offer little structural support, so the vessels rely on anchoring filaments to attach themselves to the ECM. The interstitial tissue and blood vessels are the main components of the perimysial space between fibers of muscle bundles, and this relatively noncompressible space must compress and expand to allow fluid to escape from the muscle. Muscular activity and tension increases the volume and flow of lymph in a function similar to that performed by fascia in the hemodynamics of the body by compression of blood vessels. In addition, since lymphatics are found adjacent to arterioles, any changes in diameter of arterioles through expansion and relaxation of blood flow could cause lymph formation and flow.

FASCIA-RELATED PATHOLOGIES

Although the superficial fascia plays a major role in normal glucose metabolism, problems can arise. They occur when lipolysis of triglycerides increases (in adipocytes) and produces abundant free fatty acids (FFA), which are then converted to excess glucose in the liver (A. Avram et al., 2005).

Insulin Resistance

The location of body adipose tissue appears to be a determinant factor in insulin resistance. Kelly and colleagues (2000) have used computer tomography as a diagnostic imaging method to see the fascial plane of abdominal subcutaneous adipose tissue (SAT). This plane separates the subcutaneous fat into a superficial and deep subcutaneous tissue, with the latter showing a stronger association with insulin resistance. The superficial adipose layer consists of compact fascial septa, in contrast to the deep layer with its loosely organized fascial septa. The superficial layer also contains small, tight fat lobules compared to the larger and irregular distribution of lobules found in the deep layer. These structural differences account for some of the importance of the distinct metabolic functioning and insulin resistance between the two layers.

Insulin resistance in the thigh depends on adipose tissue distribution within muscle groups. SAT, which

comprises most of the thigh adipose tissue, does not appear to be correlated with insulin resistance. Adipose tissue distribution within muscle groups and those located beneath the fascia in obese patients and type 2 diabetics appear related to insulin resistance (Goodpaster, Thaete, & Kelley, 2000). It is thought that the impairment of blood flow within the muscle due to the presence of adipose tissue and a greater localization of FFAs might contribute to insulin resistance.

Aging

An array of structural changes is commonly associated with aging: loss of elasticity due to degenerative changes in the structure of the elastic fibers, stiffening in tissues due to changes in the ECM, thickening of the basement membrane in various bodily structures, and an increase in the amount of type I fibers and mature cross-links (Barros et al., 2002; McCormick, 1994; Monnier et al., 2005). Various cross-linking reactions (enzymatic and nonenzymatic) contribute to changes in the collagen matrix; this is an ongoing process that occurs with the slowing of collagen synthesis rates as people age. Its effects are evident in the perimysium and endomysium of older people's hearts, where the collagen fibers are thick and dense and result in stiffening and inelastic properties of the affected organ (Figure 6-5; Debessa, Maifrino, & Rodrigues de Souza, 2001). Changes in the structure of the elastic fibers can be seen in the transversalis fascia of patients with direct inguinal hernias. The elastic fibers become more thickened, fragmented, and tortuous with age, and they lose their functional capacity to perform as supporting structures (Quintas, C. Rodrigues, Yoo, & A. Rodrigues, 2000).

An important contributor to chronological aging is glycation. The process whereby proteins are degraded in the body by the presence of sugars is called glycation, and the end products of such reactions are called advanced glycation end products (AGE). AGE are unwanted reactions between sugar and proteins, and they exhibit less flexibility, compact structure, and peptide cross-linking (Yeargans & Seidler, 2003). AGE accumulate on elastin and

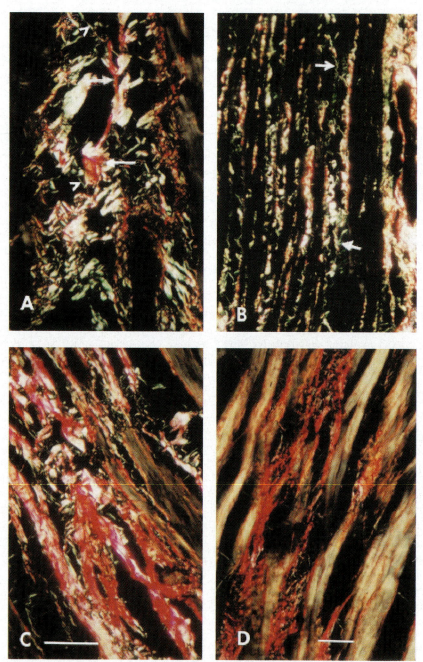

Figure 6-5 Age-Related Differences between Old and Young Collagen Fibers. The perimysium of the heart in the young group (A) showing thick yellow and red fibers (arrows) of collagen type I and green thin fibers (arrowhead) of collagen type III. The endomysium in the young group (B) shows abundant green fibers. In the old group (C and D), mostly thick collagen fibers exist in the perimysium and endomysium.

Source: Debessa et al. (2001).

collagen in the skin and contribute to skin aging through loss of the skin supporting structure. Also, AGE sensitize the skin to UV radiation and enhance photoaging and photocarcinogenesis (Wondrak, Roberts, M. Jacobson, & E. Jacobson, 2002). Tendons and intramuscular ECM become more load resistant and stiffer with aging due to accumulation of AGE. As a result, the tendon is less able to adapt to changes in load.

Scar Formation

In skeletal muscle, disruption of the epimysium from physical trauma changes the normal architecture of the underlying components. Connective tissue becomes denser and more irregular, and the number of plump fibroblasts (connective tissue cells) increases (McCombe et al., 2001). The defined boundaries of the epimysium-deep fascia interface can become obliterated, resulting in loss of effective sliding movement (Kragh et al., 2005).

The sequence of wound healing is organized into four distinct stages: hemostasis, inflammatory, proliferative, and remodeling (MacKay & Miller, 2003). When muscle degeneration occurs, myofibers undergo necrosis to set the stage for healing and regeneration. The first stage of wound repair, hemostasis, is brief and transient. Vasoconstriction is followed by vasodilation and increased capillary permeability, which causes edema. Hematoma formation occurs when platelets form a fibrin plug, allowing recruitment of inflammatory cells. The inflammatory stage takes place during the first 24 to 48 hours following injury and is characterized by some of the cardinal signs of inflammation: pain, redness, swelling, and heat. Neutrophils and monocytes are specialized white blood cells that migrate to the injured area and provide protection from infection in addition to cleaning up cellular debris. Macrophages derived from monocytes are essential to wound healing since they phagocytize debris and release growth factors and cytokines, which in turn promote angiogenesis and new tissue formation. During the healing or remodeling phase, satellite cells regenerate into myofibers under the influence of growth factors. Two weeks after injury, fibrosis

sets in and disrupts the regeneration process (Huard et al., 2002).

In scarred fascia, the following physical changes were observed over normal fascia (Koźma, Olczyk, Głowacki, & Bobiński, 2000): (1) an increase in collagen solubility, (2) an increase in the ratio of collagen type III to I, and (3) an increase in total glycosaminoglycan (GAG) types (chondroitin, dermatan, and heparan sulfates as well as HA). Collagen type III is more stretchable, contains thinner fibrils, and is not as strong as type I collagen; therefore the reduction in type I/type III ratio gives rise to a fascia with reduced mechanical strength. Similarly, changes in collagen and GAG content result in conditions observed in hypertrophic scars (Costa & Desmouliere, 1998). These changes in ECM components can hinder the functional recovery of muscle, contribute to injury recurrence, and lead to compartment syndrome (Bedair, Ho, Fu, & Huard, 2004).

Changes in HA can also contribute to loss of effective fascial and muscle function. HA is a glycosaminoglycan widely distributed throughout connective, epithelial, and neural tissues. Under conditions of homeostasis, HA exists as a structure with high molecular weight, which allows it to engage in a wide variety of physiological functions such as cell signaling, wound healing, lubrication, space filling, and adjustments in tissue and matrix water (Liao, Jones, Forbes, Martin, & Brown, 2005). When a tissue is damaged, fragments of HA with low molecular weight accumulate. Various enzymes (hyaluronidases, chondroitinases, hexosaminidases) and nonenzymatic process from reactive oxygen intermediates degrade HA with high molecular weight into smaller, fragmented products with a lower molecular mass (Liao et al., 2005; Noble, 2002). These HA degradation products act as a signal to initiate inflammation and contribute to scar formation.

McCombe and colleagues (2001) showed that the structurally defined interface of fascia and muscle creates an effective plane for sliding motion; but a scarred fascia can disrupt the planes and limit motion (Figure 6-6). The events leading from injury to healing constitute a slow process that occurs in

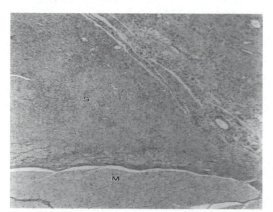

Figure 6-6 Appearance of Fascial Scarring. The normal fascia and areolar structure are obliterated due to scarring (S). Shown here is the fascial flap over disrupted epimysium of muscle (M).

Source: McCombe et al. (2001).

stages and ends in loss of function or limitation of movement of the affected fascia-muscle component.

Compartment Syndrome

Compartment syndrome (CS) arises when swollen muscle presses against the fascial sheath (surrounding it) and causes pain and swelling. The increased pressure affects the function of the affected organ and the blood vessels and nerves it contains (Golden et al., 2005). Circulation is compromised, resulting in reduced blood flow and tissue hypoxia (Altizer, 2004).

There are two types of CS—acute and chronic. Acute CS occurs suddenly; increasing pain despite medication is its most significant symptom. Causes of this syndrome are multiple; they range from crush injuries, contusions, and overuse of muscles, ligaments, and tendons to surgery, burns, and bleeding disorders. Fasciotomy is considered the best treatment for the leg and forearm; but the resulting scar tissue formation after surgery can result in a more restrictive fascia, leading to recurrence of CS symptoms. Fasciotomy is not without risk, because infections can occur.

Chronic CS is a gradual increase in pressure, due to physical stress and exercise, over a period of time. It resolves with rest but can proceed to acute CS if

muscle exertion continues. The location and occurrence of CS depends on the properties of the fascial covering that contains the tissue. As compared to fascia of the arms, the firmer fascia of the lower legs makes them more susceptible to CS (Palumbo & Abrams, 1994). In contrast, CS is a rare occurrence in the thigh because its fascial compartment has larger volume and allows for greater adjustments in pressure than do the fascial compartments in the arms and lower legs. Compartment pressure in the thigh needs to be very high to elicit damage; this is usually the result of hemorrhage from arterial injury and tissue edema that increases the pressure above a critical level (Suzuki, Morimura, Kawai, & Sugiyama, 2005).

Infections

Infections of the fascia, although not common, can be serious—as in the life-threatening necrotizing fasciitis. This condition arises through trauma, surgery, vascular disease, and diabetes. A single infective organism, *Klebsiella pneumoniae*, is the most common pathogen, although necrotizing fasciitis infections can also harbor a mixture of anaerobic and aerobic bacteria (Liu et al., 2005; Levine & Manders, 2005). The superficial fascia and fat are extensively necrotized as the invading bacteria spread through the fascial planes and release toxins and enzymes that cause the necrosis. The network of blood vessels is unable to receive oxygenated blood, and the affected tissue becomes cyanotic. Inflammation is usually extensive, involving both the superficial and deep fascia layers. Surgical fasciotomy with debridement, antibiotic therapy, and reconstruction are the main treatments of choice.

Plantar Fasciitis

Plantar fasciitis is a common medical condition of the plantar fascia, resulting in inferior heel pain. While the causes of most plantar fasciitis are unknown, it is often associated with a wide range of conditions: repetitive weight-bearing activities (running), prolonged standing, improper footwear, and obesity (Roxas, 2005). Plantar fascia is composed of strong collagen fibers that provide longitudinal arch support and shock-absorbing properties. Many elastic fibers give the aponeurosis flexibility and increased stiffness under progressive loads (Aquino & Payne, 1999). Athletic activities such as running put excessive repetitive stress on the plantar fascia, producing small tears and leading to inflammation. Sedentary adults can also succumb to plantar fasciitis through disuse of muscles that atrophy and lead to inadequate support and anatomical changes in foot structure. Pain in the inferior heel area is the most significant symptom, which varies in the degree of intensity and is commonly aggravated by weight-bearing activities. Resolution of plantar fasciitis can take months; rest and stretching exercises are a common treatment approach.

Summary

Fascia is a less recognized structural component that is important to anatomical functioning of the body. It is a continuous sheet, extending from head to toe and encompassing every organ, nerve, muscle, blood vessel, and tendon. Fascia's structural arrangement facilitates motion, protects the body by adapting to physical stresses, and assists in the movement of nutrients and wastes via the circulatory system. Like any anatomical structure in the body, fascia is susceptible to pathological conditions ranging from trauma to diseases that affect its roles and function. More research is required to precisely determine how fascia functions in all bodily processes and how to minimize and effectively treat its related pathologies.

References

Alitalo, K., Tammela, T., & Petrova, T. V. (2005, December 15). Lymphangiogenesis in development and human disease. *Nature, 438,* 946–953.

Altizer, L. (2004, November–December). *Orthopaedic Nursing, 23*(6), 385–390.

Aquino, A., & Payne, C. (1999). Function of the plantar fascia. *The Foot, 9,* 73–78.

Avram, A. S., Avram, M. M., & James, W. D. (2005). Subcutaneous fat in normal and diseased states: 2. Anatomy and physiology of white and brown adipose tissue. *Journal of the American Academy of Dermatology, 53,* 671–683.

Barros, E. M. K. P., Rodrigues, C. J., Rodrigues, N. R., Oliveira, R. P., Barros, T. E. P., & Rodrigues, A. J., Jr. (2002). Aging of the elastic and collagen fibers in the human cervical interspinous ligaments. *Spine Journal 2,* 57–62.

Bedair, H. S., Ho, A. M., Fu, F. H., and Huard, J. (2004). Skeletal muscle regeneration: An update on recent findings. *Current Opinion in Orthopedics, 15,* 360–363.

Caggiati, A. (2001). Fascial relationships of the short saphenous vein. *Journal of Vascular Surgery, 34,* 241–246.

Costa, A. M. A., & Desmouliere, A. (1998). Mechanisms and factors involved in development of hypertrophic scars. *European Journal of Plastic Surgery, 21,* 19–23.

Debessa, C. R. G., Maifrino, L. B. M., & Rodrigues de Souza, R. (2001). Age-related changes of the collagen network of the human heart. *Mechanisms of Ageing & Development, 122,* 1049–1058.

Dobrin, P. B. (1978). Mechanical properties of arteries. *Physiological Reviews, 58*(2), 397–460.

Garfin, S. R., Tipton, C. M., Mubarak, S. J., Woo, S. L.-Y., Hargens, A. R., & Akeson, W. H. (1981). Role of fascia in maintenance of muscle tension and pressure. *Journal of Applied Physiology, 51,* 317–320.

Golden, D. W., Flik, K. R., Turner, D. A., Bach, B. R., Jr., & Sawyer, J. R. (2005, December). Acute compartment syndrome of the thigh in a high school soccer player. *Physician & Sportsmedicine, 33*(12), 19–24.

Goodpaster, B. H., Thaete, F. L., & Kelley, D. E. (2000). Thigh adipose tissue distribution is associated with insulin resistance in obesity and in type 2 diabetes mellitus. *American Journal of Clinical Nutrition, 71,* 885–892.

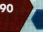

Gray's anatomy. (1995). St. Louis, MO: Mosby. Churchill Livingstone

Huard, J., Li, Y., & Fu, F. H. (2002). Muscle injuries and repair: Current trends in research. *Journal of Bone & Joint Surgery American Volume, 84,* 822–832.

Huijing, P. A. (1999). Muscle as a collagen fiber reinforced composite: A review of force transmission in muscle and whole limb. *Journal of Biomechanics, 32,* 329–345.

Kawamata, S., Ozawa, J., Hashimoto, M., Kurose, T., & Shinohara, H. (2003). Structure of the rat subcutaneous connective tissue in relation to its sliding mechanism. *Archives of Histology & Cytology, 66,* 273–279.

Kelley, D. E., Thaete, F. L., Troost, F., Huwe, T., & Goodpaster, B. H. (2000). Subdivisions of subcutaneous abdominal adipose tissue and insulin resistance. *American Journal of Physiology, Endocrinology, & Metabolism, 278,* E941–E948.

Kjaer, M. (2004). Role of extracellular matrix in adaptation of tendon and skeletal muscle to mechanical loading. *Physiological Review, 84,* 649–698.

Koźma, E. W., Olczyk, K., Głowacki, A., & Bobiński, R. (2000). An accumulation of proteoglycans in scarred fascia. *Molecular & Cellular Biochemistry, 203,* 103–112.

Kragh, J. F., Jr., Svoboda, S. J., Wenke, J. C., Brooks, D. E., Bice, T. G., & Walters, T. J. (2005). The role of epimysium in suturing skeletal muscle lacerations. *Journal of the American College of Surgeons, 200,* 38–44.

Levine, E. G., & Manders, S. M. (2005). Life-threatening necrotizing fasciitis. *Clinics in Dermatology, 23,* 144–147.

Liao, Y. H., Jones, S. A., Forbes, B., Martin, G. P., & Brown, M. B. (2005). Hyaluronan: Pharmaceutical characterization and drug delivery. *Drug Delivery, 12,* 327–342.

Light, N., & Champion, A. E. (1984). Characterization of muscle epimysium, perimysium, and endomysium collagens. *Biochemical Journal, 219,* 1017–1026.

Lin, S.-C., and Li, P. (2004). CIDE-A, a novel link between brown adipose tissue and obesity. *Trends in Molecular Medicine, 10*(9), 434–439.

Liu, Y.-M., Chi, C.-Y., Ho, M.-W., Chen, C.-M., Liao, W.-C., Ho, C.-M., et al. (2005). Microbiology and factors affecting mortality in necrotizing fasciitis. *Journal of Microbiology, Immunology, & Infection, 38,* 430–435.

MacKay, D., & Miller, A. L. (2003). Nutritional support for wound healing. *Alternative Medicine Review, 8*(4), 359–377.

Mazzoni, M. C., Skalak, T. C., & Schmid-Schonbein, G. W. (1990). Effects of skeletal muscle fiber deformation on lymphatic volumes. *American Journal of Physiology Heart and Circulatory Physiology, 259,* H1860–H1868.

McCombe, D. Brown, T., Slavin, J., and Morrison, W. A. (2001). The histochemical structure of the deep fascia and its structural response to surgery. *Journal of Hand Surgery, British and European Volume, 26B*(2), 89–97.

McCormick, R. J. (1994). The flexibility of the collagen compartment of muscle. *Meat Science, 36,* 79–91.

Monnier, V. M., Mustata, G. T., Biemel, K. L., Reihl, O., Lederer, M. O., Zhenyu, D., et al. (2005). Cross-linking of the extracellular matrix by the Maillard reaction in aging and diabetes: An update on "a puzzle nearing resolution." *Annals of the New York Academy of Science, 1043,* 533–544.

Noble, P. W. (2002). Hyaluronan and its catabolic products in tissue injury and repair. *Matrix Biology, 21*(1), 25–29.

Palumbo, R. C., & Abrams, J. S. (1994). Compartment syndrome of the upper arm. *Orthopedics, 17,* 1144–1146.

Quintas, M. L., Rodrigues, C. J., Yoo, J. H., & Rodrigues, A. J., Jr. (2000). Age-related changes in the elastic fiber system of the interfoveolar ligament. *Revista do Hospital das Clinicas, 55*(3), 83–86.

Roxas, M. (2005). Plantar fasciitis: Diagnosis and therapeutic considerations. *Alternative Medicine Review, 10*(2), 83–93.

Schleip, R., Klingler, W., & F. Lehmann-Horn. (2005). Active fascial contractility: Fascia may be able to contract in a smooth muscle-like manner and thereby influence musculoskeletal dynamics. *Medical Hypotheses, 65,* 273–277.

Schleip, R., Naylor, I. L., Ursu, D., Melzer, W., Zorn, A., Wilke, H.-J., et al. (2006). Passive muscle stiffness may be influenced by active contractility of intramuscular connective tissue. *Medical Hypotheses, 66,* 66–71.

Suzuki, T., Morimura, N., Kawai, K., & Sugiyama, M. (2005). Arterial injury associated with acute compartment syndrome of the thigh following blunt trauma. *Injury, 36,* 151–159.

Trotter, J. A. (2002). Structure-function considerations of muscle-tendon junctions. *Comparative Biochemistry & Physiology Part A, 133,* 1127–1133.

Wilson, I. F., Schubert, W., & Benjamin, C. I. (2001). The distally based radial forearm fascia-fat flap for treatment of recurrent de Quervain's tendonitis. *Journal of Hand Surgery, 26,* 506–509.

Wondrak, G. T., Roberts, M. J., Jacobson, M. K., & Jacobson, E. L. (2002). Photosensitized growth inhibition of cultured human skin cells: Mechanism and suppression of oxidative stress from solar irradiation of glycated proteins. *Journal of Investigative Dermatology, 119,* 489–498.

Yeargans, G. S., & Seidler, N. W. (2003). Carnosine promotes the heat denaturation of glycated protein. *Biochemical & Biophysical Research Communications, 300,* 75–80.

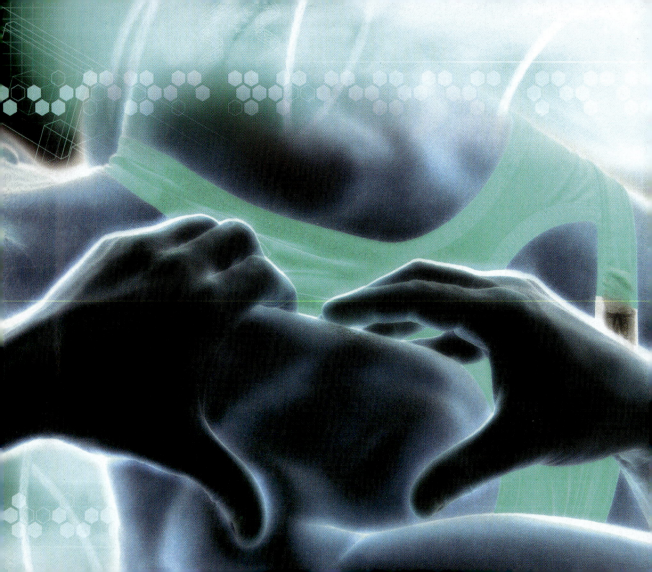

COMPREHENSIVE EVALUATION OF MYOFASCIAL INJURIES

Musculoskeletal injuries are common in both elite athletes and the general population. They are usually diagnosed and treated without a quantitative clinical differential workup. The purpose of this chapter is to provide an evidence-based summary of the diagnosis of myofascial injuries and related musculoskeletal injuries to assist health practitioners in making informed decisions to improve health outcomes. A systematic and accurate differential diagnosis of myofascial injuries (e.g., trigger points, tears) can be accomplished by following an ordered sequence of steps: clinical assessment (patient history and physical examination) and then laboratory studies progressing to imaging, with magnetic resonance imaging (MRI) being the gold standard. The information gained from using a systematic assessment can be helpful in making a diagnosis and determining the severity of an injury to the fascia as well as in guiding therapy and monitoring treatment response.

CLINICAL ASSESSMENT FOR MYOFASCIAL INJURIES

Pain that is poorly localized is often reported by patients with myofascial pain resulting from trigger points (TrPs). In addition, numbness occurring in a typical or prominent distribution may be present as sensory disturbances. The appearance of these symptoms may be due to repetitive overuse, bad posture, or rapid onset of injury or trauma (McPartland, 2004).

Physical

A significant part of a physical examination is determining the location of TrPs. This is done either by dragging the fingers perpendicular to the muscle fibers or by palpating them to detect a "tight, ropy sensation" or a knot confined to a particular location (McPartland, 2004; D. Simons, Travell, & L. Simons, 1999). When TrPs in individual muscles are located through needle insertion or palpating the muscle, sharp pain is normally reported by the individual (Simons et al., 1999). Other responses may be elicited in the same area, such as (1) sensory disturbances (e.g., burning, prickling, or tingling [paresthesias]; unpleasant sensation to normal stimuli [dyesthesias]; localized skin tenderness) and (2) autonomic disturbances (e.g., sweating, goose bumps [piloerection], and temperature changes).

To help identify active and/or latent TrPs, the following criterion should be adhered to:

1. Pressure on the tender nodule produces pain.

2. If the muscle is accessible, it is a palpable, taut band with a rope-like consistency.

3. There is a hypersensitive tender spot in a palpable, taut band.

4. Full range of motion (ROM) produces a painful limit when involved muscle is stretched.

Confirmatory observations include the following:

1. Visual or tactile identification of local twitch reaction

2. Imaging of local twitch reaction induced by needle penetration of tender nodule

3. Pain or altered sensation on compression of a tender nodule in the distribution expected from a TrP in that muscle

Electromyography (EMG) records and evaluates the physiologic properties of muscles at rest and during contraction. EMG detects an electrical potential of an active loci. Active loci are responsible for contraction knots, which form taut bands and palpable nodules (Ingber, 1993).

Lowered skin resistance to electrical current, which has been found over active TrPs when compared with surrounding tissue, may be useful in localizing TrPs. Skin resistance normalizes after treatment of TrP (Hong & Simons, 1998; Hsueh, Chang, Kuan, & Hong, 1997; Simons, 2004).

Causes

Myofascial pain can be caused by several factors, such as abnormal stress placed on the muscles due to shortened muscle subject to sudden stress, poor posture, and discrepancies of leg length. Deficiencies of vitamins C, thiamine, pyridoxine, and cyanocobalamin and minerals such as iron, calcium, and potassium are thought to play a role (Gerwin, 2005; McPartland, 2004). Medical conditions of hypoglycemia, hyperuricemia, hypothyroidism, and depression are thought to contribute to myofascial pain. The pathogenesis may be centrally acting with peripheral indications (Gerwin, 2005; McPartland, 2004).

Differentials

Because the symptoms of various diseases and disorders can mimic other types of syndromes, it is important to do an extensive and thorough physical examination and history taking. The following disorders should be distinguished from myofascial TrP pain.

Fibromyalgia

Fibromyalgia is characterized by its subtle onset of symptoms, chronic nature, and widespread muscle tenderness. In contrast, myofascial pain syndrome patients experience onset of symptoms according to sports activity or other initiating events. In addition, the muscles are taut and hard with areas of muscle tenderness (Gerwin, 2005).

Articular Dysfunction Requiring Manual Mobilization

Articular dysfunction refers to an abnormality of spinal biomechanics due to faulty movements. Some muscles have a tendency for reduced muscle tone, and these can house TrPs. There can be either joint hypomotility or hypermotility. Hypomotility requires manipulation or manual mobilization to restore function (Danto, 2003).

Nonmyofascial TrPs

Myofascial trigger points are small foci located in muscle and fascia, often with taut bands of skeletal muscle. These points are hyperirritable spots giving rise to myofascial pain. The TrP types for nonmyofascial pain include fascia, ligament, skin, scars, and periosteum. Active myofascial TrPs cause pain at rest and are tender to palpation, in contrast to the sharp burning or stinging pain of nonmyofascial TrPs.

Radiculopathy

Radiculopathy is an irritation of the nerve root caused by disk herniation or bone spurs. Besides pain, the affected limb is subject to tingling and weakness (Ceccherelli, 2005).

WORKUP AND LAB STUDIES

Specific lab tests are not available in confirming myofascial pain. They can help in diagnosing medical conditions (e.g., hypoglycemia, hyperuricemia, hypothyroidism) that predispose or contribute to myofascial pain. Such tests include complete blood count (CBC), erythrocyte sedimentation rate (ESR), and levels of certain vitamins such as C, thiamine (B_1), pyridoxine (B_6), cyanocobalamin (B_{12}), and folic acid.

Imaging Studies

Advances in medical imaging have dramatically improved the ability to diagnose injuries to muscle, tendon, and fascia. The main two modalities are magnetic resonance imaging (MRI) and ultrasound (US). Until recently MRI has been the gold standard; however, US has challenged MRI as the optimal diagnostic test for soft tissue injuries. This is largely due to recent advances in US technology and radiological techniques.

Prior to MRI, US was gaining popularity in imaging of the musculoskeletal system. However, when MRI became more widespread, US use declined. The recent development of new transducer technology has significantly improved US imaging of muscle and tendon injury at higher resolution than can be achieved with MRI.

A thorough clinical assessment usually is sufficient for deciding on the clinical management of muscle injuries. Imaging may be needed in some situations, for example, a complete muscle tear that may need surgical repair or injuries in high-caliber athletes during the competitive season of their sport.

MRI utilizes magnetic energy to make tissue "resonate" (i.e., absorb and release energy). Each tissue has a unique resonating frequency that is demonstrated on a computer image. Injured tissue also has different signal characteristics that differentiate it from its healthy counterpart. Important features of an MRI unit are high field strength (e.g., 1.5 teals), high quality, and a wide variety of coils. Coils are the hardware that is placed around the region of interest, and they usually transmit and receive radiofrequencies to and from the injured tissue.

Why Image Myofascial Injuries?

If most myofascial injuries can be diagnosed using relatively inexpensive clinical assessment tools such as palpation, lab studies, muscle testing, and EMG and treated conservatively, then what is the real value of using MRI? In the current marketplace, multimillion-dollar sports contracts are being signed by athletes; such athletes hold the status of investments whose physical condition should be closely monitored and protected (Reebok & Terrain, 2003).

The primary goal of any injured athlete is to return to full activity as soon as possible without increasing the risk for repeated and, perhaps, worse injury. MRI has significantly contributed to the speedy and effective recovery of athletes in several ways. First, MRI has made it possible to diagnose a specific injury and its severity with greater accuracy than ever before. As a result, MRI can be used to aid in the designing of a custom-made exercise and rehabilitation program (El-Khoury et al., 1996; Fleckenstein, Crues, & Reimers, 1996; Fisher et al., 1990; Meyer & Prior, 2000; Shellock et al., 1991). Moreover, MRI allows clinicians to make a distinction between nonoperative "conservative treatment" and using an invasive surgical treatment. Lastly, MRI may detect subclinical injury and help define a period of continued vulnerability (Fleckestein et al., 1996).

Normal Skeletal Muscle Anatomy and MRI Characteristics

Each skeletal muscle fiber is a single cylindrical muscle cell. An individual skeletal muscle may be made up of hundreds, or even thousands, of muscle fibers bundled together and wrapped in a connective tissue covering. Each muscle is surrounded by a connective tissue sheath called the epimysium. Fascia, connective tissue outside the epimysium, surrounds and separates the muscles. Portions of the epimysium project inward to divide the muscle into compartments. Each compartment contains a bundle of muscle fibers. Each bundle of muscle fiber, called a fasciculus, is surrounded by a layer of fascia called the perimysium. Within the fasciculus, each individual muscle fiber is surrounded and separated by a thin layer of fascia called the endomysium.

Skeletal muscle cells (fibers), like other body cells, are soft and fragile. Their connective tissue coverings furnish support and protection for the delicate cells and allow them to withstand the forces of contraction. The coverings also provide pathways for the passage of blood vessels and nerves.

Commonly, the epimysium, perimysium, and endomysium extend beyond the fleshy part of the muscle—the belly or gaster—to form a thick, ropelike tendon or a broad, flat, sheetlike aponeurosis. The tendon and aponeurosis form indirect attachments from muscles to the periosteum of bones or to the connective tissue of other muscles. Typically, a muscle spans a joint and is attached to bones by tendons at both ends. One of the bones remains relatively fixed or stable, while the other end moves as a result of muscle contraction.

On a macrostructural basis, muscles act on bones through tendons. This relationship creates a chain consisting of the following:

Muscle belly $\longrightarrow$ myotendinous junction $\longrightarrow$ tendon $\longrightarrow$ enthesis $\longrightarrow$ bone/apophysis

Any of these structures can act as the weak link and site of injury. Most sports-related injuries are the result of damage to the myotendinous (MT) junction. The MT junction may be a well-defined discrete area for some muscles or an elongated broad area in others. Anatomic studies have shown that infoldings of the contractile myofibrils of the muscle and the collagen of the tendon at the MT junction increases its surface area. Nevertheless, the MT junction has less capacity for energy absorption than either the muscle or tendon (Kaplan et al., 2001; Weishaupt, Schweitzer, & Morrison, 2001).

Characteristics of Normal Muscle Imaging

The high sensitivity and multiplanar capacity of MRI makes it the diagnostic mechanism of choice for muscles, tendons, and ligaments exhibiting hemorrhage and edema as a result of soft tissue injuries (Blankenbaker & De Smet, 2004). Normal skeletal muscle results in intermediate signal intensity on T1- and T2-weighted pulse sequences; on T1-weighted images, the muscles appear feathered or marbled due to the fat distributed between fibers. As a result, fat interspersed along fascial planes can outline muscle groups (Kaplan et al., 2001).

Characteristics of Injured Muscle Imaging

T2-weighted images best delineate soft tissue injuries, including myofascial tears, since the adjacent healthy muscle shows optimal contrast with edema and hemorrhage (Blankenbaker & De Smet, 2004).

MRI Findings in Muscle Strain

When muscle is excessively stretched or under great tension, the result can be muscle strain (Steinback, Fleckenstein, & Mink, 1993). Most strains occur at the weakest link—myotendinous junction within a muscle (Agre, 1985; De Smet & Best, 2000; Ehman & Berquist, 1986; Garret, 1996; Palmer, Kuong, & Elmadbouh, 1999; Tuite & De Smet, 1994). Muscle strains, including their severity, can be diagnosed by MRI. This technique can indicate which particular muscle is strained in addition to other confounding factors associated with the strain.

An acute muscle tear bears two notable MRI findings: (1) muscle is deformed, and (2) the existence of "high signal intensity on edema-sensitive series" as a result of edema and blood at the injury site (Nguyen, Brandser, & Rubin, 2000). An incomplete tear results in a feathery presentation due to blood and edema infiltrating between muscle bundles. This "featherlike" edema occurring at the MT junction is distinctive of muscle strains (Nguyen, Brandser, & Rubin, 2000). Since fascia encapsulates the muscle, the blood and edema are confined to the surrounding area, and they tread between fascial planes of the muscles. This produces a "rim" of blood and edema (Nguyen, Brandser, & Rubin, 2000). Initially, acute tears are seen as high signal areas on T1- and T2-weighted images, and muscle signal decreases as healing occurs (De Smet et al., 1990). High signal on T1- and T2-weighted images can be seen long after injury; this signal is thought to be secondary to repeated minimal hemorrhage (De Smet et al., 1990).

Muscle strains have been classified into three grades, as described in the following paragraphs.

Grade I Strain

Grade I strains are characterized by microscopic injury to the muscle or tendon, typically with less than 5% fiber disruption. No significant loss in strength or range of motion is observed clinically (Boutin, Fritz, & Steinbach, 2006). On MRI, there is a feathery increased T2 signal intensity centered at the MT junction with no discrete discontinuity of muscle fibers (Reebok & Terrain, 2003; Figure 7-1). Within three to five days, a rim of edema may track along muscle fascicles, creating a feathery margin (Reebok & Terrain, 2003). In addition, a rim of hyperintense perifascial fluid may track around the muscle belly or group of muscles. Perifascial fluid or edema is common, occurring in up to 87% of athletes with acute partial tears (De Smet & Best, 2000). No architectural distortion of the muscle or tendon is present with first-degree strains. Pain and imaging abnormalities resolve with appropriate rest from aggravating activities (Boutin, Fritz, & Steinbach, 2006).

Grade II Strain

Grade II strain injuries involve a partial tear of the myotendinous junction (Reebok & Terrain, 2003). The tendon fibers are irregular and thinned with mild laxity. Associated muscle edema and hemorrhage occur with extension along the fascial planes between muscle groups. A hematoma at the myotendinous junction is highly characteristic of grade II strain (Palmer et al., 1999).

The MRI appearance varies with the acuity and severity of the partial tear. In the acute setting, high signal intensity on T2-weighted or IR-FSE images reflects the extent of the edema and hemorrhage (Figure 7-2). In the setting of an old second-degree strain, the presence of hemosiderin or fibrosis may cause low signal intensity on T2-weighted images (Boutin et al., 2006). Diminished caliber of the myotendinous unit

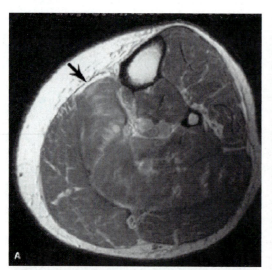

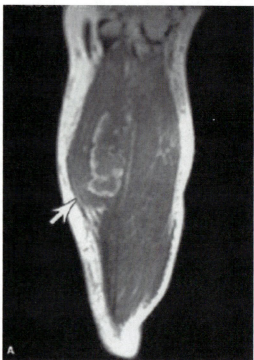

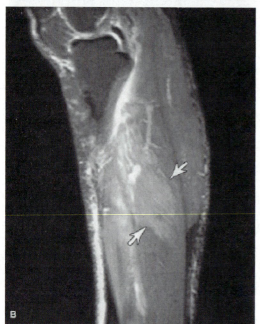

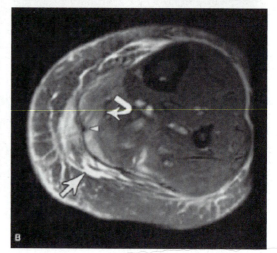

Figure 7-1 MRI of a Calf Muscle with Grade I Strain.
The medial soleus muscle shows increased signal intensity with
no muscle fiber discontinuity. Image (A) is axial T1-weighted
and (B) is sagittal fat-suppressed T2-weighted.

Source: Reebok & Terrain (2003).

Figure 7-2 Grade II Strain. (A) A coronal T1-weighted
image of the calf with a partial (grade II) tear. The medial gastrocnemius muscle (arrow) has retracted, and high signal intensity
indicates hemorrhage and fresh blood products. (B) An axial
fat-suppressed T2-weighted MRI of the calf myotendinous fiber tear
(bottom arrow) and diffuse increased signal intensity of the soleus
muscle displaying a grade I strain. The top arrow shows the plantar
tendon preserved in contiguous images.

Source: Reebok & Terrain (2003).

at the site of injury also may be observed if healing has been incomplete.

Most of these strains resolve clinically within approximately two weeks, although some of these injuries are associated with persistent pain and increased susceptibility to recurrent strain (Garrett, 1996; Palmer et al., 1999). Given that a myotendinous unit is significantly more susceptible to injury after an initial strain injury, imaging may provide objective information regarding the status of recovery. In particular, the presence of persistently altered signal intensity in strained muscles may define a period of vulnerability to reinjury, despite clinical resolution of symptoms (Greco et al., 1991).

Grade III Strain

Severe strains are characterized by complete musculotendinous disruption, with or without retraction (Boutin et al., 2006). Retraction of fibers may result in a palpable defect or a focal soft tissue mass (Boutin et al., 2006). Physical examination usually reveals loss of strength in the affected muscle group (Boutin et al., 2006).

Accurate clinical diagnosis of injury severity can be hampered in at least three ways (Boutin et al., 2006). First, clinical attempts to palpate an acute myotendinous rupture may be frustrated by patient guarding, swelling, hematoma, or the presence of a deeply situated injury. Second, muscle weakness, which is most characteristic of a complete rupture, may be masked by recruitment of synergistic muscles during clinical strength testing. Third, pain and spasm in a patient with a low-grade strain may result in the misleading impression of a high-grade tear owing to weakness in the acute clinical setting.

MRI demonstrates complete discontinuity of fibers, commonly with fiber laxity. A hematoma often is seen in the gap created by an acute tear (Figure 7-3). Surgery may be indicated occasionally for loss of function after a complete rupture in the acute setting, or for persistent pain and functional limitations that may be caused by scarring and adhesions in the chronic setting. Muscular atrophy begins to develop within 10 days after immobilization and may be irreversible by 4 months (Booth, 1987).

COMMON SPORTS-RELATED MYOFASCIAL INJURIES

Excessive stretch can cause tears or myotendinous strain. This occurs more frequently while the muscle is being activated. When strong muscular contractions combined with forced lengthening of the myotendinous unit occur, such strain injuries are common. Strains are inclined to occur under the following conditions: (1) when muscles cross two joints, (2) when muscles contain a high proportion of fast-twitch fibers, and (3) when muscles stretch during contraction (eccentric contraction). Therefore, the gastrocnemius, hamstrings, and rectus femoris are commonly involved in muscle strain injuries. In addition, strain injuries can occur with eccentric contraction of specific muscles (e.g., hip adductors) that do not extend over two joints.

Upper Extremity

Tendinous structures of the upper extremity are involved in certain common sports injuries, even though most muscle strains occur in the lower extremity.

Pectoralis Major

The pectoralis major is a thick, fan-shaped muscle of the upper front (anterior) chest wall. It stems from the anterior surface of the sternal half of the clavicle, the sternum, and down to the cartilage attachment of the sixth rib.

The functions of the pectoralis major are adduction and internal rotation of the arm. Therefore, most injuries occur when the arm is abducted upon eccentric contraction, as seen in weightlifters (Boutin et al., 2006). Direct trauma, as seen in contact sports, generally causes intrasubstance tears of the muscle (Boutin et al., 2006).

Complete tears of the pectoralis major are less common than partial tears (Connell et al., 1990). The MT junction is usually the site of partial tears and can be treated nonsurgically, whereas complete tears are

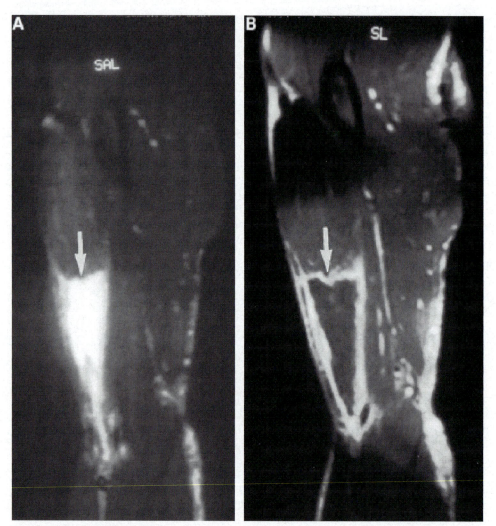

Figure 7-3 Grade III Strain. The biceps tendon at the elbow shows a third-degree strain (complete tear) with hematoma and retraction. (A) Sagittal fat-suppressed FSE T2-weighted image. (B) Fat-suppressed T1-weighted image with fluid-filled rim (arrow) distal to the biceps muscle.

Source: Boutin et al. (2002).

normally found distally at a site where ligament attaches to bone (enthesis; Figure 7-4).

With avulsion of the tendon from its insertion site, high T2 signal intensity may be seen superficial to the adjacent cortex because of periosteal stripping (Connell et al., 1990). Complete tears, especially avulsion injuries from the long bone of the upper arm (humerus), are treated surgically to facilitate rapid functional recovery. This emphasizes the

significance of MRI to distinguish between complete and partial tears (Berson, 1979; Kretzler & Richardson, 1989; Park & Espiniella, 1970; Wolfe, Wickiewicz, & Cavanaugh, 1992).

Lower Extremity

The adductors, quadriceps, medial gastrocnemius, and hamstrings are the most commonly injured muscles or groups of muscles in the lower extremity.

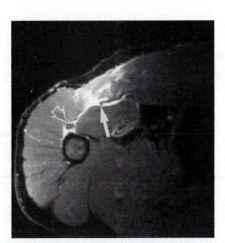

Figure 7-4 Tendon Tear of the Pectoralis Major. The pectoralis major tendon showing complete tear of the sternal portion with muscle retraction and high-signal fluid-filled gap (white arrow). Biceps tendon (outlined arrow). Axial fat-suppressed FSE T2-weighted MRI.

Source: Boutin et al. (2006).

Hamstring

The biceps femoris, semitendinosus, and semimembranosus comprise the hamstring muscles. These groups of muscles insert distally into the tibia and evolve proximally from the posterolateral ischial tuberosity (De Smet & Best, 2000). The main function of the hamstrings is to bend the knee and extend the hip. During activities involving running or jumping, the hamstrings help slow down the knee before the foot strikes the ground and therefore assists with hip extension after foot strike.

Athletes who sprint and jump are prone to hamstring muscle injuries. The cause is a sudden bending movement or flexion around a joint in a limb (Agre, 1985). In athletes whose muscles are "skeletally mature," most hamstring injuries are partial tears as opposed to complete tears (Figure 7-5) or avulsions, and the biceps femoris is the most commonly injured muscle. It is not unusual to injure more than one component of the hamstrings; this occurs with a prevalence of 25% (Garrett et al., 1989).

The transition zone between muscles and tendons in the hamstrings is long. As a result, the tendons stretch down the length of each muscle either completely or

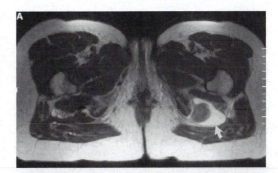

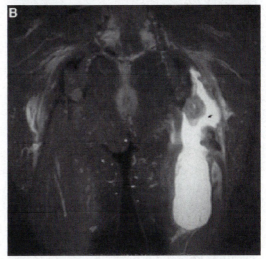

Figure 7-5 Hamstring Muscle Showing Complete Tear with Hematoma. (A) An axial T2-weighted image and (B) coronal fat-suppressed FSE MRI. The arrow points to a large hematoma in a full-thickness tear of hamstring tendon. Between the proximal and distal retracted musculotendinous unit, there is a 2- to 3-cm gap (small arrow).

Source: Boutin et al. (2006).

almost completely (Garrett et al., 1989). Therefore, when strains occur at the MT junction, the muscle belly itself, or the ends of it, can suffer injuries.

An MRI study involving 15 college athletes showed diverse locations of acute hamstring injuries at the MT junction: distal myotendinous junction (13%), proximal MT junction (33%), and intramuscular MT junction (53%). When underlying tendinosis is present, hamstring injuries such as partial or complete avulsions may occur at the tendinous origin (Sallay et al., 1996). Recovery from hamstring strains can take from 3 months to 1.5 years before patients are able to return to vigorous activities (Sallay et al., 1996), and one-fourth of athletes suffer from recurrent injuries. There is twice the risk of even more severe injury within two months from even minor hamstring injuries (Ekstrand & Gilquist, 1983).

Quadriceps

Running and soccer commonly cause quadriceps injuries when eccentric contraction occurs in attempts to control knee flexion. Most injuries occur at the rectus femoris muscle MT junction. Two types of strain injuries of the rectus femoris have been identified: (1) "proximally at the MT junction of the deep tendon of the indirect head of the rectus femoris," and (2) "more distally at the MT junction of the direct head" (Hughes et al., 1995). These injuries can occur together or separately.

Adductors

Groin pain is a common symptom among athletes due to strains in the adductor compartment. This type of injury commonly involves eccentric contraction of the adductors in an effort to stabilize the hips as the adductors contract. Soccer and hockey players are prone to this type of injury, which accounts for 10% of all injuries in hockey players (Lynch & Renstrom, 1999; Nicholas & Tyler, 2002). Most injuries implicate the adductor longus muscle at the MT junction.

Medial Gastrocnemius

Tendons and muscles such as the popliteus, gastrocnemius, and plantaris muscles, located at the posterior aspect of the knee, can be subject to strain injuries (Benson, Sathy, & Port, 1996; Fleiss, 1992; Gaulrapp, 1999; Wine & Phadeke, 1996).

A condition called tennis leg is a common muscular strain that occurs in the calf and affects the gastrocnemius muscle's medial head (Figure 7-6) at the MT junction (Helms, Fritz, & Garvin, 1995). The condition is characterized by acute onset of sharp pain followed by ecchymosis and calf swelling. Clinical diagnosis may include the following: herniation of

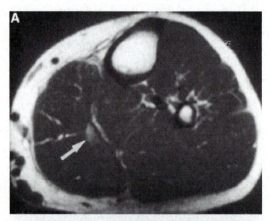

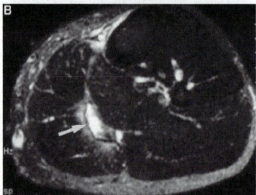

Figure 7-6 Plantaris Tendon Rupture with Adjacent Gastrocnemius Strain. A hematoma resides in the region of the torn plantaris tendon (arrow) between the soleus and gastrocnemius muscles. (A) Axial T1-weighted and (B) fat-suppressed FSE T2-weighted MRI.

Source: Boutin et al. (2006).

the fascia, tendonitis due to overuse, nerve entrapment, stress fracture, thrombosis of the vein, chronic exertional compartment syndrome, and popliteal artery entrapment syndrome (Liu & Chen, 1989).

An accurate diagnosis can be done by MRI to establish severity of the injury (Bianchi et al., 1998). A study of 23 injuries to the distal gastrocnemius muscle done by MRI revealed that 96% of the cases involved the MT junction, and the medial head was affected more frequently compared to the lateral head (86% versus 14%, respectively). In addition, partial or low-grade tears were more regular than complete tears (Weishaupt, Schweitzer, & Morrison, 2001).

Conservative treatment is required, with pain relief occurring in about two weeks and return to sports after a minimum of three weeks (Gaulrapp, 1999).

Basic mechanisms of muscle injury and the MRI appearance of the more common injuries and their mimics were discussed to provide the reader with basic tools to recognize these entities in everyday practice. Regardless of the disorder affecting muscle, MRI may help in honing the clinical differential diagnosis; defining the location, extent, and severity of a disorder; predicting the prognosis or possible complications associated with a disorder; directing the type and location of an intervention, such as surgery (when indicated); and assessing treatment response or failure after medical or surgical therapy.

MAGNETIC RESONANCE IMAGING

Magnetic resonance imaging (MRI) is increasingly being used to evaluate muscle injuries because of its unparalleled anatomic resolution and high sensitivity in detecting acute and chronic soft tissue abnormalities. These features allow detection of characteristic injury patterns that lead to accurate diagnoses and grading of severity. The precise assessment of muscle injuries with MRI plays an important role in determining the treatment plan (surgical versus conservative) and prognosis of injured athletes.

The advantages of MRI are as follows:

1. Excellent tissue contrast
2. Ability to visualize deeper tissues
3. Less reliance on operator skill, although proper protocols and prescription of sequences are essential
4. Very sensitive to bone marrow changes (e.g., stress reactions)
5. Excellent visualization of intra-articular structures

ULTRASOUND

Ultrasound (US) imaging utilizes ultrasonic energy to produce "echoes." These echoes are unique to different tissues and are used to characterize and/or study internal structures and tissues. Similar to MRI, the generated computer image is a result of the tissue interrogated, and injured tissue produces different echoes. There are many kinds of US units and probes. The key features are high resolution (minimum of 10–12 megahertz), which is a characteristic of the imaging probe, as well as advanced software that enhances the images. In general, the highest frequency possible for the depth of imaging necessary is best. Extended field-of-view imaging is helpful to demonstrate the overall anatomy and extent of an abnormality, providing a global anatomic overview of a region of interest with a single sweep of the transducer (Peetrons, 2002). Power Doppler can be useful to demonstrate the presence or absence of pathological blood flow surrounding an abscess, increased vascularity in cases of inflammation (myositis), or irregular vessels (neovascularity).

The advantages of US are as follows:

1. Excellent resolution in the near field (i.e., the tissue closest to the probe)
2. Ability to "dynamically" evaluate the musculoskeletal system in real time. Those movements causing or leading up to a particular injury can be diagnosed.
3. Use of "Doppler" US, which evaluates increase in blood flow (i.e., hyperemia)
4. Ability to directly image injured/painful area with patient interaction
5. Earlier visualization of calcifications in soft tissues
6. Usually more accessible and less expensive
7. Claustrophobia is a nonissue.

Imaging Characteristics of Normal Muscle

Muscles are composed of multiple parallel bundles of muscle fibers, each surrounded by a fascial sheath referred to as the perimysium (Figure 7-7). The perimysium forms septa, which coalesce to form a tendon. An intramuscular portion of the tendon is visible on cross-sectional images as a linear curvilinear, echogenic structure within the muscle. At either end of the long axis of the muscle, the tendon continues to its origin or insertion onto bone. Surrounding the entire muscle is a connective tissue aponeurosis.

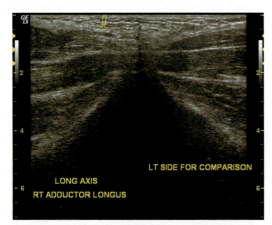

Figure 7-7 Image Representing the Left Adductor Muscles. This image depicts the perimysium as the thin white lines within the muscle, and the muscle itself has a pennate appearance. The epimysium is the overlying superficial thin white line. Three muscle bundles then terminate centrally to the muscle tendon junction. To compare, on the right adductor longus there is a low-grade partial tear at the muscle tendon junction of the superficial fibers. Notice the loss of the normal striations of the muscle echotexture as well as blurring of the epimysium and overlying epimysium. Note: To see images 7-7 through 7-22 larger online, go to www.delmarlearning/companions.

The pennation structure of a muscle belly is well visualized using ultrasound. Unipennate muscle structures such as the hamstring can be seen to have only a single perimysium located at the periphery of the muscle (Peetrons, 2002). Bipennate or circumpennate muscles, such as the rectus femoris, demonstrate an echogenic perimysium within the muscle (Peetrons, 2002). The muscle fibers are hypoechoic, while the septa and tendon are hyperechoic.

On dynamic ultrasound imaging, muscle thickness increases during contraction and appears to decrease in echogenicity, which is probably attributed to the increased thickness of the muscle due to contraction.

Imaging Characteristics of Injured Muscle

Muscle strains are characterized by tearing at the weakest portion of the muscle known as the MT junction. The myofascial attachment (attachment of the muscle fibers to the perimysium or aponeurosis) is another location prone to traumatic injury (Peetrons, 2002). Muscles with the highest predisposition for strain injuries are those that cross two joints, those with eccentric action, those with a higher proportion of type II muscle fibers, and those with fusiform shape (Bencardino et al., 2000; Mallone, 1988; Shellock, Fukunaga, Mink, & Edgerton, 1991).

Grade I Strain

The US in Figure 7-8 shows a hypoechoic or mixed echogenicity region adjacent to the MT junction with loss of normal-looking muscle architecture.

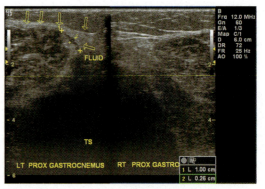

Figure 7-8 Grade I Strain of the Gastrocnemius Muscle. On the left, there is a low-grade partial tear of the lateral fibers of the proximal gastrocnemius muscle. The caliper represents the outer borders of the tear (grade I strain); in the central aspect of the calipers, there is hypoechoic region representing fluid in the tear. As well, the overlying fascia and epimysium are thickened relative to the right side as demonstrated by the corresponding arrows. This represents fluid and blood tracking along the facial layer of the superficial muscle. The image on the right demonstrates a normal appearance of the proximal gastrocnemius.

The MT is often small on cross-sectional images, but it may be quite long.

Grade II Strain

Grade II strains are clinically shown to be partial tears that place a limit on motor function. US will demonstrate an anechoic or hypoechoic defect in the muscle fibers (Figures 7-9 and 7-10), often showing torn fragments of muscle floating in a hematoma. At the myotendinous (MT) junction adjacent to the fascia, pooling of blood is evident. This usually results in a posterior acoustic enhancement denoting the fluid nature of the collection, but it can appear as a pseudomass.

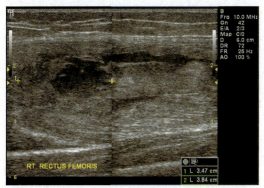

Figure 7-9 A Partial Tear within the Rectus Femoris Muscle in the Mid Belly. The intramuscular tear represented by the hypoechoic and anechoic regions is outlined by the calipers. This represents a grade II muscle injury.

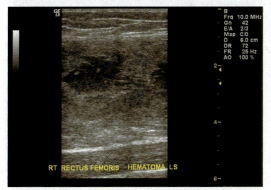

Figure 7-10 A Transverse Image of the Rectus Femoris Grade II Muscle Tear. The hypoechoic central region represented by darker grey corresponds to the intramuscular hematoma from the tear.

Grade III Strain

Grade III strains are characterized as complete tears, usually with retraction (Figure 7-11; Bencardino et al., 2000; Peetrons, 2002). A mass of retracted muscle may be evident at physical examination (Peetrons, 2002). Sonographically, the muscle and tendon are discontinuous and may demonstrate a wavy or masslike contour. In the acute setting, a hematoma is invariably present.

Ultrasound-Guided Musculoskeletal Intervention

Real-time US imaging allows the radiologist to dynamically insert needles into the musculoskeletal system in order to inject diagnostic and/or therapeutic medication. This includes intra-articular and extra-articular structures (e.g., bursa, tendon sheaths, intramuscular). Ultrasound-guided intervention is also being utilized for treatment of these conditions:

1. Carpal tunnel syndrome
2. Plantar fasciitis
3. Morton's neuroma

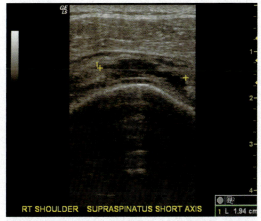

Figure 7-11 Transverse Image of the Supraspinatus Muscle Tendon Junction Demonstrating a Full-Thickness Tear Outlined by the Calipers. This image depicts a grade III muscle tendon strain. The dark region represents the fluid/hematoma in the gap created by the tear. The superficial region superiorly represents the overlying deltoid muscle, which is normal.

4. Calcific tendinopathy

5. Cyst/ganglion aspiration

Studies have demonstrated very poor accuracy of musculoskeletal injections without imaging guidance. For elite and professional athletes, US should be used not only to diagnose but also to guide therapy in soft tissue injuries. It should be noted that musculoskeletal US is operator dependent and has a long and challenging learning curve, especially for US-guided intervention.

The following illustrations are representative examples of soft tissue injuries as demonstrated with US and MRI.

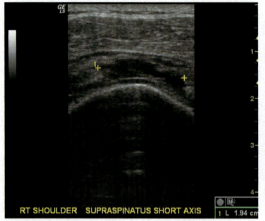

Figure 7-12 Twenty-one-year-old Professional Baseball Pitcher with Progressive Shoulder Pain. Transverse US image of the supraspinatus tendon demonstrates a full-thickness tear as outlined by the calipers (measuring 1.9 cm). The black area represents fluid in the gap created by the tear.

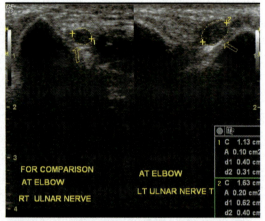

Figure 7-14 Twenty-six-year-old Female Left-Handed Javelin Thrower with Medial Elbow Pain. Transverse US images of bilateral elbows. On the left of the elbow, the ulnar nerve is thicker, indicating ulnar neuritis. No subluxation was elicited on dynamic evaluation.

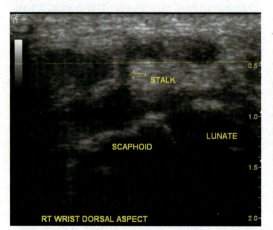

Figure 7-13 Sixteen-year-old Female Elite Tennis Player with Dorsal Wrist Pain and Swelling. Transverse US image of the dorsum of the wrist shows a ganglion cyst with a neck emanating from the scapholunate joint.

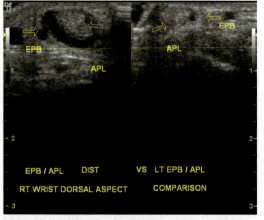

Figure 7-15 Thirty-year-old Elite Cross-Country Skier with Dorsal Right Thumb Pain. Transverse US images of bilateral wrists at extensor compartment 1. On the right there is a dark rim around the abductor pollicus longus and extensor pollicus brevis tendons, representing tenosynovitis. The right APL and EPB tendons are also thickened relative to the left side, indicating tendinopathy.

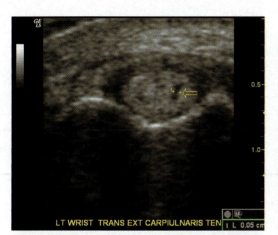

Figure 7-16 Twenty-nine-year-old Male Left-Handed Professional Squash Player with Progressive Ulnar Wrist Pain. Transverse US image of the left wrist at the level of extensor compartment 6. The extensor carpi ulnaris tendon is thickened with a dark rim. These findings represent ECU tendinopathy and tenosynovitis. There is also a dark region within the ECU tendon measuring 5 mm, as outlined by the calipers. This corresponds to a small interstitial tear within the tendon. This finding was not seen on MRI.

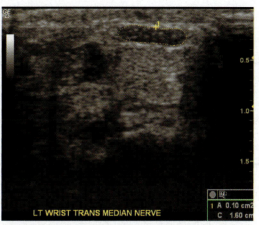

Figure 7-18 Twenty-six-year-old Male Elite Cyclist with Progressive Left Volar Wrist Pain with Numbness. Transverse US image of the wrist at the level of the carpal tunnel. The elliptical cursor outlines a thickened median nerve. It measures 16 mm², which represents carpal tunnel syndrome (upper limit of normal is 12 mm²). The nerve is darker than surrounding tissue, indicating edema and fluid within the median nerve.

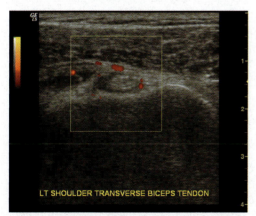

Figure 7-17 Thirty-two-year-old Male Left-Handed Quarterback with Anterior Shoulder Pain. Transverse US image of the shoulder at the level of the bicipital groove and long head of the biceps tendon. The biceps tendon is thickened with a dark rim around the tendon. This represents tendinopathy and tenosynovitis. The box represents Doppler interrogation to assess blood flow. The red areas demonstrate hyperemia in the biceps sheath and surrounding soft tissue.

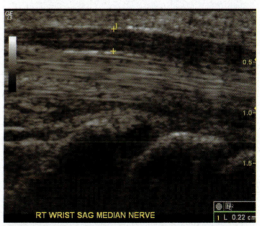

Figure 7-19 Longitudinal Ultrasound Image of the Wrist at the Level of the Carpal Tunnel. The most superficial structure outlined by the calipers represents a thickened median nerve. Again, note a darker nerve indicating edema within the nerve fibers.

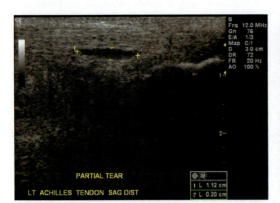

Figure 7-20 Twenty-nine-year-old Male Sprinter with Sudden Onset of Achilles Pain. Longitudinal US image of the Achilles tendon demonstrates a dark area outlined by calipers. This represents a small interstitial tear within the Achilles tendon.

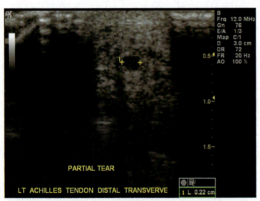

Figure 7-21 Transverse Ultrasound Image of the Achilles Tendon. This image shows a dark region, outlined by calipers, representing the interstitial tear.

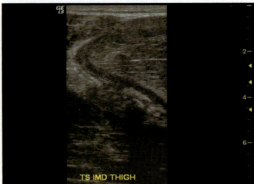

Figure 7-22 Thirty-one-year-old Male Track Athlete with Acute Hamstring Pain While Sprinting. Transverse US image through the mid hamstring shows a curvilinear dark region in the midline between the semimembranosis and semitendinosis muscles. This represents an acute intermuscular fascial tear. On dynamic evaluation, there was restricted movement between the two muscles.

References

Agre, J. C. (1985). Hamstring injuries. Proposed aetiological factors, prevention and treatment. *Sports Medicine, 2*(1), 21–33.

Bencardino, J. T., Rosenberg Z. S., Brown, R. R., Hassankhani, A., Lustrin, E. S., & Beltran, J. (2000). Traumatic musculotendinous injuries of the knee: diagnosis with MR imaging. *Radiographics, 20,* S103–S120.

Benson, L. S., Sathy, M. J., & Port, R. B. (1996). Forearm compartment syndrome due to automated injection of computed tomography contrast material. *Journal of Orthopaedic Trauma, 10,* 433–436.

Berson, B. L. (1979). Surgical repair of pectoralis major rupture in an athlete: Case report of an unusual injury in a wrestler. *American Journal of Sports Medicine, 7,* 348–351.

Bianchi, S., Martinoli, C., Abdelwahab, I. F., Derchi, L. E., & Damiani, S. (1998). Sonographic evaluation of tears of the gastrocnemius medial head. *Journal of Ultrasound Medicine, 17,* 157–162.

Blankenbaker, D. G., & De Smet, A. A. (2004). MR imaging of muscle injuries. *Applied Radiology, 33*(4), 14–26.

Summary

As a general principle, ultrasound is the imaging modality of choice in injuries to extra-articular and superficial structures, whereas MRI is preferred in evaluating intra-articular and deep tissues. However, in many cases, both modalities act synergistically to accurately diagnose musculoskeletal abnormalities. This approach is of even more importance in treating the injuries of elite or professional athletes.

Booth, F. W. (1987). Physiologic and biochemical effects of immobilization on muscle. *Clinical Orthopaedics 219,* 15–20.

Boutin, R. D., Fritz, R. C., & Steinbach, L. S. (2006). Imaging of sports-related muscle injuries. *Radiology Clinics of North America, 40,* 333–362.

Connell, D. A., Potter, H. G., Sherman, M. F., & Wickiewicz, T. L. (1990). Injuries of the pectoralis major muscle: Evaluation with MR imaging. *Radiology, 210,* 785–791.

Danto, J. B. (2003). Review of integrated neuromusculoskeletal release and the novel application of a segmental anterior/posterior approach in the thoracic, lumbar, and sacral regions. *Journal of the American Osteopathic Association, 103,* 583–596.

De Smet, A. A., & Best, T. M. (2000). MR imaging of the distribution and location of acute hamstring injuries in athletes. *American Journal of Roentgenology, 174,* 393–399.

De Smet, A. A., Fisher, D. R., Heiner, J. P., & Keene, J. S. (1990). Magnetic resonance imaging of muscle tears. *Skeletal Radiology, 19,* 283–286.

Ehman, R. L., & Berquist, T. H. (1986). Magnetic resonance imaging of musculoskeletal trauma. *Radiology Clinics of North America, 24,* 291–319.

Ekstrand, J., & Gillquist, J. (1983). Soccer injuries and their mechanisms: A prospective study. *Medicine & Science in Sports & Exercise, 15,* 267–270.

El-Khoury, G. Y., Brandser, E. A., Kathol, M. H., Tearse, D. S., & Callaghan, J. J. (1996). Imaging of muscle injuries. *Skeletal Radiology, 25,* 3–11.

Facco, E., & Ceccherelli, F. (2005). Myofascial pain mimicking radicular syndromes. *Acta Neurochirurgica Supplement, 92,* 147–150.

Fisher, M. J., Meyer, R. A., Adams, G. R., Foley, J.M., Potchen, E. (1990). Direct relationship between proton T2 and exercise intensity in skeletal muscle MR images. *Investigative Radiology, 25,* 480–485.

Fleckenstein, J. L., Crues, J. V., & Reimers, C. D. (1996). *Muscle imaging in health and disease.* New York: Springer-Verlag.

Fleiss, D. J. (1992). Magnetic resonance imaging of a rupture of the medial head of the gastrocnemius muscle: A case report. *Journal of Bone & Joint Surgery American Volume, 74,* 792.

Garrett, W. E., Jr. (1996). Muscle strain injuries. *American Journal of Sports Medicine, 24*(Suppl. 6), S2–S8.

Garrett, W. E., Jr., Rich, F. R., Nikolaou, P. K., & Vogler, J. B., III. (1989). Computer tomography of hamstring strains. *Medicine & Science in Sports & Exercise, 21,* 506–514.

Gaulrapp, H. (1999). "Tennis leg": Ultrasound differential diagnosis and follow-up. *Sportverletz Sportschaden, 13,* 53–58.

Gerwin, R. D. (2005, September). A review of myofascial pain and fibromyalgia—factors that promote their persistence. *Acupuncture Medicine, 23*(3), 121–134.

Greco, A., McNamara, M. T., Escher, R. M., Michael, R., Trifilio, G., & Parienti, J. (1991). Spin-echo and STIR MR imaging of sports-related muscle injuries at 1.5 T. *Journal of Computer Assisted Tomography, 15,* 994–999.

Helms, C. A., Fritz, R. C., & Garvin, G. J. (1995). Plantaris muscle injury: Evaluation with MR imaging. *Radiology, 195,* 201–203.

Hong, C. Z., & Simons, D. G. (1998). Pathophysiologic and electrophysiologic mechanisms of myofascial trigger points. *Archives of Physical Medicine & Rehabilitation, 73,* 256–263.

Hsueh, T. C., Cheng, P.T., Kuan, T. S., & Hong, C. Z. (1997). The intermediate effectiveness of electrical nerve stimulation and electrical muscle stimulation on myofascial trigger points.

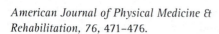

American Journal of Physical Medicine & Rehabilitation, 76, 471–476.

Hughes, C., Hasselman, C. T., Best, T. M., Martinez, S., & Garrett, W. E., Jr. (1995). Incomplete, intrasubstance strain injuries of the rectus femoris muscle. *American Journal of Sports Medicine, 23,* 500–506.

Ingber, D. E. (1993). Cellular tensegrity: Defining new rules of biological design that govern the cytoskeleton. *Journal of Cell Science, 104,* 613–627.

Kaplan, P. A., Dussault, R. D., Helms, C. A., & Anderson, M. W. (2001). Tendons and muscles. In Saunders; first ed. *Musculoskeletal MRI* (pp. 55–87). Philadelphia: WB Saunders.

Kretzler, H. H., Jr., & Richardson, A. B. (1989). Rupture of the pectoralis major muscle. *American Journal of Sports Medicine, 17,* 453–458.

Liu, S. H., & Chen, W. S. (1989). Medial gastrocnemius hematoma mimicking deep vein thrombosis: A report of a case. *Taiwan I Hsueh Hui Tsa Chih, 88,* 624–627.

Lynch, S. A., & Renstrom, P. A. (1999). Groin injuries in sport: Treatment strategies. *Sports Medicine, 28,* 137–144.

Mallone, T. R. (1988). Basic science of musculotendinous structure. In W. E. Garrett Jr., P. W. Duncan, & T. R. Mallone (Eds.), *Muscle injury and rehabilitation* (pp. 1–42). Baltimore, MD: Williams & Wilkins.

McPartland, J. M. (2004). Travell trigger points—molecular and osteopathic perspectives. *Journal of the American Osteopathic Association, 104,* 244–249.

Meyer, R. A., & Prior, B. M. (2000). Functional magnetic resonance imaging of muscle. *Exercise & Sport Science Reviews, 28,* 89–92.

Nguyen, B., Brandser, E. A., & Rubin, D. A. (2000). Pains, strains and fasciculations. *MRI Clinics of North America, 89,* 391–408.

Nicholas, S. J., & Tyler, T. F. (2002). Adductor muscle strains in sport. *Sports Medicine, 32,* 339–344.

Palmer, W. E., Kuong, S. J., & Elmadbouh, H. M. (1999). MR imaging of myotendinous strain. *American Journal of Roentgenology, 173,* 703–709.

Park, J. Y., & Espiniella, J. L. (1970). Rupture of pectoralis major muscle: A case report and review of literature. *Journal of Bone & Joint Surgery American Volume, 52,* 577–581.

Peetrons, P. (2002). Ultrasound of muscles. *European Radiology, 12,* 35–45.

Reebok, L. D., & Terrain, M. (2003). Magnetic resonance imaging of sports-related muscle injuries. *Topics in Magnetic Resonance Imaging, 14,* 209–220.

Sallay, P. I., Friedman, R. L., Coogan, P. G., & Garrett, W. E. (1996). Hamstring muscle injuries among water skiers: Functional outcome and prevention. *American Journal of Sports Medicine, 24,* 130–136.

Shellock, F. G., Fukunaga, T., Mink, J. H., & Edgerton, V. R. (1991). Acute effects of exercise on MR imaging of skeletal muscle. *American Journal of Roentgenology, 156(4),* 765–768.

Shellock, F. G., Fukunaga, T., Mink, J. H., & Edgerton, V. R. (1991). Exertional muscle injury: Evaluation of concentric versus eccentric actions with serial MR imaging. *Radiology, 179,* 659–664.

Simons, D. G. (2004). Review of enigmatic MTrPs as a common cause of enigmatic musculoskeletal pain and dysfunction. *Journal of Electromyography & Kinesiology, 14,* 95–107.

Simons, D. G., Travell, J. G., & Simons, L. (1999). *Myofascial pain and dysfunction: The trigger point manual: The lower extremities.* (Vol. 2). Baltimore, MD: Williams & Wilkins.

Steinback, L. S., Fleckenstein, J. L., & Mink, J. H. (1993). MR imaging of muscle injuries. In B. S. Weissman (Ed.), *Syllabus: A categorical course in musculoskeletal radiology* (pp. 225–237). Oak Brook, IL: RSNA Publications.

Tuite, M. J., & De Smet, A. A. (1994). MRI of selected sports injuries: Muscle tears, groin pain, and osteochondritis dissecans. *Seminars in Ultrasound, CT, & MRI, 15,* 318–340.

Weishaupt, D., Schweitzer, M. E., & Morrison, W. B. (2001). Injuries to the distal gastrocnemius muscle: MR findings. *Journal of Computer Assisted Tomography, 25,* 677–682.

Wine, S., & Phadeke, P. (1996). Isolated popliteus muscle rupture in polo players. *Knee Surgery, Sports Traumatology, Arthroscopy, 4,* 89–91.

Wolfe, S. W., Wickiewicz, T. L., & Cavanaugh, J. T. (1992). Ruptures of the pectoralis major muscle: An anatomic and clinical analysis. *American Journal of Sports Medicine, 20,* 587–593.

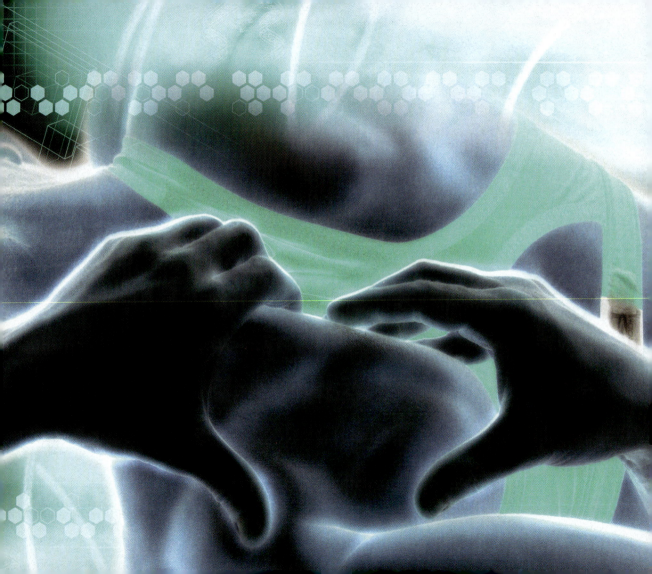

MANUAL AND REHABILITATIVE TECHNIQUES USED FOR SOFT TISSUE INJURIES

Soft tissue injuries involve physical damage to muscle, fascia, tendons, ligaments, and skin. Minor injuries that do not require immediate or surgical intervention can be treated according to the principles of rest, ice, compression, and elevation (RICE). Serious injuries usually require surgical procedures followed by manual rehabilitative techniques to improve dynamic stability dysfunction at a joint or region.

MOVEMENT DYSFUNCTION

The myofascial system has an intricate and coordinated interaction with the articular system, connective tissue, and neural system. A dysfunction in any of these components will result in a loss of dynamic stability and muscle balance and ultimately manifest itself as a source of musculoskeletal pain.

Biomechanical dysfunction in movement can present at a segmental level in the translational movements and functional movements at a single motion segment (e.g., injured articular joint that is responsible for accessory and translational joint motion). However, dysfunction can occur at a multisegmental level in the functional movements across several motion segments (e.g., abnormal myofascial system and motor unit recruitment via neural dynamics). Multisegmental dysfunction will be the primary focus of discussion in this chapter, even though both segmental and multisegmental functions are critical for optimal biomechanical movement.

Multisegmental (myofascial) dysfunction can result in displacement of the instantaneous center of motion, which is associated with changes in length and recruitment of myofascial tissue and reactivity of the nervous system. To fully encapsulate the role of the myofascial system, an overview of the segmental axis of rotation and its determinants will be presented. Every joint moves to some extent in all three planes of motion. At any particular range in motion, there exists a point about which the joint rotates or pivots: the instantaneous axis of rotation (IAR). The path of the IAR is primarily determined by a functional interrelationship between the following components: passive subsystem (osseous and connective tissue structures), the active subsystem (dynamic contractile myofascial tissues), and the neural subsystem (motor control and proprioceptive factors).

The IAR is acted upon by force couples in all three axes of a joint. If there is an imbalance between any of the force vectors (synergistic and antagonistic muscles, passive connective tissue restraints) acting around the respective joint, it can result in displacement of the IAR. The imbalance in force vectors can be attributed to extrinsic or intrinsic factors. Extrinsic load changes, such as running on an angled surface, or intrinsic changes due to shortening of the iliotibial band will contribute to valgus loading of the knee and external tibial torsion. Hence, faulty joint articulation will lead to microtrauma in the tissues around the joint. If this situation persists, it can lead to movement dysfunction and pain.

Changes in the IAR can be accounted for by a give or restriction phenomenon. *Give* is defined as hypermobility or a lack of active muscle control, which compensates for an articular or myofascial restriction in order to maintain normal range of motion. Give or excessive segmental translational motion may be the result of various factors, such as connective tissue changes (insidious or traumatic laxity of ligaments, capsule, menisci, or labrums); or neurophysiological responses (motor control deficits and inhibition of local stability muscles or pathoneurodynamics). Restriction or loss of segmental translational motion may be the result of various factors such as connective tissue changes (joint restriction, adhesion formation); or neurophysiological (guarding, muscle spasm). A segmental, articular, and translational restriction is associated with a lack of extensibility of the connective tissue, resulting in abnormal displacement of the path of instantaneous center of motion (PICM). A restriction may be multisegmental or myofascial and is associated with a lack of extensibility of contractile myofascial or neural tissue, resulting in dysfunctional flexibility.

Segmental and articular give and restriction as well as multisegmental (myofascial) give and restriction can be clinically identified at an intra-articular, inter-articular, or regional level. They present as segmental dysfunction in the passive connective tissues (displaced PICM) or as multisegmental dysfunction in the active contractile tissues (motor

Table 8-1 Give and Restriction Interactions

Level	Characteristics
Articular segmental (intra-articular dysfunction)	– Occurs within the same joint – Occurs in different or opposing directions – Associated with abnormal accessory or translational movement – Give and restriction primarily involve connective tissue changes – Relates to a displaced path of the instantaneous center of motion (PICM) – Articular dysfunction: segmental, translational, or type II (articular or translational give and restriction can be confirmed by manual palpation assessment)
Articular segmental (inter-articular dysfunction)	– Occurs between adjacent joints – Usually occurs in the same direction – Relates to a displaced PICM and to changes in the relative flexibility of muscles – May have some characteristics of both articular and myofascial dysfunction
Myofascial multisegmental (regional dysfunction)	– Occurs between adjacent regions – Occurs in the same direction – Associated with abnormal physiological or functional movements – Give and restriction primarily involve contractile tissue changes – Relates to changes in relative flexibility – Myofascial dysfunction: multisegmental or type I (myofascial give and restriction can be confirmed with movement analysis and muscle length and recruitment tests)

control deficits or relative flexibility faults). Give and restriction interactions at all three levels are described in Table 8-1.

As previously mentioned, multisegmental dysfunction can result in abnormal movement about several motion segments. Muscle contraction generates tension across motion segments at both ends; if there is inadequate stability or control at any segment, this leads to compensatory excessive movement at adjacent segments. It is not unusual to have

all combinations of restrictions present simultaneously, or to have hypermobility or laxity without any noticeable restriction.

PRINCIPLES OF REHABILITATION

Upon sustaining an injury, patients should be evaluated for rehabilitation to assess and identify the injury and its impact on normal daily activities. Various health-care professionals must collaborate and be involved in a multidisciplinary team. Effective treatment depends on accurate diagnosis, and treatment must be garnered to reduce pain, promote healing, and restore normal function. The main component of the treatment plan is to control initial pain and swelling using RICE therapy, followed later by strengthening and flexibility exercises to minimize muscle atrophy and restore normal range of motion.

Rest, Ice, Compression, and Elevation (RICE)

Basic treatment strategies should be initiated during the first 72 hours following soft tissue injuries. This modality reduces the metabolic demands of the tissue to protect it from further injury by decreasing pain and inflammation (Association of Chartered Physiotherapists, 1998). The edema and swelling that occur following an injury limit tissue function. At this early stage of injury, the basic principle of the RICE therapy is to limit ischemia to the affected area and prevent hematoma formation (T. Jarvinen, Kaarianen, M. Jarvinen, & Kalimo, 2000).

Rest

Resting the injured tissue prevents further damage by decreasing its metabolic requirements. Inflammation and edema are reduced, in turn inhibiting progressive injury (Reed, 1996). Mild trauma may require 24 hours of rest, and severe injuries may need up to 7 days (Association of Chartered Physiotherapists, 1998). While rest is beneficial to a certain extent, prolonged periods of immobilization can lead to significant muscle atrophy and loss of strength (T. Jarvinen et al., 2000). Complete immobilization also results in significant water loss of tissues, especially in the interfascial planes. During recovery, controlled motion is advised to maintain functional adaptation of a particular limb in addition to preventing intra-articular adhesions from becoming stiff (Donatelli & Owens-Burkhart, 1981). Rehabilitation

should be undertaken within the limits of pain; that is, there will be some discomfort, but excessive pain is an indication of further damage.

Ice

Administering cryotherapy (therapeutic use of cold) such as by applying ice should occur within 48 hours following an acute trauma to reduce pain, inflammation, and swelling by constricting blood vessels. This vasoconstriction prevents further trauma to the area and reduces hematoma and hemorrhage (Reed, 1996).

To prevent frostbite, wrap the ice in a towel and apply for no more than 20 minutes duration at 2-hour intervals (Merrick, Rankin, Andres, & Hinman, 1999; Paddon-Jones & Quigley, 1997; Stitik & Nadler, 1998). Areas composed of abundant subcutaneous fat may require 30 minutes of application time, whereas bony areas with little fat should be restricted to 5 to 10 minutes.

Compression

Applying wraps or bandages to the injured area limits swelling from fluid accumulation. Compression should be applied with uniform pressure across the entire site immediately after injury and maintained for 72 hours. Wraps may need to be reapplied to maintain constant pressure and in a distal to proximal direction to minimize an increase in local blood flow (Association of Chartered Physiotherapists, 1998).

Elevation

While maintaining compression for the first 72 hours, the affected area should be elevated above the heart level to allow drainage of fluid via the lymphatics. This also limits edema and hematoma formation (Association of Chartered Physiotherapists, 1998; T. Jarvinen et al., 2000). While it is more practical to elevate the arms and legs than the hips and back, support aids such as pillows and slings can be utilized for any of those body parts.

REHABILITATION STRATEGY FOR RESTORING DYNAMIC STABILITY AND MUSCULAR STRENGTH

Movement dysfunction often arises from incorrect recruitment and poor motor control. Hence the central nervous system's modulation of low-threshold motor units and its integration of local and global muscles are not concise, and muscle imbalances develop over time. The priority for clinicians is to diagnose the pathology and treat the pain mechanisms, inflammation, and pathology with a wide range of treatments such as low-level laser, ultrasound, frequency-specific microcurrent, acupuncture, muscle energy techniques, and appropriate pharmaceuticals and or nutraceuticals.

After a clear diagnosis has been established, the clinician can start designing a rehabilitation program that addresses instability by focusing his or her attention on the following key principles.

Local Stability System— Control of the Neutral Joint Position

It is important to retrain the tonic, low-threshold motor units to increase local muscle stiffness. In addition, retraining of the functional low-threshold integration motor units of the local and global stabilizer muscles is required for the effective control of the neutral joint position.

Global Stability System— Control the Direction of Stability Dysfunction

Use low loads on the local and global stabilizer muscles to control and limit the range of motion at the segment or region of give, and then actively move the restriction. Control of direction directly unloads mechanical provocation of pathology and therefore is the key strategy for symptom management.

Global Stability System— Control of Imbalance

Rehabilitating the global stabilizers will result in the global stability system actively controlling the full available range of joint motion. These muscles are required to actively shorten and control limb load through the full passive inner range of joint motion. As previously discussed, dynamic instability of a multijoint muscle often demonstrates a lack of extensibility due to overuse or adaptive shortening; compensatory overstrain or give occurs elsewhere in the kinetic chain in an attempt to maintain function. Hence the clinician must either lengthen or inhibit the activity of the global mobilizers in order to eliminate the need for compensating to keep proper function.

The rehabilitation program designed to correct movement dysfunction can be divided into seven stages:

1. Controlling neutral joint position
2. Regaining dynamic control of direction of stability dysfunction
3. Retraining control of global stability muscles throughout joint range
4. Regaining extensibility and inhibiting overactivity in the global mobility muscles
5. Training stability during overload training
6. Training stability during slow spinal and girdle movements
7. Training functional stability during high-speed movements

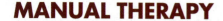
MANUAL THERAPY

Manual therapy has become an invaluable tool for managing soft tissue injuries. Pioneers like Guy Voyer and Michael Leahy laid the foundation for integrating mind-body manual therapy. The various techniques described in this section have provided clinicians with the necessary means to restore functional recovery of the injured tissue.

Stretching

The two types of stretching, pompage and myofascial, were created by Dr. Guy Voyer.

Pompage (French for "pumping") draws synovial fluid into the joint via a pumping action. This tends to reduce inflammation and pain, thus improving range of motion. Injuries such as sprains, anterior cruciate ligament (ACL) tears, and tendon ruptures all benefit.

Myofascial stretching focuses on the connections between muscles and tendons as well as bones and ligaments. Stretching, which includes ELDOA (Etierement Longitudinaux avec Decoaptation Osteo Articulaire, a stretching method developed by Voyer), puts tension on the myofascial chains to increase muscle tone and proprioception as well as improve circulation and kinesthetic awareness (Voyer, 2003).

Articular Pumping

Articular pumping is a manual therapeutic technique used to break and reduce fibrous adhesions by using active and passive motions to restore gliding between fascial planes (Voyer, 2001). It targets the entire joint of nerves, fascia, blood vessels, and synovial fluid. This results in increased fluidity and circulation, which in turn improves removal of metabolic wastes via lymph drainage. Range of motion is improved along with reduced tissue stiffness.

Articular pumping is best used within 24 to 48 hours post surgery since applying force to the fascia during

healing improves the strength and plasticity of the tissue by improving remodeling and repair.

Active Release Technique® (ART)

Active release technique® (ART) is a soft tissue technique using a hands-on approach that allows the therapist to diagnose and treat soft tissue injuries. Like articular pumping, ART® is used to establish motion between fascial planes and thus reduce fibrous adhesions (Leahy, 1998). ART® can be applied to muscles, tendons, ligaments, fascia, and nerves to treat repetitive strain injuries, post-surgical cases, joint dysfunction, tissue hypoxia, and adhesions.

ART® is time consuming but very practical because it requires no equipment other than the clinician's hands. Accurately locating adhesions by touch remains the greatest obstacle to learning ART®. Once a lesion is found, it is manipulated using specific hand contacts.

Certain guidelines must be adhered to when using ART® (Leahy, 1998):

1. Use specific hands-on contacts depending on the area being treated.

2. Work longitudinally to break tissue adhesions. This direction of motion will prevent muscle fibers from sliding or rolling under the contact.

3. Use active motion when possible to give the patient a sense of control and maximize motion between tissues.

4. Use slow motion to improve patient tolerability.

5. Use patient tolerance to determine the limit of pressure and the number of passes.

6. Use tissue tolerance as a guide to determine whether to delay or reduce treatment frequency.

7. Work with lymphatic and venous flow.

8. Treat on alternate days to avoid tissue intolerance.

Manual Resistance Technique (MRT)

Manual resistance technique (MRT) involves manual resistance to isometric or isotonic exercise performed by a patient, followed by stretching or relaxation (Liebenson, 2007). This therapy results in stretch of the fascia and shortened muscle or relaxation of an overactive muscle. Concentric, eccentric, and isometric contractions are all encompassed in MRT. The main employment is to work the muscular part in order to increase the capacity of joint adjustments and restore normal range of motion.

Advantages of MRT over ART®, deep-tissue massage, and trigger point therapy are the faster response to therapy and minimal pain involved in reducing muscle tension. Training weak muscles can also benefit from MRT, and patient control over movements is more precise when manual therapy is performed.

Before doing stretching movements, it is important that the neural and muscular tissues are relaxed. This enables the clinician to accurately diagnose the problem as being neuromuscular in nature and avoid damaging the contractile units in the muscle. Patients may require deep-breathing exercises and moist heat application to help them attain relaxation.

Proprioception

Proprioception involves sensing the position of a body part relative to other neighboring body parts. It involves the interaction of sensory and motor neurons. Mechanoreceptors signal changes in the original shape of the soft tissue, and nociceptive receptors signal painful stimuli. These receptors are found in tissues surrounding structures such as the skin, joint, and muscle.

Four types of mechanoreceptors have been classified, each displaying different levels of threshold, shapes, and adaptive properties:

1. Type 1—found in the proximal joints

2. Type 2—nerve endings found through the distal joints

3. Type 3—the Ruffini corpuscle located in the individual joint ligaments

4. Type 4—the nociceptive free nerve endings located in joint capsules, ligaments, and subcutaneous fat layers

Any mechanical deformation is sensed by the mechanoreceptors and transmitted by efferent and afferent pathways to provide information on the caliber of stretch, compression, and tension of a particular joint.

It is important to begin proprioceptive exercises early in the course of the treatment to determine if any damaged proprioceptors require neurological retraining. In addition, early treatment is required to restore normal gait pattern without pain in addition to attaining the ABCs of proprioception of "agility, balance, and coordination." (Houglum, 2005).

Proper progression of proprioceptive exercises is important to maintain efficacy and avoid injury. Progression must not be done too quickly, and the receptors must be stressed appropriately to restore proprioceptive function.

Isometric Exercise

Isometric refers to exercise in which the length of the muscle does not change. It involves muscle contraction without a change in the joint angle. The advantages of isometrics are faster workouts and maximum contraction of a particular muscle; disadvantages are reduced muscular endurance and increased blood pressure. When muscles are exercised against a resistance, there is a substantial rise in blood pressure although it appears to be mainly due to exercise duration (Kubo, Kanehisa, & Fukunaga). In addition, isometrics when used in squat training has shown a negative effect on the tendon–aponeurosis complex in knee extensors (Kubo, Kanehisa, & Fukunaga). The increased stiffness in the tendon negatively affected the pre-stretch during stretch–shortening cycle exercises.

Isotonic Exercise

Isotonic refers to muscle contraction in which the tension remains constant as the muscle shortens or lengthens. This form of exercise can be used on a broad range of major muscle groups by doing a variety of exercises. The main benefits of using this type of exercise during rehabilitation are that it increases muscle strength and neuromuscular performance (Taaffe, Duret, Wheeler, & Marcus, 1999). Other benefits include improved physical conditioning, increased bone density, and effective capillary blood flow to the exercised muscle (Lamotte, Strulens, Niset, & Van de Borne, 2005).

Plyometrics

Plyometric exercise involves lengthening of the muscle–tendon unit followed by shortening (stretch–shortening cycle) through rapid acceleration and deceleration (Chmielewski, Myer, Kauffman, & Tillman, 2006). These exercises involve skipping, bounding, hopping, and lunging. Plyometric exercises are best done during the final stages of rehabilitation because they improve athletic performance by enhancing power, speed, and rhythm in addition to conditioning the muscles to handle the added strain of eccentric contractions. The patient progresses through a series of low- to moderate- to high-intensity exercises as tolerated. The patient should warm up first, so that maximum power can be created through rapid concentric and eccentric muscle movements.

Summary

While minor injuries can be treated using the basic principles of rest, ice, compression, and elevation (RICE), rehabilitation of serious injuries can be

successfully treated using manual techniques. Manual therapies employed to help restore functional activity of the affected organ include hands-on manipulation to reduce fascial adhesions and restrictions, as in soft tissue release, or articular pumping to target the entire joint area.

Background knowledge of movement dysfunction theory and concepts can be invaluable in implementing certain rehabilitation programs. No single particular treatment technique is suitable for all patients. More importantly, all rehabilitation should be performed within the patient's limits of pain.

Chapter 9 presents manual techniques of rehabilitation using the shoulder and anterior cruciate ligament (ACL) injury as case studies.

References

Chmielewski, T. L., Myer, G. D., Kauffman, D., & Tillman, S. M. (2006). Plyometric exercise in the rehabilitation of athletes: Physiological responses and clinical application. *Journal of Orthopaedic & Sports Physical Therapy, 36,* 308–19.

Donatelli, R., & Owens-Burkhart, H. (1981). Effects of immobilization on the extensibility of periarticular connective tissue. *Journal of Orthopaedic & Sports Physical Therapy, 3*(2), 67–72.

Gibbons, S. (2001). *Movement dysfunction, dynamic stability and muscle balance of the lumbar spine and trunk: Local muscle system, kinetic control.* Mede House.

Houglum, P. (2005). *Therapeutic Exercise for Musculoskeletal Injuries*-2nd Edition. Champaign, IL: Human Kinetics.

Jarvinen, T. A., Kaariainen, M., Jarvinen, M., & Kalimo, H. (2000). Muscle strain injuries. *Current Opinion in Rheumatology, 12,* 155–161.

Kerr, K., Daley, L., Booth, L., & Stark, J. (1998). *Guidelines for the physiotherapy management* of soft tissue injury with PRICE during the first 72 hours. England: Chartered Society of Physiotherapists and Association of Chartered Physiotherapists in Sports Medicine.

Kubo, K., Yata, H., Kanehisa, H., & Fukunaga, T. (2006). Effects of isometric squat training on the tendon stiffness and jump performance. European Journal of Applied Physiology, 96, 305–314.

Lamotte, M., Strulens, G., Niset, G., & Van de Borne, P. (2005). Influence of different resistive training modalities on blood pressure and heart rate responses of healthy subjects. Isokinetics & Exercise Science, 13, 273–277.

Leahy, M. (1998). Development of active release techniques, soft-tissue management system. Colorado Springs, CO: Champion Health Associates.

Liebenson, C. (2007). Rehabilitation of the spine: A practitioner's manual (3rd ed.). Philadelphia: Lippincott Williams & Wilkins.

Merrick, M. A., Rankin, J. M., Andres, F. A., & Hinman, C. L. (1999). A preliminary examination of cryotherapy and secondary injury in skeletal muscle. Medicine & Science in Sports & Exercise, 31, 1516–1521.

Paddon-Jones, D. J., & Quigley, B. M. (1997). Effect of cryotherapy on muscle soreness and strength following eccentric exercise. International Journal of Sports Medicine, 18, 588–593.

Reed, B. V. (1996). Wound healing and the use of thermal agents. In S. L. Michlovitz (Ed.), Thermal agents in rehabilitation, 3rd ed. (pp. 3–9). Philadelphia: FA Davis.

Stitik, T. P., & Nadler, S. F. (1998). Sport injuries. Part 1: When and how to use cold most effectively. Consultant, 38, 2881–2884, 2887–2888.

Taaffe, D. R., Duret, C., Wheeler, S., & Marcus, R. (1999). Once-weekly resistance exercise improves muscle strength and neuro-muscular performance in older adults. Journal of the American Geriatrics Society, 47, 1208–1214.

Voyer, G. (2001). Somatotherapy Interactive Seminars Inc.–Articular Pumping. Practice Manual by Jane Stark.

Voyer, G. (2003). The ELDOA.

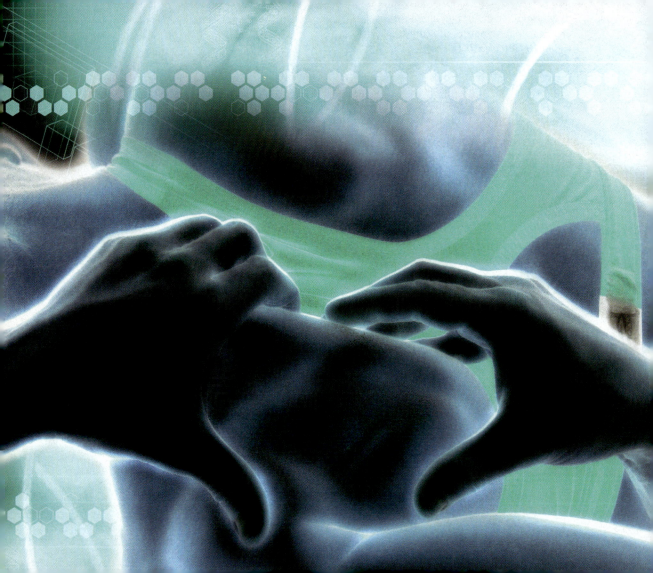

CONSERVATIVE REHABILITATION PROTOCOLS FOR FASCIA INJURIES

Two common sports injuries (adhesive capsulitis and anterior cruciate ligament) are presented here using the manual rehabilitative treatment as discussed in the previous chapter. Treatment protocols can vary depending on the therapist and capabilities of the patient.

TREATMENT AND REHABILITATION OF ADHESIVE CAPSULITIS: MULTIPHASE APPROACH

A clinical examination of the shoulder joint complex must be performed to establish a differential diagnosis in order to determine the physical limitations or problems causing the shoulder complex disorder. A rehabilitation trainer must thoroughly assess the range of motion (ROM), muscle strength, laxity, and proprioception as well as the athlete's throwing program, exercise schedule, and throwing mechanics. Once these areas have been assessed, a comprehensive rehabilitation program can be constructed (Wilk, Meister, & Andrews, 2002).

The nonoperative treatment and rehabilitation program used for adhesive capsulitis for the over-head-throwing athlete will involve a multiphase approach that is progressive and sequential. The overhead-throwing athlete should follow these nine rehabilitation principles during the course of treatment:

1. Never overstress the healing tissue.
2. Prevent negative effects of immobilization.
3. Emphasize external rotation muscular strength.
4. Establish muscular balance.
5. Emphasize scapular muscular strength.
6. Improve posterior shoulder flexibility (internal rotation ROM).
7. Enhance proprioception and neuromuscular control.
8. Gradually return to throwing activities.
9. Use established criteria to progress.

The four phases of treatment are described in the following sections.

PHASE I— ACUTE TRAUMA, INFLAMMATION, AND PHAGOCYTOSIS

Acute trauma results in immediate inflammation. This is an early response to tissue injury characterized by edema, vasodilation, and emigration of leukocytes. Acute inflammatory response leads to rapid phagocytosis, a process of engulfing foreign debris, bacteria and viruses.

Time	Goals	Modalities
0–48 hrs	1. Minimize injury.	Ice.
	2. Minimize inflammation.	15 minutes to injury site.
	3. Prevent further injury.	Repeat 2–3× daily for first 48 hrs Low-Level Laser 635-nm wavelength.
		Frequency—3 Hz to reduce inflammation
		A low-level laser should be held at the area of focus no longer than 20 seconds at a time and moved around surrounding areas of tenderness. The clinician should determine which fascial chain has been affected by the injury, and from that point, treat the respective anatomical areas.
		(continued)

Nutritional Protocol

Disclaimer: The following doses used for each supplement are based on the RDA or experimental studies and are designed to mitigate inflammation, enhance muscle growth, improve wound healing, or maintain health. Consult with a qualified practitioner or health-care professional.

Arginine	Carnosine	Copper	Fish Oil	Bovine Colostrum	Bromelain (EC)*
17–25 grams (Appleton, 2002)	450 mg (Antonini et al., 2002)	0.4–0.9 mg (Turnlund et al., 2004)	1 gram of DHA/EPA (Trebble et al., 2003)	20 grams (Antonio, Sanders, & Van Gammeren, 2001)	750–2000 milligrams 1 hr before meals (Maurer, 2001)

*EC = enteric coated. Dosages given are oral daily doses unless otherwise indicated.

There are various modalities used to treat acute trauma and these modalities are administered at appropriate times.

PHASE II—INITIATE AND ESTABLISH HEALING

Collagen cross-linking begins to occur during phase II. This process results in the formation of tissue adhesion, which in turn can result in the following:

1. Altered pain afferents with efferent reflexes
2. Altered proprioception afferents with efferent reflexes
3. Altered instantaneous axis of rotation (IAR) with kinetic muscular stress
4. Altered muscle function

The glenohumeral joint is only one link in the fascial chain. The whole body must be integrated with trained movements to allow for functional carryover to sport.

Time	Goals	Modalities
3–14 days	1. Diminish pain and inflammation.	Low-Level Laser
	2. Normalize motion.	635-nm wavelength
	3. Retard muscular atrophy.	Frequency—3 Hz to reduce inflammation for days 3–5
	4. Reestablish dynamic stability (muscular balance).	Frequency—25 Hz to promote fascia and muscle regeneration for days 6–14
	5. Control functional stress/strain.	Frequency—42 Hz—lymphatic regeneration and promote removal of metabolic by-products from injury for days 6–14
	6. Restore proprioception.	Frequency—125 Hz—reoxygenation for days 6–14

(continued)

Nutritional Protocol					
Arginine	**Carnosine**	**Copper**	**Fish Oil**	**Bovine Colostrum**	**Bromelain (EC)***
17–25 grams (Appleton, 2002)	450 mg (Antonini et al., 2002)	0.4–0.9 mg (Turnlund et al., 2004)	1 gram of DHA/EPA (Trebble et al., 2003)	20 grams (Antonio, et al., 2003)	750–2000 mg 1 hr before meals (Maurer, 2001)

*EC = enteric coated. Dosages given are oral daily doses unless otherwise indicated.

Myofascial Mobility and Articular Pumping

The goals of articular pumping are as follows:

1. Restore proper muscle recruitment pattern.

2. Restore lymphatic drainage to reduce edema.

3. Promote full ROM in the glenohumeral joint.

4. Promote synovial fluidity between the respective fascial chains.

Tables 9-1 through 9-4 summarize the rehabilitation protocols of the glenohumeral joint using articular pumping.

Table 9-1 Articular Pumping of the Glenohumeral Rehabilitation Joint: Protocol 1	
Rehab Protocol 1	Long-axis traction (passive) is applied to shoulder at 90° abduction and 25–30° extension in neutral tension.
Position of the Patient	• Patient is seated facing away from the therapist with her arm kept in 90° abduction with 25–30° extension.
	• Patient's right arm is supported by the therapist's forearms.
	• Patient's right elbow is kept in flexion.
Position of the Therapist	• Therapist positions his left leg against the right side of the patient with his knee and tibia pushed laterally against the patient's thorax to stabilize her upper body.
	• Left hand—connects both the right and left third fingers together to be in contact with the superior aspect of the humerus.
	• Right hand—loops under the patient's arm to support the elbow.
Instructions during the Inhalation Phase	The therapist applies long-axis traction of the arm (Figure 9-1) by leaning laterally away from the patient while the patient remains relaxed. The patient may use her opposite hand to pull up to prevent rotation of the shoulder girdle.
	(continued)

Table 9-1 Articular Pumping of the Glenohumeral Joint:
Rehabilitation Protocol 1 (continued)

Instructions during the Exhalation Phase	The therapist moves in the direction of the release of the myofascial tissue while the patient remains relaxed.
Instructions during the Relaxation Phase	The therapist releases the applied myofascial tension on the humerus.

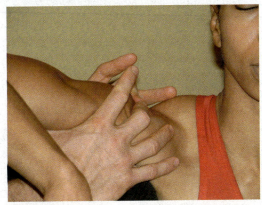

Figure 9-1 Using both hands, the therapist palpates the tubercule of the patient's humerus while applying long-axis traction along the length of the humerus.

Table 9-2 Articular Pumping of the Glenohumeral Joint:
Rehabilitation Protocol 2

Rehab Protocol 2	• Articular pumping of the posterior-inferior aspects of the shoulder capsule is performed.
	• Long-axis traction (active/passive with internal rotation of the shoulder starting at 90° abduction in external rotation).
Position of the Patient	• Patient is seated facing away from the therapist with her arm kept in 90° abduction with external rotation.
	• Patient's right arm is supported by the therapist's knee and left forearm.
	• Patient's right elbow is kept in flexion.
Position of the Therapist	• Therapist positions his left leg against the right side of the patient with his knee and tibia pushed laterally against the patient's thorax to stabilize her upper body.
	• Left hand—supports the wrist of the patient.

(continued)

Table 9-2 Articular Pumping of the Glenohumeral Rehabilitation Joint: Protocol 2 (continued)

	• Right hand—loops under the patient's arm to support the forearm and elbow.
	• The third finger palpates the greater tubercule of the humerus.
Instructions during the Inhalation Phase	The therapist applies long-axis traction to the patient's shoulder (Figure 9-2) by leaning his body away from the patient while resisting but allowing internal rotation of the arm.
Instructions during the Exhalation Phase	The therapist maintains long-axis traction while the arm internally rotates (Figure 9-3).
Instructions during the Relaxation Phase	The therapist releases long-axis traction and returns the patient's upper arm to external rotation (Figure 9-4).

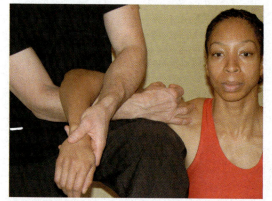

Figure 9-2 The therapist's left hand supports the patient's wrist while his right hand loops under her arm to support the forearm, which is held in external rotation.

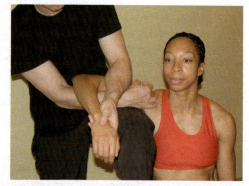

Figure 9-3 The patient internally rotates her shoulder using approximately 20% of her strength while the therapist applies long-axis traction resisting the internal rotation of the patient's arm.

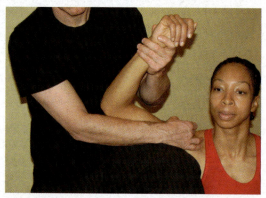

Figure 9-4 The therapist releases long-axis traction and returns the patient's arm to its original position of external rotation.

Table 9-3 Articular Pumping of the Glenohumeral Joint: Rehabilitation Protocol 3	
Rehab Protocol 3	Long-axis traction (active/passive) is applied with internal rotation of the shoulder starting at 90° abduction in external rotation.
Position of the Patient	• Patient is seated facing away from the therapist with her arm kept in 90° abduction with internal rotation (Figure 9-5). • Patient's right arm is supported by the therapist's left forearm. • Patient's right elbow is kept in flexion.
Position of the Therapist	• Therapist positions his left leg against the patient's right side with his knee and tibia pushed laterally against the patient's thorax to stabilize her upper body. • Left hand—supports the patient's wrist. • Right hand—loops under the patient's arm to support the forearm and elbow. • The third finger palpates the greater tubercule of the humerus.
Instructions during the Inhalation Phase	The therapist applies long-axis traction to the shoulder by leaning his body away from the patient while resisting but allowing internal rotation of the arm.
Instructions during the Exhalation Phase	The therapist maintains long-axis traction while the patient's arm externally rotates (Figure 9-6).
Instructions during the Relaxation Phase	The therapist releases long-axis traction and returns the patient's upper arm to internal rotation (Figure 9-7).

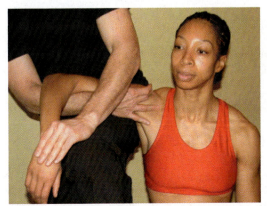

Figure 9-5 The therapist's left hand supports the patient's wrist while the right hand loops under the patient's arm to support the forearm, which is held in internal rotation.

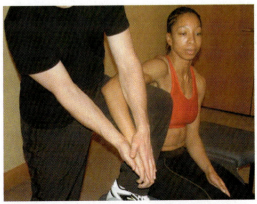

Figure 9-6 The patient externally rotates her shoulder using approximately 20% of her strength while the therapist applies long-axis traction resisting the external rotation of the patient's arm.

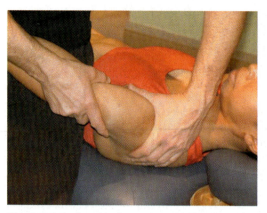

Figure 9-7 The therapist releases long-axis traction and returns the patient's arm to its original position of internal rotation.

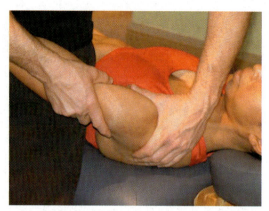

Figure 9-8 The therapist's right hand grasps the outer lateral surface of the patient's upper arm while the left hand covers the anterior aspect of the shoulder. The therapist applies tension in the inferior direction, causing decoaptating of the patient's glenohumeral joint.

Table 9-4 Articular Pumping of the Glenohumeral Joint: Rehabilitation Protocol 4

Rehab Protocol 4	• Deepest part of the glenohumeral articulation.
	• Long-axis traction (passive) of the shoulder starting at 45° abduction with slight flexion.
Position of the Patient	• Patient is supine with her left arm in slight abduction.
Position of the Therapist	• The patient's left arm is supported between the therapist's right hand and body.
	• Left hand—palmar surface covers the anterior aspect of the patient's shoulder.
	• Right hand—supports the lateral surface of the patient's humerus with the fingers close to the joint line.
Instructions during the Inhalation Phase	The therapist applies long-axis traction to the glenohumeral joint in the inferior direction (Figure 9-8).
Instructions during the Exhalation Phase	The therapist maintains myofascial tension along the patient's upper arm.
Instructions during the Relaxation Phase	The therapist allows the patient's humerus to relax and return to its original position in the glenoid fossa (Figure 9-9).

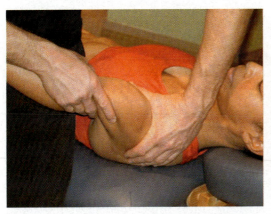

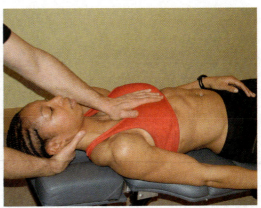

Figure 9-9 The therapist maintains decoaptation and eventually allows the fascia to relax, and the patient's humerus moves back to its original position.

Figure 9-10 The therapist releases pressure on the patient's sternum in a fluidic manner during the inhalation phase.

Table 9-5 Articular Pumping of the Pretrachial Fascia	
Position of the Patient	The patient is supine with her arms lying by her sides.
Position of the Therapist	• Therapist is seated at the patient's head. • Cephalad hand—supports the patient's head. • Caudal hand—The thenar and hypothenar eminence of the hand lies over the sternoclavicular joint. The third finger points to the xiphoid process.
Instructions during the Inhalation Phase	The therapist maintains contact with the patient's sternum through the inhalation phase; but when the patient's neck goes into flexion, the therapist releases contact on the sternum in a fluidic manner (Figure 9-10).
Instructions during the Exhalation Phase	The therapist's caudal hand follows the downward movement of the sternum while waiting for the patient's neck to go into cranial extension (Figure 9-11). At this point, the therapist allows the patient to breathe again.
Instructions during the Relaxation Phase	The therapist releases tension between the occiput and the sternum.

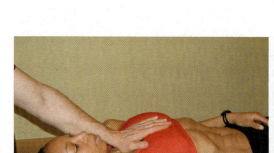

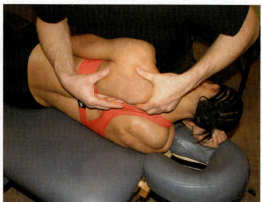

Figure 9-11 The therapist places his hand on the patient's sternum and pushes in a downward vector during patient exhalation. The therapist continues to push downward on the sternum until the end of the exhalation phase.

Figure 9-12 The therapist places the ulnar border of both hands under the spinal border of the patient's scapula while his thumbs rest on top.

Table 9-6 Articular Pumping of the Scapula

Position of the Patient	The patient is lying on her side, facing the therapist, with her arms by her sides.
Position of the Therapist	• The therapist is standing in front of the patient, situated across her shoulder girdle. • Both hands—palpate the spinal border of the scapula and place the ulnar aspects of the last three digits under the spinal border of the scapula while the thumbs rest on top (Figure 9-12).
Instructions during the Inhalation Phase	The therapist holds the medial border of the scapula to make sure that the serrato-thoracic articulation will be closed upon inhalation (Figure 9-13). Therefore, the serrato-scapula will be open.
Instructions during the Exhalation Phase	Under normal conditions, the serrato-thoracic articulation will be open and the serrato-scapula articulation will close. However, during the inspiration phase, the therapist positions his fingers medially such that during exhalation the serrato-thoracic joint will open so that the spinal border will fall posterior to the fingers (Figure 9-14). At this point, the scapulo-serratus joint opens even more.
Instructions during the Relaxation Phase	The therapist opens the patient's serrato-thoracic joint and then closes the serrato-scapular joint. This is subsequently followed by closing both the serrato-thoracic and serrato-scapular articulations, which is then followed by release.

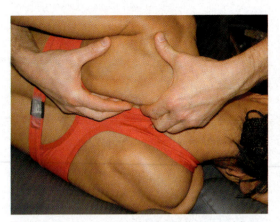

Figure 9-13 When the patient inhales, the therapist stabilizes the medial border of the scapula to prevent the opening of the serrato-thoracic junction.

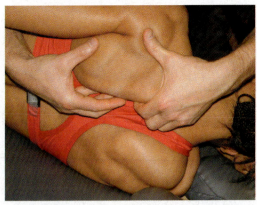

Figure 9-14 When the patient exhales, the therapist maintains the fingers medially so that during the exhalation phase, the serrato-thoracic junction opens. The therapist will then move the scapula by opening the serrato-thoracic joint and then closing the serrato-scapular joint.

Active Release Technique® and/or Sound-Assisted Soft Tissue Mobilization (SASTM)

Frequency: Days five and eight
Goal: Reduce myofascial adhesions.
Anatomical Sites Treated:

- Anterior, inferior, and posterior capsule
- Rotator cuff (RTC) muscles, including the subscapularis
- Triceps major and minor
- Anterior and posterior deltoid at the infraspinatus
- Latissimus dorsi
- Rhomboids, levator scapulae

Articular Range of Motion: Muscle Activation Technique (MAT)

Goal: Assess muscle weakness and imbalances.
Anatomical Sites Assessed:

- Scapulae abductors (serratus anterior) and adductors (rhomboids major and minor)
- Scapulae elevators (trapezius, levator scapulae, subclavius)
- Scapular depressors (pectoralis minor)
- Humeral adductors (pectoralis major, latissimus dorsi, and teres major)
- Humeral abductors (deltoid anterior, middle, and posterior, and supraspinatus)
- Humeral external rotators (infraspinatus and teres minor)
- Humeral internal rotators (subscapularis)

Considerations in ROM Assessment:

- If a muscle imbalance is evident, it is crucial to restore dynamic motion in the glenohumeral joint.
- Look for asymmetrical motion.
- Follow the law of reciprocal inhibition.

○ Decrease in the range of motion (ROM) in the agonist may come from the protective hypertonicity of the antagonist.

○ Tightness represents joint instability in extreme ranges.

○ Check for loss in internal rotation.

Shoulder Stretch (posterior capsule)

Optimal flexibility of the inferior and posterior joint capsule will enable the humeral head to roll and spin properly against the glenoid fossa during abduction and flexion. A tight or adhesive capsule seen with adhesive capsulitis can interfere with proper humeral rotation and can contribute to upward migration of the humeral head beneath the acromion process, resulting in impingement. Optimal flexibility in both the inferior and posterior capsule can be accomplished by using the stretches listed below in a rehabilitation program. Capsule stretches can be done daily and should occur after performing a light, 5–10 minute warm-up (e.g., low-level aerobic activity) or at the end of a general exercise session. During each stretch, gently apply light pressure until a comfortable stretch is felt.

The following are types of stretching exercises:

1. Horizontal adduction with scapular stabilization in supine position

2. Behind-the-back elbow push-off

3. Horizontal adduction stretch with distraction in standing position

4. Horizontal adduction stretch can be performed at 90° of shoulder abduction. The arm is horizontally adducted while the scapula is stabilized to enhance posterior shoulder stretch.

5. Behind-the-back stretch with baseball bat or golf club

6. Internal rotation stretch with the arm placed in the throwing position and passively stretched into internal rotation to stretch the external rotators

Additionally, it is recommended to have the athlete stretch his or her pectoralis minor muscle and strengthen the lower trapezius muscle as well as scapular retractor and protractor muscles.

Perform Range of Motion Exercises (passive, active-assisted, active) at a Pain-free Level

An essential goal during the first phase of rehabilitation is to normalize shoulder motion, particularly shoulder internal rotation and horizontal adduction. It is common for the overhead-throwing athlete to experience a noticeable decrease in internal rotation. This may be accounted for by soft tissue tightness, which may be caused by muscle inflexibility due to significant and repetitive eccentric muscle forces during arm deceleration (Wilk et al., 2002).

Increase Range of Motion and Restoration of Function

Functional Exercises:

○ Corrective isometrics/manual therapy

○ Isolated strengthening exercises

○ Isolated flexibility exercises

Frequency: Days 9 and 14
Goal: Reduce soft tissue adhesions.
Anatomical Sites Treated:

○ Anterior, inferior, and posterior capsule

○ RTC muscles, including the subscapularis

○ Triceps major and minor

○ Anterior and posterior deltoid at the infraspinatus

○ Latissimus dorsi

○ Rhomboids, levator scapulae

Additional primary goals of this phase in the rehabilitation program are to restore muscle strength, reestablish baseline dynamics stability, and restore proprioception. In this early phase of rehabilitation, the goal is to reestablish muscle balance (Wilk, Arrigo, & Andrews, 1995; 1997). The focus should be on improving the strength of the weak muscles such as the supraspinatus and scapular muscles (trapezius, serratus anterior, rhomboids; Wilk et al., 1995; 1997). If the athlete is extremely sore or in pain, submaximal isometric exercises should be used; conversely, if the athlete exhibits minimal soreness, isotonic exercises can be started.

Proprioceptive Neuromuscular Facilitation (PNF)

An injury to the shoulder resulting in adhesive capsulitis can negatively affect the balance between mobility and stability of the glenohumeral joint, which is required for optimal athletic performance. Shoulder stability is dependent on a complex interaction between static and dynamic factors. As shown in recent studies, shoulder proprioceptive receptors may play an important role in maintaining dynamic joint stability (Jerosch, Steinbeck, Clahsen, Schmitz-Nahrath, & Grosse-Hackmann, 1993; Lephart, Pincivero, Giraldo, Fu, 1997). When shoulder motion reaches its terminal range, it relies on the early input of proprioceptive information to detect its strain limit and avoid injury. Shoulder proprioception is derived from the sense of position and movement without visual cues. Two types of mechanical receptors are responsible for providing the proprioceptive information: (1) the load- and tensile-sensitive receptors in muscle spindles, and (2) the Golgi tendon organ and the stretch-sensitive receptors in the fibrous capsule and ligaments. Specific drills designed to restore the neurosensory properties of the shoulder capsule and to enhance the sensitivity of the afferent mechanoreceptors (Lephart, Pincivero, Giraldo, & Fu, 1997; Lephart, Warner, Borsa, Fu, 1994) are provided later in this section.

Most recently, research indicates that during proprioceptive neuromuscular facilitation (PNF) techniques, muscle electrical activity increases and co-contraction of agonist and antagonist muscles takes place (Shrier, 1999). PNF stretching activates an eccentric contraction of the targeted muscle group, which also appears to have an analgesic effect, permitting greater ROM and relaxation to occur (Magnusson, Simonesen, Aagaard, Dyhre-Poulsen, McHugh, & Kjaer, 1996). Specific drills that restore neuromuscular control during this initial phase are rhythmic stabilization and reciprocal isometric contractions for the internal and external rotator muscles of the shoulders. Additionally, PNF patterns are used with rhythmic stabilization and slow-reversal hold to reestablish proprioception and dynamic stabilization (Lephart et al., 1994; Lephart et al., 1997; Sullivan, Markos, & Minor, 1982; Wilk & Arrigo, 1992).

PNF exercises are believed to build strength through functional planes of motion by incorporating both spiral and diagonal planes of motion that demand neuromuscular coordination. It is important to note that during PNF techniques, the targeted muscle often undergoes an eccentric contraction during the stretch; this can increase the risk of injury to the targeted tissue.

For shoulder abduction and external rotation, position the shoulder in the scapular plane (approximately 20–30° forward of the coronal plane).

Neuromuscular Control: Proprioceptive and Kinesthetic Awareness

Goals:

1. Reestablish afferent pathways from the mechanoreceptors at the injury site to the central nervous system (CNS).

2. Facilitate supplementary afferent pathways as a compensatory mechanism for proprioceptive deficits that resulted from joint injury.

Instructions:

1. Place the patient's upper arm into a predetermined position and then instruct the patient to reproduce the joint position as accurately as possible.

2. Initially the patient can use visual cues, progressing to the removal of visual cues through the use of a blindfold.

3. Joint position sense trials can be performed within mid ranges of motion to stimulate musculotendinous mechanoreceptors, as well as in end ranges of motion in positions of vulnerability to stimulate capsuloligamentous afferents.

4. Utilize passive reproduction of joint position, progressing to active reproduction of joint position (Figures 9-15 through 9-17).

Dynamic Joint Stability

Goal: Reestablish the synergistic coactivation of force couples present at the shoulder. Facilitating this coactivation of the force coupled at the glenohumeral joint, restores dynamic stability, as the re-

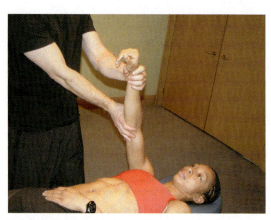

Figure 9-16 The therapist moves the patient's upper arm into a horizontal flexion position.

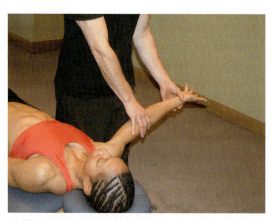

Figure 9-17 The therapist moves the patient's upper arm into a horizontal extension position.

sulting vector forces centralize and compress the humeral head within the glenoid fossa. Also, contraction of the rotator cuff pulls on the glenohumeral joint capsule, applying tension, which results in increased stability.

Weight-Bearing Shift Exercises

Instructions:

1. Have the patient assume a tripod position on a firm surface (Figure 9-18).

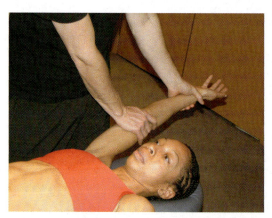

Figure 9-15 The therapist elevates the patient's upper arm into an overhead position.

2. Once she is able to maintain the above position with ease, progress to holding the tripod stance on an unstable surface (Figure 9-19).

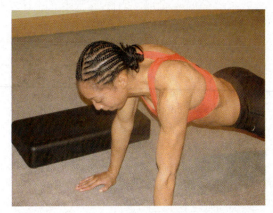

Figure 9-18 The patient assumes a tripod stance with both hands on the ground, which is a stable surface.

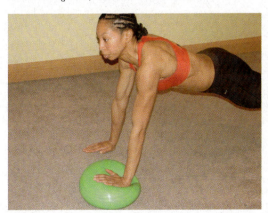

Figure 9-19 The patient can progress to a more unstable surface by placing one hand on a Dyna Disc and keeping her opposite hand on the ground.

Preparatory and Muscle Reactivation

Goals:

1. Reestablish the preparatory activation that provides joint stability through an increase in muscle stiffness.

2. Stimulate the reflexive contraction that results when a force acts upon the shoulder joint.

Rhythmic Stabilization against Perturbation

Instructions:

1. The patient lies supine with her elbow extended and the limb projecting upward in the scapular plane.

2. Instruct the patient to maintain this position while the clinician applies repeated joint perturbations in randomized directions (Figures 9-20 through 9-22).

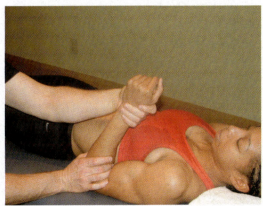

Figure 9-20 The patient attempts to resist the therapist's attempt to move her lower arm into flexion.

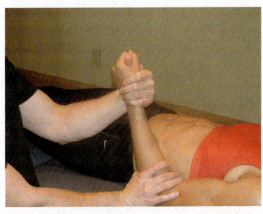

Figure 9-21 The patient attempts to resist the therapist's attempt to move her lower arm into extension.

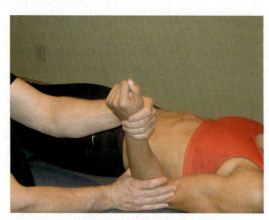

Figure 9-22 The patient attempts to resists the therapist's attempt to move her lower arm into external rotation.

Functional Motor Patterns

Goal: Strengthen and coordinate the serratus anterior as well as auto-mobilize the capsule. Be sure to allow passive retraction. Good patient instruction is important here. The auto-mobilization technique is vital to restoring ROM and capsular freedom.

Scapular stabilization exercises:

1. Rotator scapula RS for the glenohumeral joint GHJ (short lever) and scapula. This is to restore proprioception in the GHJ capsule. Perform short-lever GHJ RS supine with HMP placed anterior and posterior on the GHJ. When RS is finished, remove HMP, approximately 10 minutes.

2. Start with eyes open and supported. Progress with patient ability to eyes closed and unsupported.

3. Quadrupeds with plus to strengthen and coordinate the serratus anterior as well as auto-mobilize the capsule. Be sure to allow passive retraction. Good patient instruction is important here. This auto-mobilization tech-

nique is vital to restoring ROM and capsular freedom.

4. Seated scapular pinches, 10 seconds × 10, four times daily ("elbows in the back pockets"). Be sure to have elbows go down and back into the hip pockets to stimulate the lower trapezius.

5. Supine cervical retractions 10 seconds × 10, three times daily. Chin tuck and push head straight back into the floor. Once chin tuck is established, be sure *not* to extend the cervical spine. Perform chin tuck and straight retraction of the cervical spine.

Instructions:

1. Keep the elbow fully extended and retract the scapulas.

   a. Let your body sink down so that your shoulder blades come together.

2. Keep the torso, spine, and lower extremities rigid.

3. Protract the scapulae as if to push yourself off of the floor.

   a. Do not flex the thoracic spine.

Note: Your motion may be limited to start.

Active Isometric Strengthening Exercises Shoulder Internal Rotation, Standing

Instructions:

1. Keep the elbow tucked into the side as you attempt to internally rotate the humerus.

2. Isometrically contract the shoulder for 10 seconds for 10 sets.

Shoulder External Rotation

Instructions:

1. Keep the elbow tucked into the side as you attempt to externally rotate the humerus

2. Isometrically contract the shoulder for 10 seconds for 10 sets. Use multiple angles. The shoulder position and intensity may be adjusted to allow for a pain-free muscle contraction to occur. All isometrics should be performed with a scapular set (retracted/depressed scapula).

3. Perform all isometrics with a 10-second hold for 10×, four times daily for each motion.

Standing Three-Way Stretch

Instructions:

1. From a standing position, the first movement in each of the three movements is to retract the scapulae and squeeze them together. Then raise the arms with the thumbs up in forward flexion with the elbows fully extended (Figure 9-23).

2. In position 2 the scapulae are again retracted and then the arms are raised in the scapular plane with the thumbs up and the elbows fully extended (Figure 9-24).

3. In position 3 the scapulae are again squeezed together before raising the arms into abduction with the thumbs up and the elbows fully extended.

    Perform all isometrics with a 10-second hold for 10×, four times daily for each motion.

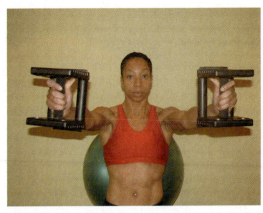

Figure 9-23 The patient, in a standing position with her back against a Swiss ball, retracts the scapulae and squeezes them together. The patient then raises her arms in a forward flexion position with the elbows fully extended.

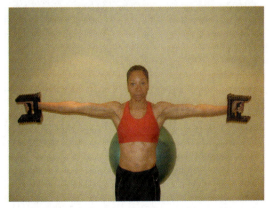

Figure 9-24 The patient continues to retract her scapulae and moves her arms in the scapular plane with the thumbs pointed up and the elbows fully extended.

Dynamic Blackburn

Instructions:

1. Place your hands on the buttocks with the fingers and thumbs slightly interlocked and retract the scapulae (squeeze the shoulder blades together; Figure 9-25).

2. Depress the scapulae by reaching for your feet with both hands. Keep the hands together (Figure 9-26).

3. While keeping the hands together, lift them off your buttocks (Figure 9-27).

4. Slowly release the hands, allowing them to separate. Begin to externally rotate the humeri so that the palms are now facing the floor (Figure 9-28).

5. Continue to abduct the humeri, but also continue to externally rotate the humeri (Figure 9-29). In this step you will reach 90° of abduction, and the thumbs should be pointing to the ceiling.

6. Continue to abduct and externally rotate the humeri. The thumbs should still be pointing upward, and the humeri is at 100° of abduction (Figure 9-30). This is the end ROM for this exercise.

Perform all isometrics with a 10-second hold for 10×, four times daily for each motion.

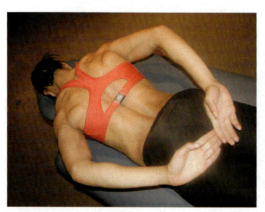

Figure 9-25 The patient places her hands on her gluteus with the fingers and thumbs interlocked while retracting her scapula.

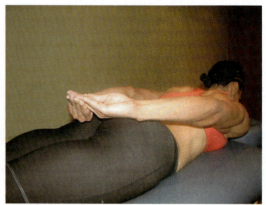

Figure 9-27 The patient lifts her hands off the gluteus.

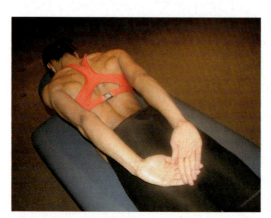

Figure 9-26 The patient depresses her scapula.

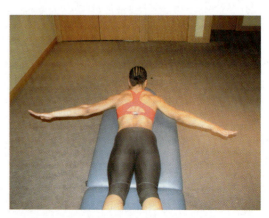

Figure 9-28 The patient slowly releases her hands, allowing them to separate, and begins to externally rotate the humerus.

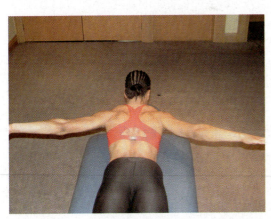

Figure 9-29 The patient continues to externally rotate and abduct her humeri. At this point, the thumbs should be pointed upward.

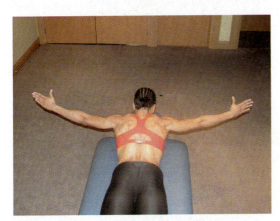

Figure 9-30 The patient continues to externally rotate and abduct the humeri while pointing the thumbs upward. The end ROM for this exercise occurs when the humeri is at 100° abduction.

Seated Scapular Pinches

Instructions:

1. Keep your elbows down and back into your "hip pockets" to stimulate the lower trapezius.

2. Isometrically retract your scapulae for 10 seconds for 10 sets.

Supine Cervical Retractions

Instructions:

1. Tuck your chin and push your head back against the floor. Once the chin is tucked, be sure not to extend the cervical spine.

2. Perform chin tuck and straight retraction of the cervical spine.

Add forearm-strengthening exercises (elbow and wrist):

1. Hammer curls

2. Eccentric elbow flexion

3. Pronation/supination

4. Radial/ulnar deviation

5. Hand-gripping exercises

6. Wrist roller

PHASE III— INTERMEDIATE PHASE

Time Period: Days 15–25

Goals:

1. Increase the volume of the shoulder strengthening program.

2. Continue to improve flexibility.

3. Facilitate neuromuscular control.

Instructions:

Continue with rotator cuff/capsule stretches, range-of-motion exercises, scapular stabilization, and accessory exercises with tubing and/or dumbbells. During this phase, the rehabilitation program is progressed to more aggressive isotonic strengthening exercises with emphasis on the restoration of muscle imbalance.

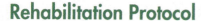

Rehabilitation Protocol

During this phase of the rehabilitation program the athlete will continue with rotator cuff/capsule stretches, range-of-motion exercises, scapular stabilization, and accessory exercises with tubing and/or dumbbells. However, there will be a stronger emphasis on training the local and global muscle groups to enhance the stability of the kinetic chain and restoring any existing muscle imbalances using aggressive isotonic strengthening exercises.

- ○ Add RTC proprioceptive exercises.
- ○ Add triceps stretch/inferior capsule stretch.
- ○ Add the following scapular stabilization exercises:
  - ○ Side-lying abduction to increase external rotation strength.
  - ○ Modified empty.
  - ○ Prone rowing into external rotation.
  - ○ Add pectoralis minor and anterior capsule stretch on doorway.
  - ○ Add total body conditioning with a focus on muscular strength and endurance.

The scapula provides proximal stability to the shoulder joint, enabling distal segment mobility. To optimize the restoration of the biomechanics of the scapula to normal, several authors have emphasized the importance of scapular strength and neuromuscular control. Isotonic exercise techniques are used to strengthen the scapular muscles. A neuromuscular control drill designed by Wilk and Arrigo (1992) to enhance the proprioceptive and kinesthetic awareness of the scapula should be initiated at this phase.

PNF Exercises

For shoulder abduction and external rotation, position the shoulder in the scapular plane (approximately 20–30° forward of the coronal plane).

D2 Flexion-Extension Pattern

These exercises are typically used in the rehabilitation of overhead-throwing athletes due to the similarity between the exercise plane of motion and the throwing and serving movement pattern.

Scapular Stabilization Exercises

The following scapular exercises are to be added to the existing ones.

Field Goal

Instructions:

1. Place a Swiss ball under the chest (Figure 9-31).
2. Keep arms relaxed and hanging downward (Figure 9-32).
3. Start by actively retracting the scapulae (pinch the shoulder blades together).
4. While maintaining scapular retraction, extend the shoulders to 90°. The elbows should be flexed to 90° as shown in Figure 9-33.
5. Maintain 90° of shoulder extension and scapular retraction (Figure 9-33).
6. Start externally rotate the shoulder with the thumbs pointed upward (Figure 9-33).
7. Slowly reverse the motion and return to the original starting position.

Subscapularis Pull (tube)

Instructions:

1. Start with the elbow fully extended and the thumb pointed upward (Figure 9-34).

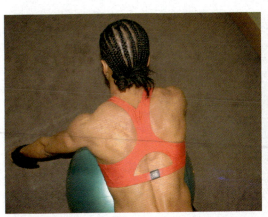

Figure 9-31 The patient places a Swiss ball under her chest and keeps the arms relaxed in a hanging down position. Next, the patient will retract her scapula.

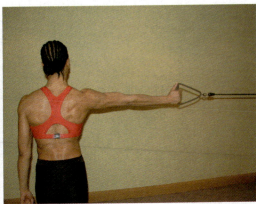

Figure 9-34 The patient starts with her elbow fully extended and thumb pointing upward.

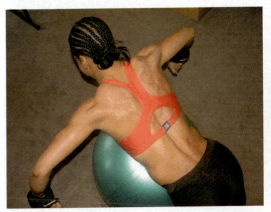

Figure 9-32 While maintaining scapular retraction, the patient will extend her shoulders to 90° while keeping the elbows flexed.

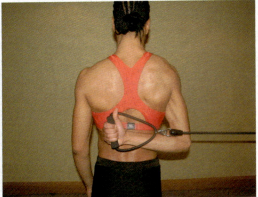

Figure 9-35 The patient pulls the tube behind the back, causing internal rotation of the upper arm, and attempts to touch the thumb to the inferior angle of the opposite scapula.

2. Pull the tube behind the back; this will create internal rotation of the upper arm (Figure 9-35).

3. Attempt to touch the thumb to the inferior angle of the opposite scapula. Range of motion is more important than resistance, so use a thin or light-resistance tubing.

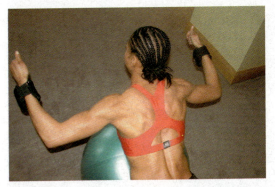

Figure 9-33 The patient continues to keep her shoulders in 90° extension while externally rotating the shoulders with her thumbs pointed upward.

Shoulder Plyometric Exercises

Plyometrics play a vital role in rehabilitation of the shoulder. Plyometrics incorporate stretch–shortening contractions. The benefits of plyometric training can be summarized as follows:

1. Recreate the type of eccentric—concentric contraction experienced during athletic activity; followed by the reactive (reflexive) contraction from increased stimulation of the muscle spindle
2. Neural adaptation by increasing muscle spindle sensitivity
3. Increased muscle stiffness

The following exercises involve pitching, chest passing, and trunk rotation (Figures 9-36 and 9-37).

PHASE IV—ADVANCED STRENGTHENING PHASE AND RETURN TO PRIOR ACTIVITY LEVEL

Goals:

1. Initiate aggressive strengthening drills.
2. Enhance power and endurance.
3. Perform functional drills.
4. Gradually initiate throwing activities.

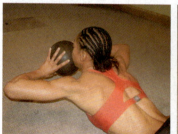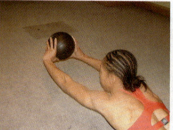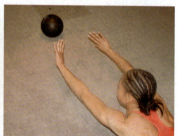

Figure 9-36 The patient performs overhead medicine ball throws while lying on the ground.

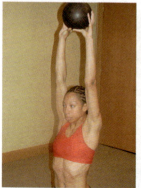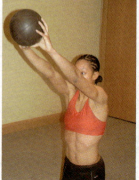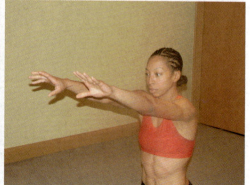

Figure 9-37 The patient performs overhead medicine ball throws while standing.

Rehabilitation protocols have traditionally focused on isolated absolute strength gains, isolated muscles, and single planes of motion. However, all functional activities are multi-planar (MP) and require acceleration, deceleration, and dynamic stabilization (Caraffa, Cerulli, Projetti, Aisa, Rizzo, 1996; Swanik, Straub, 2004; (Hewett, Lindenfeld, Riccobene, Noyes, 1999). Movement may appear to be one-plane dominant but the other planes require dynamic stabilization in order for optimal neuromuscular efficiency to take place (Ford, Myer, Hewett, 2003). Hence training must focus on training the entire kinetic chain at this stage of the rehabilitation protocol by utilizing all planes of movement while establishing high levels of functional strength and neuromuscular efficiency (Junge, Rösch, Peterson, Graf-Baumann, & Dvorak, 2002). In this advanced stage of the rehabilitation program, the athlete will continue using the manual resistance stabilization and plyometric drills used in the previous protocol.

Rehabilitation Protocol

Add Core Stabilization Exercise Drills:

○ Supine position
○ Single leg lifts
○ Single leg slide
○ Double leg lifts
○ Double leg slide

Prone Position:

○ Gluteal squeeze
○ Cobra

Add Core Strength Exercise Drills:
Medicine Ball Progression:

○ Crunch
○ Curls
○ Hip extension
○ Pullovers

○ Reverse crunch
○ Knee-ups
○ Russian twists

Cable Progression:

○ Wood chop
○ Lifts

Dumbbell Progression:

○ MP lunge/curl/press
○ Squat press
○ MP step-press

Add dynamic stabilization exercise drills:

○ Throwing a 2-pound plyoball
○ Push-up into a plyoball

Using a Medicine Ball the following drills can be performed:

○ Soccer throws
○ Chest pass
○ Oblique throws
○ Overhead throws

Add plyometric drills:

○ Standing one-handed throws in a functional throwing position
○ Wall dribbling
○ Plyometric step-and-throws

Add specific endurance exercise drills:

○ Wall arm circles
○ Upper-body cycle
○ Isotonic exercises using lower weights with higher repetition

Add an interval throwing program.

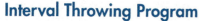

Interval Throwing Program

Before initiating such a program, it is suggested that the athlete perform "shadow" throwing, or mirror throwing, which is the action of mimicking the throwing mechanics into a mirror, but not actively throwing. The purpose of this is for the athlete to focus on the proper throwing biomechanics before throwing a baseball.

The interval throwing program can be started once the following criteria have been satisfied:

1. Satisfactory clinical exam
2. Nonpainful ROM
3. Satisfactory isokinetic test results
4. Appropriate rehabilitation progress

The purpose of the interval-throwing program is to gradually increase the quantity, distance, intensity, and type of throws needed to facilitate the gradual restoration of normal biomechanics.

Preparation for Returning to the Prior Activity Level (work, recreational, or sport)

The final facet of functional rehabilitation is to include activities that mimic athletic function. By mimicking the type of activities and forces experienced by the athlete, the return-to-play transition may be less stressful on the athlete. It is important to incorporate specificity when implementing functional activities. Therefore, the athlete should be trained in sport-specific positions of function. The position of function for a baseball player or tennis player is a position of vulnerability in abduction and external rotation. In contrast, the position of vulnerability for a football offensive lineman is just below shoulder level, anterior to the thorax. Functional rehabilitation should reflect such positions. Add total body conditioning with emphasis on strength and endurance.

After the throwing athlete returns to full strength and endurance, throwing may be resumed. Velocity is not an important part of the early stage of return to throwing. Stress should be placed on the proper biomechanics of throwing in the early stages of the exercise program. The velocity of the ball can be gradually increased once the throwing mechanics and fluidity of motion are satisfied. A long-toss/short-toss program can be implemented at this stage (Table 9-7).

ACL REHABILITATION PROGRAM FOLLOWING ACL RECONSTRUCTION

A variety of opinions and choices are available for a clinician to consider when designing a rehabilitation

Table 9-7 Return-to-Throwing Phase of the Rehabilitation Program

Phases	Long Toss	Intensity	Short Toss	Intensity	Stretch
1	90 ft, 10–20 throws	50%	30 ft, 15–20 throws	50%	10 min[1]
2	90–120 ft, 10–12 throws	50%	60 ft, 15–20 throws	50%	10 min[1]
2	90–120 ft, 10–12 throws	50%	60 ft, 25–30 throws	50%	10 min[1] (continued)

Table 9-7 Return to Throwing Phase of the Rehabilitation Program (continued)

2	90–120 ft, 10–12 throws	50%	60 ft, 30–40 throws	50%	10 min[1]
3	120–150 ft, 10–12 throws	50%	60 ft, 15–20 throws	75%	10 min[1]
3	120–150 ft, 10–12 throws	50%	60 ft, 25–30 throws	75%	10 min[1]
3	120–150 ft, 10–12 throws	50%	60 ft, 35–40 throws	75%	10 min[1]
4[2]			60 ft, 10–20 throws	75%	10 min
5[3]			60 ft, 10–20 throws Rest: 10 throws, Rest: 5 throws	75%	
5[3]			60 ft, 15 throws, Rest: 15 throws, Rest: 10 throws	75%	
5[3]			60 ft, 15 throws Rest: 15 throws	75%	
6[3]			60 ft, 20–30 throws	75% to full	
6[3]			60 ft, 30–40 throws	75% to full	
6[3]			60 ft	75% to full	

[1] Applies to long toss
[2] Begin on mound
[3] Begin on mound, including breaking balls
Notes: Simulate game situation with work and rest intervals.
- Approximately 15 throws per inning; 10-minute rest.
- Progress innings as tolerated, checking endurance and throwing speed.
- The athlete should begin the program with approximately 10 to 15 minutes light warm-up.
- Throws at a distance of about 30 ft. It may be helpful to mimic the throwing motion before throwing the ball.
- The long-toss exercises are very gentle, high lobs thrown at a distance of 90 to 150 feet. The throw should be done in a rainbow fashion with minimal cocking effort. It is important to follow through smoothly.
- The short-toss exercises, the most important phase of the program, progress from a distance of 30 to 60 feet.
- Level throwing should be attempted before throwing from the mound (Jaffee & Moorman, 2001).
Source: M. B. Jaffe and C. T. Moorman. (2001). Shoulder conditioning for the throwing athlete: The off-season program. *Sports Medicine and Arthroscopy Review, 9,* 19–23.

program of the knee after plastic surgery of the anterior cruciate ligament (ACL). When the patient is an athlete, one of the most frequent questions concerns the time of abstention after the operation. The answer depends on factors such as the nature of the injury, grade of the lesion, specific demands of the sport, level of the athlete, and when in the year's practicing cycle the injury occurred.

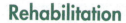

Rehabilitation

It is generally acknowledged that rehabilitation is critical to successful ACL treatment. Although many specific aspects of rehabilitation protocols remain highly controversial, current evidence (DeMaio, Noyes, & Mangine, 1992; Irrgang, 1993) supports the concept that intensive rehabilitation can help to prevent early arthrofibrosis and to restore strength and function earlier (Paulos & Stern, 1993; Shelbourne & Nitz, 1990; Shelbourne & Wilckens, 1990; Shelbourne, Wilckens, Mollabashy, & DeCarlo, 1991). The importance of early restoration of full extension in patients who have a bone–patellar ligament–bone graft has been emphasized (Rubenstein et al., 1995). Electrical muscle stimulation has been reported to be a useful adjunct in some patients (Snyder-Mackler, Delitto, Bailey, & Stralka, 1995). The most intensive programs have been recommended particularly for patients who are predisposed to stiffness (as noted earlier), such as those who had a semiacute procedure, those who had an ACL injury combined with injuring at least one other ligament (Noyes, Mangine, & Barber, 1992), and those in whom patellofemoral entrapment is developing or has already developed (Forman & Jackson, 1993; Fu, Irrgang, & Harner, 1993; Paulos & Meislin, 1993).

The limits of stress, strain, frequency, and duration beyond which an intensive rehabilitation protocol can induce damage to a healing joint by putting too much mechanical stress on its structures remain controversial. It has been found that healing graft complexes are probably weak and compliant for many months and that grafts remodel over many years (Rougraff, Shelbourne, Gerth, & Warner, 1993). Certain exercise protocols have been particularly worrisome for surgeons and therapists due to the abundant information suggesting that resisted quadriceps exercises put some strain on the ACL (Beynnon et al., 1995), particularly in the last few degrees of extension of the knee if the limb is not bearing weight. These extension exercises, with or without the use of ankle weights, have been called open-chain exercises. To protect the anterior cruciate graft during quadriceps exercises, it has been suggested that the patient should instead stand, thus loading the knee joint axially during motion. This position may protect the graft by using the contours of the joint to stabilize the knee. These exercises have been called closed-chain exercises. A clinical test of a closed-chain exercise (two-legged squat), however, was not found to strain the ACL any differently than did an open-chain limb-extension exercise (Beynnon, Johnson, & Fleming, 1993). It is not known whether strains induced by rehabilitation exercises always have negative effects on grafts by causing them to stretch, or whether some strain is actually necessary to stimulate remodeling of the graft.

Reconditioning

Reconditioning is the process of reestablishing and improving an athlete's overall physical qualities following injury or surgery. It addresses the athlete's need to continue fitness and strength training for the first four months postop. Reconditioning and performance training are basically the same, with the understanding that the training protocol will need to be adjusted according to the athlete's tolerance and healing response.

Strength and Conditioning around the Knee

After knee surgery, managing an athlete's physical qualities is more than just following an ACL protocol. It is developing a plan to train the entire body from postop to return-to-comp—from strength development to cardiovascular conditioning to movement quality training. It is an individualized plan that focuses less on the knee and more on the athlete's overall physiological profile. Of course, the surgery creates limitations that require special strategies to make appropriate strength gains. Still, an excellent strategy is available. Successfully managing an athlete encourages using familiar movements to motivate them. To do this requires exercising *around the knee*, rather than focusing on traditional rehabilitation techniques that target isolated muscles of the lower extremity.

For example, an upper-body cycle ergometer is often implemented during rehabilitation to condition an athlete's cardiovascular system, but this is not *exercising around the knee*. It is exercising *without* the knee. Using functional and sport-specific movement patterns offers a level of familiarity and predictability. For the athlete, this translates into a higher-quality effort and helps to restore confidence. For example, deep-water training within two to three weeks postop can effectively address core strength endurance and cardiovascular conditioning. Many of the movements may be new, but they encourage athletic coordination in a nonloading environment. This program's hidden agenda is hundreds of repetitions to improve knee joint ROM and reduce postop edema. By four weeks postop, the patient may be working as hard in the water as an uninjured athlete. Using winged water walkers (W3s) for forward- and backward-resisted pool running is excellent for hip strength and anaerobic conditioning. The goal is for the athlete's cardiovascular system to be well conditioned by three or four months postop, so he or she will require less of this training in later stages of the "comeback." Now the athlete can focus more time on sport specificity, weight training, and various movement-specific qualities. Spinning bike, elliptical cross-trainers, and treadmill programs are also developed for every phase of the comeback. The emphasis here is cardiovascular and strength endurance training. Due to lower joint stress, this training can be done very well during the first few months.

Total body training that encourages upper and core strength should be implemented as well during the reconditioning phase. Much of this work should be performed in the standing position to emphasize the athletes' inherent athletic ability, allowing stabilization and control during athletic conditioning.

Working *around the knee* with progressive cardiovascular programs or other total body training does not have to compromise the integrity of the surgery. This practice should be consistently encouraged.

Pool Training

The pool is used consistently following injury or surgery for athletes. It provides a safe environment to completely or partially reduce the compression forces on the knee joint.

The hydrostatic pressure naturally compresses the muscles and joints. When this pressure is paired with active ROM at the knee and active neuromuscular coordination through exercise, the result is reduced inter-articular swelling and increased strength endurance of the upper and lower extremity.

Flotation equipment is used to improve the quality of the exercises, but it should not limit or interfere with the movements. In deep water (with flotation), there is no limit to the ROM that can be achieved; it comes from active movements versus passive. Subtle ground contact forces can be introduced in chest- and waist-deep water.

This is an effective way to progressively load the joint and build the athlete's confidence. An athlete's weight is decreased by 75% at shoulder level and 50% at waist level. Restoring speed of movement also builds the athlete's confidence, and water provides a smooth and consistent resistance to achieve this goal. While it is true that increased speed of movement in water causes increased resistance, the movement quality and speed achievable provide an excellent transition from the middle stages of reconditioning to performance training on the ground.

Program Outline

○ Early Rehab: used specifically to improve range of motion (ROM) after 2+ weeks postop (wounds must be closed)

○ Focus: movement quality, slow–medium speed, improve ROM, decrease edema

○ 2–3× per week: 30 min

○ Flotation assistance: barbells and waist belt

○ Water exercises: 1, 2, 3 plus arm emphasis lap swimming

- ○ Early reconditioning: 4–8 weeks postop

- ○ Focus: movement quality, medium to fast speed, core strength endurance, cardiovascular conditioning

- ○ 2× per week: 45+ min

- ○ Flotation assistance: barbells and ankle floatation for increased resistance.

- ○ Water exercises: 1, 2, 4

- ○ Middle to late reconditioning: 9–16 weeks postop

- ○ Focus: Winged water walkers—leg-strength endurance, anaerobic and aerobic conditioning

- ○ 2× week: 45+ min

- ○ Flotation assistance: waist belt initially, then remove to advance the athlete

- ○ Water exercises: 1, 2

Focus: Range of motion training/hip mobility, core strength endurance, aerobic conditioning

Equipment: A pool (4 feet deep minimum), floatation belt, floatation barbells

Frequency: Perform 2–3 times per week for 3 weeks.

Workouts

Swim laps, perform the exercises in Tables 9-8 and 9-9 in order (30 sec ON, 30 sec OFF) and then repeat. The movement is meant to be smooth first, then fast (almost explosive).

CARDIOVASCULAR AND STRENGTH ENDURANCE TRAINING SERIES

By using the elliptical cross-trainer, treadmill, and bike and rowing ergometers, athletes can maintain or increase their cardiovascular qualities in the

Table 9-8 Lap Swim Workout		
Lap Swimming	Swim 2–3 laps (then move on to the next exercise).	
1. Lateral Leg Press		Reach legs to side, cross under body to other side. Reach with heels—straight leg.
2. Forward/Backward Leg Press	30 sec ON 30 sec OFF	Lie on back, pull knees to chest and under body, until lying on stomach. Switch again until lying on back.
3. Surface Running (30 sec each direction) You may want to take cuffs off the ankles.		Side lying on the surface—run with circles to the right and then left.
Repeat the above program 3–4 times. (Increase the time to 45 sec to provide more conditioning.)		
Lap Swimming	Swim 3+ laps to finish the workout.	(continued)

Table 9-8 Lap Swim Workout (continued)

Lap Swimming	Swim 2–3 laps (then move on to the next exercise).	
1. Lateral Leg Press		Reach legs to side, cross under body to other side. Reach with heels—straight leg.
2. Forward/Backward Leg Press	30 sec ON 30 sec OFF	Lie on back, pull knees to chest and under body, until lying on stomach. Switch again until lying on back.
4. Lateral X/C—left side		Cross-country skiing movement with the legs angled 45° to the side.
4. Lateral X/C—right side		
Repeat the above program 3–4 times. (Increase the time to 45 sec to provide more conditioning.)		
Lap Swimming	Swim 3+ laps to finish the workout.	

Table 9-9 Workout Using Winged Water Walkers

Focus: Hip strength endurance; high-intensity anaerobic
Equipment: A pool, winged water walkers (W3s), waist belt (no belt = max challenge)

Warm-up: Lap Swimming	Swim 2–3 laps.	
Alternate between forward and backward movements. Backward running works the legs more!	Workout 1: 3-min rest between sets	Cardiovascular (CV)—Anaerobic: 1. Run: 4 × 25 yards: Leave every 2 min for a 25-yd rep. REST 3 min. Repeat set 2–3 more times. Finish with fast running: No W3s on feet. (4 × 5 sec—for the feeling of speed)
	Workout 2: Use a belt.	CV—aerobic 1. Jog 4–5 min (switch positions anytime). Rest 2 min. Repeat 5–7× (or 30+ minutes).

period from four weeks to four months postop. If the intent is to increase strength endurance above what the exercise does initially, then specific exercises can be added to the program.

The relationship between the resistance selected on the equipment and the associated joint loading needs to be considered. Early in the reconditioning phase, all of the cardio training equipment is usually effective if the resistance is low enough. The key is to progressively increase the resistance and challenge both heart rate and leg strength endurance without causing undue stress to the joint. These programs should be implemented one to three times per week to best prepare and improve an athlete's level of fitness prior to sport-specific training.

The following are some variables to control and coordinate based on the desired outcome and the phase postop:

- Speed: affects rpm, strides per minute, mph
- Resistance: affects load on the joint, heart rate, and leg fatigue
- Duration: gradual, but consistent changes produce the best results
- Heart rate: affects whether an aerobic or anaerobic outcome is desired

The following sections provide examples of cardio training with leg strength endurance emphasis. These programs can be introduced by four weeks postop.

Elliptical Cross-Trainer: Hill Running

Goal: Moderate joint loading
Focus: Provide a workout that introduces increased resistance for short-duration bouts and has planned recovery intervals to keep joint loading in balance.

Definitions

Flat Running: low resistance, medium strides per min, upright stance.

Hill Running: moderate+ resistance, medium–fast strides per min, forward lean, hold center console or center handles.

Forward lean position: Place feet into the back of the foot plates and stay on the toes. Lean slightly forward as if running up a hill.

Workout

- Warm-up: 8–12 min on a bike, low resistance, fast cadence
- Elliptical workout

Set 1: (total = 7 minutes)

- 3 min flat running
- Then: 30 sec hill running, followed by 30 sec flat running. Repeat this 3 more times.
- Rest: 2 minutes (walking or spinning on a bike)

Repeat this program 2–4 sets (total = 18–36 min) based on fitness and strength levels.

Treadmill Retrograde Hill Walk

Goal: Moderate joint loading

Focus: Provides an early strength endurance and cardio training opportunity with less impact than speed walking and running. Forward hill walking is excellent for strengthening the posterior chain: gastrocnemius/soleus, hamstrings, gluts, and lower back. Backward (retrograde) walking strengthens the anterior tibialis, quads, and low back.

Definitions

Treadmill hill: inclined 15–20×.

Forward hill walk: Med+ speed to get heart rate (HR) elevated, long strides, lean slightly forward for more hamstring emphasis.

	Protocol	Comments
Total = 24–32 min	1 SET = 3 min flat running, then (repeat 3×): 30 sec hill running. 30 sec flat running. Rest 2 min after set: walk and shake legs. Perform 3–4 sets total.	Be sure to change the resistance on the machine from flat running to hill running. Be sure to move feet to the back of foot plates when running the hills. The resistance must increase when you run the hills. Often your speed increases as well to keep the momentum going.

	Protocol
Total = 27–36 min	1 SET = 3 min flat running, then (repeat 3×): 45 sec hill running 45 sec flat running Rest 2 min after set: walk and shake legs. Perform 3–4 sets total.
Total = up to 40 min+	1 SET = 3 min flat running, then (repeat 3×): 60 sec hill running 60 sec flat running Rest 2 min after set: walk and shake legs. Perform 3–4 sets total.

Backward hill walk: Slow speed, short strides, slightly flexed position at the ankle/knee/hip to increase quad emphasis. Maintain a slight forward lean.

Transition: Fwd walking–slow the speed down–quick turn to backward position, then after set time–quick turn to forward position–increase speed for set time. Repeat.

Workout

- ○ Warm-up: 8–12 min on a bike, low resistance, fast cadence.
- ○ Treadmill:

Set 1: (total = 7 minutes)

- ○ 3 min flat running.
- ○ Then 30 sec hill running, followed by 30 sec flat running. Repeat 3 more times.
- ○ Rest: 2 minutes (walking or spinning on a bike).

Repeat this program 2–4 sets (total = 18–36 min) based on fitness and strength levels.

Treadmill Parameters (walking):

Speed:

- ○ Slow = 1.5–2.5 mph
- ○ Med = 2.6–5.5 mph

Incline:

- ○ High = 12 to 20 degrees

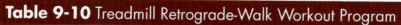

Table 9-10 Treadmill Retrograde-Walk Workout Program

Protocol	Comments
8–12 min on a bike: low resistance, then go on to workout.	Forward: use arm swing to help rhythm. Backward: place hands on hips, lower hips slightly.
Treadmill Hill Workout: 60 sec forward at med+ speed/high incline. 30 sec backward at slow speed/high incline. Repeat: 3× more (takes 5:30 min). Rest: 2 min (step off the treadmill, or walk slow with a low incline). Then repeat: 3–4× (follow the same routine as above).	Be careful when turning around; hold the handlebars for stability. Rest: spin on a bike easy, hydrate.
Total = up to 38 min	

Protocol

8–12 min on a bike: low resistance, then go on to workout.

Treadmill Hill Workout:
2 min forward at medium–fast speed with high incline.
45 sec backward at slow speed with high incline.
Repeat: 3× more (takes 11 min).

Rest: 2 min (step off the treadmill, or walk slow with a low incline).

Repeat: 2–3×.

Total = 40+ min

Bike Conditioning Programs

Goal: Low to moderate joint loading

Focus: Provides progressive conditioning for an athlete beyond typical cycle routines that are used for warm-up purposes only. Throughout the reconditioning process, bike programs are effective for increasing strength endurance and cardiovascular training. The key is to continuously increase the difficulty in order to get progressive results.

Definitions

Cadence (rpm): slow = 40–60 rpm, moderate = 61–80 rpm, fast = 81+ rpm

Resistance: low = for warm-up only; medium = will cause fatigue; high = hard work

Flat: medium resistance and moderate-to-fast cadence

Hill: medium-to-high resistance, but you must be able to work at moderate-to-fast cadence. This means push harder on the pedals.

Workouts

Two workout programs for bike conditioning are provided in Table 9-11.

Table 9-11 Two Bike Conditioning Workouts

Workout 1	Protocol	Comments
Total = 24–32 min	1 SET = 3 min flat riding, then (repeat 3×): 30 sec hill riding 30 sec flat riding 2 min: slow cadence and low resistance, then repeat the set. (Perform 3–4 sets total.)	Be sure to change the resistance on the bike from flat riding to hill riding. One goal is to have a fast cadence for all 30-sec bouts on both the flat and the hill.
Workout 2	**Protocol**	**Comments**
Total = 29–38 min	1 SET = 3 min flat riding, then (repeat 3×): 45 sec hill riding 45 sec flat riding 2 min: slow cadence and low resistance, then repeat the set. (Perform 3–4 sets total.)	Be sure to change the resistance on the bike from flat riding to hill riding. One goal is to have a fast cadence for all 45-sec bouts on both the flat and the hill.

ACL REHABILITATIVE CASE STUDY— JANUARY 2007

The patient (athlete) is a thirteen-year-old male basketball player who ruptured his left anterior cruciate ligament (ACL) while playing basketball in November 2006. He had no history of knee, foot, or ankle problems prior to the injury. The patient was placed in a standard protective brace with 10–15° of maximum flexion and given crutches to use for the next two weeks. He was then allowed to walk without the crutches but remained in the protective brace.

No standard postsurgical physical therapy—including ultrasound, electrical stimulation, and manual manipulation—was recommended for the patient. His only therapy to that point was icing every day. The patient was seen three to four weeks post surgery and given permission to begin a rehabilitative-strengthening program. Evaluation of the athlete at four and a half weeks post surgery found the left knee still visibly swollen. He had approximately 80–90° of passive knee flexion, a significant difference in rotation at the knee from right to left, zero translation in the repaired knee, and a difference of about 10° of lesser dorsi flexion from left to right ankle.

The vastus medialis was flaccid and underdeveloped on both lower limbs. Manual muscle testing showed a bilateral weakness in both gluteus medius muscles, vastus medialus muscles, rectus femoris, and adductor longus muscles. The patient then began the first phase of his rehabilitative program, which required him to undergo four supervised sessions per week and 20 minutes of solo work per night.

Phase I Protocol

The patient's phase I protocol consisted of six segments:

1. General conditioning warm-up including a 12- to 15-minute bike warm-up in which the patient began pedaling with the bicycle seat providing about 70° of knee flexion; the seat was progressively lowered until until he was getting about 85–90° of knee flexion. He then performed a series of osteoarticular closed- and open-chain warm-up drills for the ankles, knees, and hips.

2. The patient then had the left knee pumped (Voyer pompage technique) using a series of 8–10 pumping techniques that pumped the anterior, posterior, lateral, and medial quadrants of the left knee. The emphasis was to pump the knee in flexion and internal rotation, flexion and external rotation, extension and external rotation, and extension and internal rotation. The knee was also pumped in translation (medial and lateral), rotation, and decoaptation (Figures 9-38 and 9-39).

3. Allowing the patient to target the quadriceps from the point of origin, he then performed passive prone stretches (Figure 9-40); the patient then performed a series of solo kneeling stretches targeting the quadriceps segmentally while performing retroversion of the pelvis (Figures 9-40 through 9-42).

4. Segmental reinforcement exercises were then performed to precisely isolate the gluteus maximus and medius muscles. The patient then was given an isometric wall squat, with strong retroversion in four positions, to activate and reinforce each of the quadriceps muscles. Each position was held for 20-30 seconds under tension (Figures 9-43 and 9-44).

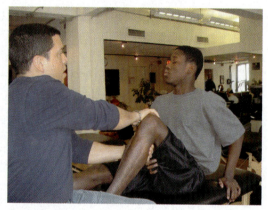

Figure 9-38 Patient's left knee is pumped in flexion and internal rotation.

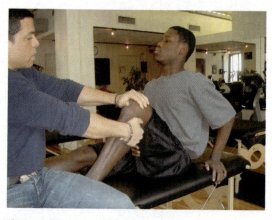

Figure 9-39 Patient's left knee is pumped in extension and external rotation.

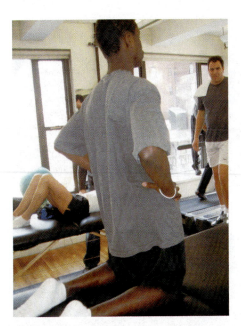

Figure 9-40 Patient statically stretches the left quadriceps from the point of origin of the vastus intermedius by keeping both his knees and feet apart.

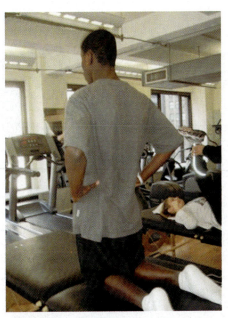

Figure 9-42 The patient statically stretches the left quadriceps from the point of origin of the vastus medialis by keeping his knees pressed together and feet apart.

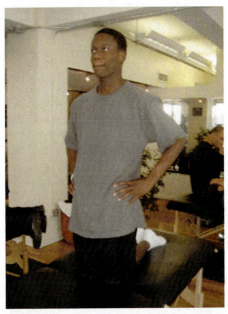

Figure 9-41 Patient statically stretches the left quadriceps from the point of origin of the lateral fibers of the vastus intermedius by keeping his knees apart and feet pressed together.

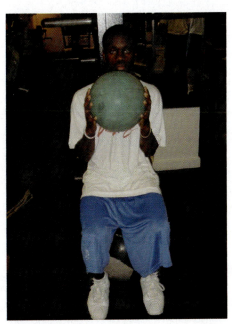

Figure 9-43 Patient isometrically contracts the vastus intermedius by keeping both his knees and feet apart.

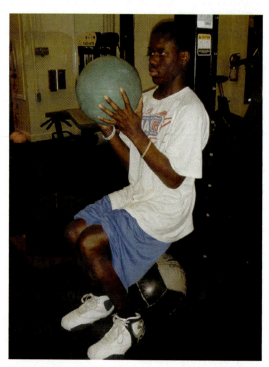

Figure 9-44 Patient isometrically contracts the vastus medialis by keeping his knees pressed together and feet apart.

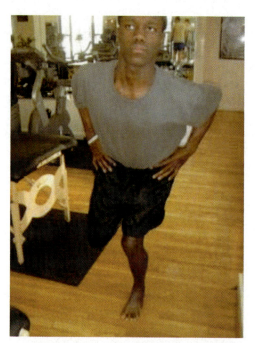

Figure 9-45 Patient trains the general proprioception for the whole knee joint.

5. Specific proprioception was then given to improve the intelligence of the joint and increase the neuromuscular activation of the general knee (Figures 9-45 and 9-46). Care was taken to make sure that the lower limb muscles had been activated and the laws of proprioceptive progression were followed.

6. Specific ELDOA (Etierement Longitudinaux avec Decoaptation OsteoArticulaire). Postures were assigned to free the lumbar sacral joint and increase myofascial mobility (Figure 9-47).

The patient was given a 20-minute series of stretches for the quadriceps, iliopsoas, biceps femoris, and gastrocnemius muscles and a general proprioceptive drill for the knee to perform every day at home. He was also instructed to drink two

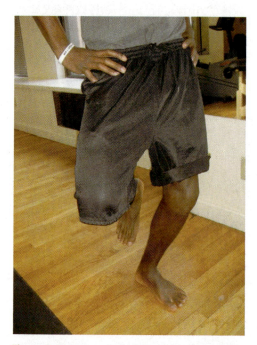

Figure 9-46 Patient specifically trains the infrapatellar proprioception.

Patient	Practitioner
• Decubitus. • Arms in the same frontal plane as the trunk. • Hands are kept shoulder width apart. • Legs must rest on a vertical support, a wall, the practitioner, a partner,... to relax the abdominal muscles.	• Control the breathing of the patient; ensuring adequate depth, rate, etc of respiration. • Practitioner rigourously monitors all the postures at all times.

Action
• Extend the arms (elbows). • External rotation of the upper limb. • Total extension of the elbow and wrist. • Push arms away from the body very strongly. • Ankle in dorsiflexion with two components of inversion (adduction and supination). • Knees in extension, heels not touching the wall. • Push legs away from the body very strongly. • Flatten the lumbar spine. • Axial extension from the coccyx to the vertex. • Put everything (heels, coccyx, lumbosacral joint, vertex and the heel of the hand) into tension at the same time.

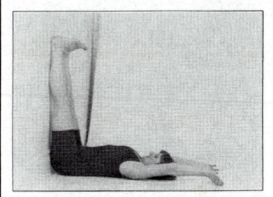

Figure 9-47 ELDOA postures.

liters of water minimum per day. After four supervised sessions, the patient was instructed not to use the brace any longer. When the passive prone flexion was tested at 100°, the left knee maintained smooth translation and rotation as compared with the unrepaired right knee.

At the two-week mark, hypertrophy of the left quadriceps muscles was visible. The patient was able to free-squat with 95° of flexion and no translation at the hips or pelvis. This phase was continued for approximately 3-1/2 weeks. Phase II of the performance rehabilitation was started, and the patient was supervised during three weekly sessions and given homework to do daily.

Phase II Protocol

The phase II protocol also included six segments:

1. General conditioning warm-up and osteo-articular warm-up drills. The only new drills to be added were tibialis heel walks, during which the patient walks forward or backward while on his heels and maintaining maximum dorsi flexion.

2. The patient then performed four positions of seated knee flexion to target the different muscles of the quadriceps at his maximum flexion. Each position was held for 15 seconds (Figures 9-48 through 9-50).

3. The reinforcement was now advanced, including a split-squat level I exercise. The patient performed 20–30 repetitions at a slow tempo of a level I split squat (Figure 9-51). Static four-position isometric squats were now increased from 40 to 60 seconds each. Single-leg calf raises were

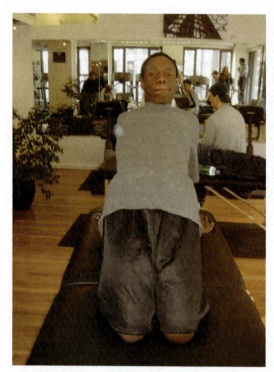

Figure 9-48 Patient isolates and stretches the vastus intermedius by keeping his knees and feet apart while in a kneeling (knee) flexion.

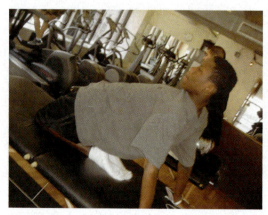

Figure 9-49 Patient isolates and stretches the vastus lateralis by keeping his knees apart and feet together while in a kneeling (knee) flexion.

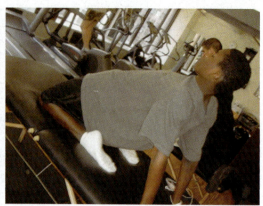

Figure 9-50 Patient isolates and stretches the vastus medialis by keeping his knees pressed together and feet apart while in a kneeling (knee) flexion.

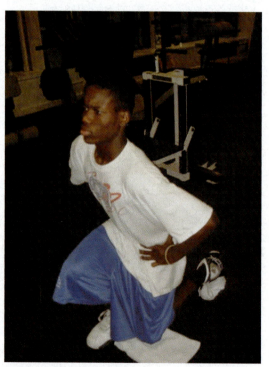

Figure 9-51 Patient dynamically recruits the vastus intermedius using a split-squat exercise.

added to work below the joint and begin reinforcing the gastrocnemius muscles. Manual prone leg curls were added to begin reinforcing the ischial tuberosity complex. The curls were performed with a strong retroversion of the pelvis and no eccentric component. Finally, the patient began to perform a backward-loaded sled drag to reinforce the quadriceps vastus medialis oblique (VMO specifically) dynamically.

4. Post-reinforcement proprioception remains critical during this stage to continue to improve the neuromuscular intelligence of the joint. Proprioception for the general knee is continued, and proprioception for the ACL and infrapatellar tendon is added (see Figure 9-46).

5. Specific myofascial stretches for the iliopsoas, biceps femoris, gluteus maximus, rectus femoris, vastus medialis, and gracilis are supervised at the end of each session.

6. The patient continues specific ELDOA postures each evening to ensure proper spinal alignment and myofascial mobility. The patient had homework of myofascial stretching, proprioception, and ELDOA to perform daily on his own. At 9-1/2 weeks post surgery, the patient has done well. He has almost full flexion bilaterally in the quadriceps and can do a full squat with zero translation of the hip and pelvis.

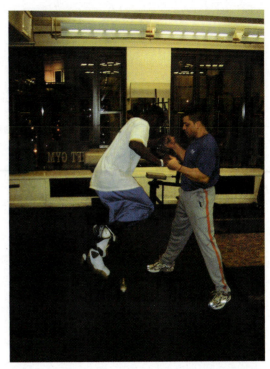

Figure 9-52 Patient performs open-chain plyometric single-leg jumps. Patient performs single-leg jumps back and forth and from side to side.

Phase III Protocol

The phase III goals will be to help the athlete progress to the point of open-chain movements, including rope skipping and single-leg jumping drills (Figure 9-52). This will be accomplished using exactly the same six segments of performance rehabilitation used in the prior two phases. The reinforcement exercises will change to include level II split squats, which will place more tension on the distal portion of the quadriceps.

Phase III will also include single-leg, partner-assisted squats with a pelvic retroversion, and it will begin to incorporate eccentric manual leg curls. The proprioception segment will be done before the reinforcement segment now, because the athlete is strong enough to hold the positions without danger of reinjury. The open-chain jumping is performed after the reinforcement, and the myofascial stretches are performed last in the session. The athlete will be allowed to return to the basketball court for shooting only. He will be required to perform the entire general warm-up and all of the proprioceptive drills before entering the basketball court. The ELDOA postures are to be performed by the athlete as homework each evening.

Phase IV Protocol

Phase IV of this patient's performance rehabilitation will begin to incorporate bilateral squatting and single-leg jumping with higher eccentric loads and times under tension. The training will also begin to incorporate upper-body reinforcement training and be geared toward improving relative strength and eventually power as measured by a one-repetition maximum. The goal is to have the athlete begin running the court at about 13 weeks post surgery and return to competitive basketball at about 16 weeks post surgery with a better, structurally balanced, stronger, and more supple physical foundation.

Over the years, there has been much debate regarding the safety and efficacy of the full squat for the athlete who has undergone an ACL surgical repair. The science lends itself to the benefits of the athlete who can safely and correctly do a full squat after the appropriate goals have been achieved in his or her performance rehabilitation. The following goals must be attained:

1. Movement of the knee in all planes, including flexion, extension, translation, and rotation
2. A balanced reinforcement of all the necessary muscle groups of the lower body
3. Suppleness and ROM in all appropriate muscle groups of the lower body
4. Proprioception of the specific parts of the knee, hip, ankles, and foot

5. Proper spinal alignment through ELDOA and myofascial stretching
6. Finally, the correct technique of squatting must be taught in its entirety while respecting the fascial connections and the kinetic chains.

When these prerequisites can be accomplished, the full squat can benefit the athlete who has rehabbed an ACL repair by managing the co-contraction of the hamstring and the quadriceps via the stretch reflex of the ACL. The squat becomes important as a global proprioceptive tool and improves the stability of the entire knee under load. Improving the stability of the knee under load is critical for the athlete who undergoes high eccentric loading in his or her respective sport (e.g., downhill skiing or basketball).

The ultimate goal for this athlete should be to correctly perform a single-leg squat five times with body weight, or a front squat with their respective bodyweight for 10 perfect repetitions.

Summary

Manual therapy is a useful modality to reduce pain, increase range of motion, and restore functional capacity of injured tissue. The two common forms of injuries presented here—adhesive capsulitis and ACL—employ different manual techniques to restore strength, muscular endurance, proprioception, and coordination, all directed toward a common goal of return to full activity.

References

Antonini, F. M., Petruzzi, E., Pinzanni, P., Orlando, C., Pogessi, M., Serio, M., et al. (2002). The meat in the diet of aged subjects and the antioxidant effects of carnosine. *Archives of Gerontology & Geriatrics, 8* (Suppl.), 7–14.

Antonio, J., Sanders, M. S., & Van Gammeren, D. (2001). The effects of bovine colostrum supplementation on body composition and exercise performance in active men and women. *Nutrition, 17,* 243–247.

Appleton, J. (2002). Arginine: Clinical potential of a semi-essential amino acid. *Alternative Medicine Review, 7*(6), 512–522.

Beynnon, B. D., Fleming, B. C., Johnson, R. J., Nichols, C. E., Renstrom, P. A., & Pope, M. H. (1995). Anterior cruciate ligament strain behavior during rehabilitation exercises in vivo. *American Journal of Sports Medicine, 23,* 24–34.

Beynnon, B. D., Johnson, R. J., & Fleming, B. C. (1993). The mechanics of anterior cruciate ligament reconstruction. In D. W. Jackson, S. P. Arnoczky, S. L-Y. Woo, C. B. Frank, & T. M. Simon (Eds.), *The anterior cruciate ligament: Current and future concepts* (pp. 259–272). New York: Raven Press.

Caraffa, A., Cerulli, G., Projetti, M., Aisa, G, & Rizzo, A. (1996). Prevention of anterior cruciate ligament injuries in soccer. A prospective controlled study of proprioceptive training. *Knee Surgery, Sports Traumatology, Arthroscopy, 4*(1), 19–21

Chimera, N. J., Swanik, K. A., **Swanik, C. B., Straub, S. J.** (2004). Effects of plyometric training on muscle-activation strategies and performance in female athletes. *Journal of athletic training, 39*(1), 21–24

DeMaio, M., Noyes, F. R., & Mangine, R. E. (1992). Principles for aggressive rehabilitation after reconstruction of the anterior cruciate ligament. *Orthopedics, 15,* 385–392.

Ford K. R., Myer G. D., & Hewett T. E. (2003). Valgus knee motion during landing in high school female and male basketball players. *Medicine and science in sports and exercise 35*(10), 1745–1750

Forman, S. K., & Jackson, D. W. (1993). Cyclops lesions. In D. W. Jackson, S. P. Arnoczky, S. L-Y. Woo, C. B. Frank, & T. M. Simon (Eds.), *The anterior cruciate ligament: Current and future concepts* (pp. 365–372). New York: Raven Press.

Fu, F. H., Irrgang, J. J., & Harner, C. D. (1993). Loss of motion following anterior cruciate ligament reconstruction. In D. W. Jackson, S. P. Arnoczky, S. L-Y. Woo, C. B. Frank, & T. M. Simon (Eds.), *The anterior cruciate ligament: Current and future concepts* (pp. 373–380). New York: Raven Press.

Hewett T. E., Lindenfeld T. N., Riccobene J. V., & Noyes F. R. (1999). The effect of neuromuscular training on the incidence of knee injury in female athletes: A prospective study. *The American Journal of Sports Medicine, 27*(6): 699–706.

Irrgang, J. J. (1993). Modern trends in anterior cruciate ligament rehabilitation: Nonoperative and postoperative management. *Clinics in Sports Medicine, 12,* 797–813.

Jaffe, M. B., & Moorman, C. T. (2001). Shoulder conditioning for the throwing athlete: The off-season program. *Sports Medicine & Arthroscopy Review, 9,* 19–23.

Jerosch, J., Steinbeck, J., Clahsen, H., M. Schmitz-Nahrath, & Grosse-Hackmann, A. (1993). Function of the glenohumeral ligaments in active stabilisation of the shoulder joint. *Knee Surgery, Sports Traumatology, Arthroscopy, 1,* 152–158.

Junge A., Rösch D., Peterson L., Graf-Baumann T., & Dvorak J. (2002). Prevention of soccer injuries: A prospective intervention study in youth amateur players. *The American Journal of Sports Medicine, 30*(5), 652–659.

Lephart, S. M., Pincivero, D. M., Giraldo, J. L., & Fu, F.H. (1997). The role of proprioception in the management and rehabilitation of athletic injuries. *American Journal of Sports Medicine, 25,* 130–137.

Lephart, S. M., Warner, J. J. P., Borsa, P. A., & Fu, F.H (1994). Proprioception of the shoulder joint in healthy, unstable and surgically repaired shoulders. *Journal of Shoulder & Elbow Surgery, 3,* 371–380.

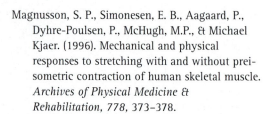

Magnusson, S. P., Simonesen, E. B., Aagaard, P., Dyhre-Poulsen, P., McHugh, M.P., & Michael Kjaer. (1996). Mechanical and physical responses to stretching with and without preisometric contraction of human skeletal muscle. *Archives of Physical Medicine & Rehabilitation, 778,* 373–378.

Maurer, H. R. (2001). Bromelain: Biochemistry, pharmacology and medical use. *Cellular & Molecular Life Sciences, 58,* 1234–1245.

Noyes, F. R., Mangine, R. E., & Barber, S. D. (1992). The early treatment of motion complications after reconstruction of the anterior cruciate ligament. *Clinical Orthopaedics, 277,* 217–228.

Paulos, L. E., & Meislin, R. (1993). Patellar entrapment following anterior cruciate ligament injury. In D. W. Jackson, S. P. Arnoczky, S. L-Y. Woo, C. B. Frank, & T. M. Simon (Eds.), *The anterior cruciate ligament: Current and future concepts* (pp. 357–363). New York: Raven Press.

Paulos, L. E., & Stern, J. (1993). Rehabilitation after anterior cruciate ligament surgery. In D. W. Jackson, S. P. Arnoczky, S. L-Y. Woo, C. B. Frank, & T. M. Simon (Eds.), *The anterior cruciate ligament: Current and future concepts* (pp. 381–395). New York: Raven Press.

Rougraff, B., Shelbourne, K. D., Gerth, P. K., & Warner, J. (1993). Arthroscopic and histologic analysis of human patellar tendon autografts used for anterior cruciate ligament reconstruction. *American Journal of Sports Medicine, 21,* 277–284.

Rubinstein, R. A., Jr., Shelbourne, K. D., VanMeter, C. D., McCarroll, J. R., Rettig, A. C., & Gloyeske, R. L. (1995). Effect on knee stability if full hyperextension is restored immediately after autogenous bone–patellar tendon–bone anterior cruciate ligament reconstruction. *American Journal of Sports Medicine, 23,* 365–368.

Shelbourne, K. D., & Nitz, P. (1990). Accelerated rehabilitation after anterior cruciate ligament reconstruction. *American Journal of Sports Medicine, 18,* 292–299.

Shelbourne, K. D., & Wilckens, J. H. (1990). Current concepts in anterior cruciate ligament rehabilitation. *Orthopaedic Review, 19,* 957–964.

Shelbourne, K. D., Wilckens, J. H., Mollabashy, A., & DeCarlo, M. (1991). Arthrofibrosis in acute anterior cruciate ligament reconstruction: The effect of timing of reconstruction and rehabilitation. *American Journal of Sports Medicine, 19,* 332–336.

Shrier, I. (1999). Stretching before exercise does not reduce the risk of local muscle injury: A critical review of the clinical and basic science literature. *Clinical Journal of Sport Medicine, 9,* 221–227.

Snyder-Mackler, L., Delitto, A., Bailey, S. L., & Stralka, S. W. (1995). Strength of the quadriceps femoris muscle and functional recovery after reconstruction of the anterior cruciate ligament: A prospective, randomized clinical trial of electrical stimulation. *Journal of Bone & Joint Surgery, 77-A,* 1166–1173.

Sullivan, P. E., Markos, P. D., & Minor, M.A.D. (1982). *An integrated approach to therapeutic exercise: Theory and clinical application.* Reston, VA: Reston Publishing.

Trebble, T., Arden, N. K., Stroud, M. A., Wootton, S. A., Burdge, G. C., Miles, E. A., et al. (2003). Inhibition of tumour necrosis factor: Alpha and interleukin 6 production by mononuclear cells following dietary fish-oil supplementation in healthy men and response to antioxidant co-supplementation. *British Journal of Nutrition, 90,* 405–412.

Turnlund, J. R., Jacob, R. A., Keen, C. L., Strain, J. J., Kelley, D. S., Domek, J. M., et al. (2004). Long-term high copper intake: Effects on indexes of copper status, antioxidant status, and immune function in young men. *American Journal of Clinical Nutrition, 79,* 1037–1044.

Wilk, K. E., & Arrigo, C. A. (1992). An integrated approach to upper extremity exercises. *Orthopaedic & Physical Therapy Clinics of North America, 1,* 337–360.

Wilk, K. E., Arrigo, C. A., & Andrews, J. R. (1995). *Functional training for the overhead athlete.* La Crosse, WI: Sports Physical Therapy Home Study Course.

Wilk, K. E., Arrigo, C. A., & Andrews, J. R. (1997). Current concepts: The stabilizing structures of the glenohumeral joint. *Journal of Orthopaedic & Sports Physical Therapy, 25,* 364–379.

Wilk, K. E., Meister, K., & Andrews, J. R. (2002). Current concepts in the rehabilitation of the overhead throwing athlete. *American Journal of Sports Medicine, 30,* 136–151.

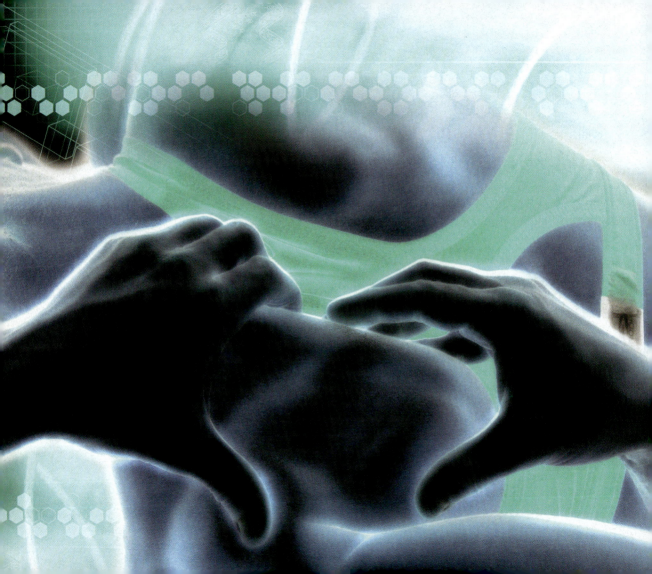

THE ROLE OF ENERGY MEDICINE IN THE THERAPEUTIC TREATMENT OF FASCIA

Energy medicine, also known as energy therapy or biofield therapeutics, is based on the premise that the human body is composed of various energy fields and that people fall ill when the energy in those fields becomes blocked, out of balance, or otherwise disturbed. Energy therapists attempt to restore health by first detecting and then removing the blockages.

Dr. James Oschman is a world authority on energy and complementary medicine and author of the groundbreaking publication, *Energy Medicine: The Scientific Basis.* He has focused many of his inquiries on the potential role of energy therapies for athletic training and protection from injury. This chapter briefly summarizes the role of energy in stimulating the healing response and repair of injuries to the living matrix. From there, it looks at the usage of some contemporary therapies such as low-level laser, frequency-specific microcurrent (FSM), percussion therapy, and so forth as used by practitioners with the goal of accelerating the healing response in connective tissue.

Modern biomedical research has revealed various cellular and molecular processes involved in the healing response (Marchesi, 1985; Miyake & McNeil, 1985; Lin & Hopf, 2003). When looking at the body's response to repair any injury it sustains, it is important to consider the integration of several areas such as self-organization (Kauffman, 1994), intercommunication (Ho, Popp, & Warnke, 1994), immunity (Ayala, Chung, Grutkoski, & Song, 2003), systems theory (Weinberg, 2003), and the role of consciousness (Ho, 1997). Recent advances in both complementary medicine and clinical research have shed new light on the nature of the energetic signals that can stimulate the healing response in a living organism.

ELECTROMAGNETIC HEALING OF FRACTURED BONE

Becker and Basset demonstrated that passing current through a bone fracture stimulated repair. Becker (1967) was able to show that a 100 mA–50 mA/cm^2 current was capable of stimulating the activity of osteoblasts, hence accelerating the healing of osseous fractures (Becker, 1967). Contemporary medicine uses electromagnetic pulse therapy to induce current flows through bone fractures that fail to heal. For example, a 10 V field introduced into a coil of wire adjacent to the body will induce an electric field of 1 mV/cm or more that can be measured with electrodes inserted into the bone (Rubin, McLeod, & Lanyon, 1989). The usage of electrical current to stimulate healing in bone has jump-started the potential usage of induced currents in other soft tissues. Since then researchers have extended their findings, and it is now known that each type of cell and tissue responds to a particular frequency of stimulation—for example, nerves, 2 Hz; bone, 7 Hz; ligaments, 10 Hz; skin and capillaries, 15 Hz, 20 Hz, and 72 Hz (Siskin & Walker, 1995).

Using electrical and magnetic stimulation takes advantage of the body's bioelectric system, which in turn influences healing of fascia by attracting repair cells like fibroblasts, changing the permeability of cell membranes and thus affecting secretions and orienting cell structures. When a tear or adhesion occurs in skin or underlying fascia, a current of energy is generated between the skin and inner fascia that in turn can be mimicked by electrical stimulation and hence accelerate the healing of injured fascia. Magnetic therapy works via a similar rationale; the use of magnets has been reported to increase blood flow and enhance cell growth by transferring energy to repair cells.

COMPLEMENTARY MEDICINE

Complementary medicine includes a variety of practices such as acupuncture, aromatherapy, jin shin jyutsu, homeopathy, massage, cranial sacral, healing touch, therapeutic touch, polarity therapy, reiki, structural integration, zero balancing, and so on. There has been a developing trend of using gentle pressure, hands-on techniques that seem to produce profound changes to the entire tissue matrix through the induction of electric fields emitted by a practitioner's hands (McCraty, Atkinson, Tomasino, & Tiller, 1998). This seems to imply that the fascial system is extremely sensitive to the energy fields that can stimulate or suppress various cellular and molecular processes.

The influence of massage therapy and biomedicine on the living matrix in controlling cellular expression throughout the living organism is only one exciting feature of the living matrix. The ability of the living matrix to act as a communication network must be explained before beginning to explore the role of frequency specific microcurrent (FSM), low-level laser, percussion therapy, and acupuncture in the treatment of fascial and other connective tissue injuries. The living matrix has the ability to generate and conduct vibrations because of the following properties, which are commonly found in all components of the living matrix:

- **Semiconduction**—all of the components are semiconductors. They are capable of conducting and processing vibrational information. Semiconductors are also capable of converting energy from one form to another (J. Oschman & L. Oschman, 1994).

- **Piezoelectricity**—all of the components are piezoelectric. Waves of mechanical vibration that move through the living matrix are capable of producing electrical fields, and vice versa (J. Oschman & L. Oschman, 1994).

- **Crystallinity**—the living matrix is arranged in crystalline lattices. This includes lipids in cell membranes, collagen molecules of connective tissue, actin and myosin molecules of muscle, and components of the cytoskeleton (J. Oschman & L. Oschman, 1994).

○ **Coherence**—the living matrix produces vibrations referred to as Frolich oscillation, which occur at particular frequencies in the microwave and visible light portions of the electromagnetic spectrum (J. Oschman & L. Oschman, 1994).

○ **Hydration**—is a dynamic component of the living matrix. On average, each matrix protein has 15,000 water molecules associated with it. Water molecules possess the property of polarity and hence have a dipole. The living matrix organizes the dipolar water molecules in a way that constrains or restricts their ability to vibrate, rotate, or wiggle about in different spatial planes. Water molecules are free to vibrate or spin only in particular directions (J. Oschman & L. Oschman, 1994).

○ **Continuity**—is spread throughout the organism. While it is possible to distinguish individual organs, tissues, cells, and molecules, the living matrix is a continuous and unbroken whole (J. Oschman & L. Oschman, 1994).

According to the continuum communication model, the living matrix is capable of conducting and generating vibrational signals throughout the three-dimensional web of fascia encasing the body (J. Oschman & L. Oschman, 1994). Disease, health disorders, and pain arise when part of the vibrational information is restricted, possibly due to scars and restrictions or adhesions set up throughout the fascial network; hence, the flow of information is altered. A failure in the transmission of information through the body can be recorded by the connective tissue; consequently, future vibrational signals can

be altered by the signatures of the stored information (J. Oschman & L. Oschman, 1994).

Frequency-Specific Microcurrent Therapy

Note: Adapted from David Young, N.D., certified microcurrent specialist (McMakin, 2004).

Tissue of the body consists of cells, organelles, neurotransmitters, hormones, electrolytes, and a variety of other structures and biochemicals. At a deeper, subatomic level, tissue is composed of bits of energy that are vibrating at great speeds. Conditions that have affected the fascia over time can form patterns that are held in the crystalline structure of the gel substance that forms the cell matrix and the interconnections between all of the cells and membranes in the body. This in turn can account for the somatic recall behavior displayed by fascia and hence affect organ and biomechanical function.

Oschman (1997) proposed that the "cell is filled with a microtrabecular lattice that forms the ground substance within the cell." All of the organelles are suspended and interconnected by the microtrabeculae (J. Oschman, 1997). Glycoproteins extend across the cell surface from the cell interior to the exterior (J. Oschman, 1997). These proteins connect with the filamentous network within the cell (J. Oschman, 1997). The filamentous network is a crystalline gel lined by water molecules, and it conveys and stores current, charge, and vibrational information (Monnier, Mustata, Biemel, Reigh, Lederer, Zhenyu et al., 2005). FSM is based on the idea that individual components of the tissue tensegrity matrix (glycoproteins, cytoskeleton, microtubules, electrons, integrins, etc.) act as semiconductors and are capable of transmitting energy in the form of specific vibrational frequencies (J. Oschman, 1997). The individualized and specific vibrational characteristics of each atom and each type of tissue can vary depending on a patient's health conditions. Trauma, inflammation, stress, and environmental influences can change the vibrational frequency of an electron in the affected fascia. As the vibrations of the electrons change, it is believed that the electrons may also change to a different "orbit" from what was normal for that tissue type (McMakin, 2004). A change in the orbit occupied by an electron will result in a change in the electrical activity, causing a disruption from homeostasis.

The goal of FSM is to introduce an identical vibrational frequency into the damaged fascia. The desired effect is to neutralize those frequencies that are incorrect for the damaged and/or affected tissues. As the frequencies of electrons in damaged tissues are neutralized and the electrons return to their normal orbital vibrations, the physiological condition of the tissues will begin to normalize (McMakin, 2004). FSM units are capable of generating a microamp setting from as low as 20 microamps to as high as 600 microamps (McMakin, 2004). This range in current allows the clinician to adjust the treatment to the specific type of fascia: superficialis (superficial) versus profundis (deep) afflicted, the type of condition (fascial tear versus adhesion or restriction in the fascial web), and the energetic nature of the fascia itself.

The speed of recovery varies according to the type of patient and the extent and type of tissue damage sustained by the individual. Patients may experience notable clinical changes to the fascia in releasing myofascial restrictions after a period of one treatment; however, in other cases the changes may not be noticeable for up to 24 hours.

If a patient is experiencing chronic myofascial pain regardless of chronology, the improvement will persist without any nutritional intervention after minimal treatment (Lamotte, Strulens, Niset, & Van de Borne, 2005). If the patient has nutritional deficiencies, improvement will last between 1 and 14 days (McMakin, 2004). To increase the therapeutic duration of the microcurrent treatment, more scheduled treatments must take place. Conditions such as oxidative stress, dysbiosis, leaky gut, mineral deficiencies, biochemical instability, deconditioned muscles, and emotional and constitutional stress must be addressed. The application of microcurrent will result in a rapid recovery. Using nutrition, nutritional supplementation, pharmacological aids, and exercise will allow the state of recovery to persist.

The majority of chronic conditions demonstrate a significant change after the first six treatments. The wide range in the number of treatments before a patient experiences relief from any fascia adhesion can be explained as follows: if the electrons have been at the wrong frequencies for an extended time, after treatment the electrons may try to go back to those wrong frequencies (i.e., rebound), perhaps within four to seven days (McMakin, 2004). Thus the net result is usually an average of six treatments for the notable changes to become long lasting (McMakin, 2004). FSM treatment should be repeated at appropriate intervals until the cause-and-effect principle becomes permanent (McMakin, 2004).

Among the many benefits of receiving FSM are increased cellular activity due to a greater production of ATP by up to 500% (McMakin, 2004), increased protein synthesis, release of toxins from damaged tissue, reestablishment of normal communication between the brain and affected tissue, and enhanced tissue recovery by stimulating the regeneration of injured tissue. This treatment also stimulates lymphatic flow, relieves myofascial adhesions, changes scar tissue, reduces inflammatory cytokines, and so on (McMakin, 2004).

Microcurrent applied to injured tissue supports the natural current flow in the tissue, allowing cells in the traumatized fascia to regain their capacitance (McMakin, 2004). Trauma to the fascia can affect the electrical potential of the fascia and the resonant frequency of the electrons in the fascia. The injured fascia will typically have a higher electrical resistance than that of surrounding tissue. This decreases electrical conductance through the injured area and decreases cellular capacitance, resulting in a hampered repair to the damaged connective tissue (McMakin, 2004). When FSM is applied, resistance is reduced, allowing bioelectricity to flow through and reestablish normal cellular functioning and hence tissue function.

The long-lasting effects of FSM on the body are not without their drawbacks. Unfortunately, side effects such as nausea, fatigue, drowsiness, temporary increase in pain, and flu-like feeling may (or may not) occur during or up to 90 minutes after treatment and can last from 4 to 24 hours (McMakin, 2004). Taking antioxidants and liver support supplementations immediately prior to treatment will help neutralize and process those toxins faster (Werb & Gordon, 2005). Drinking two quarts of water two hours immediately following treatment will greatly facilitate and accelerate liver detoxification (McMakin, 2004). The potential to experience increased pain after FSM treatment can be accounted by reestablishing the brain-to-damaged-tissue communication pathway, which is important in sending additional signals to jump-start the healing process. The brain may become reawakened to the pain in that tissue and will once again participate in sending signals to the rest of the body to heal damaged fascia. Hence, the patient may experience a slight increase in pain in the area of injury for a few days to a few weeks (Barros, Rodrigues, Rodrigues, Oliveira, Barros, & Rodrigues, Jr., 2002).

The following points are for practitioners who may be interested in learning more about how to use FSM:

○ Black graphite gloves are used to conduct the current from the FSM unit through the fascial planes. The gloves allow the clinician to feel the patient's musculature and place the current at the site of focal fascial adhesions or restrictions (McMakin, 2004).

○ Pads are used as an adjunct in delivering current to the patient's body. The pads deliver frequencies to the whole body system, not just the muscles (McMakin, 2004).

○ Changing the frequency of the FSM unit is important in targeting different types of conditions established in the fascia. In many cases, the tissue will suddenly soften and become less painful when the correct combination of frequencies is chosen. This

softening and the pain relief that comes with it seems to be long lasting and in some cases permanent (McMakin, 2004).

○ The nerve is polarized by establishing a direct current running through the fascial planes and connecting the positive to negative.

Low-Level Laser Therapy

The living matrix is a continuous physical, energetic, and informational network that distributes regulatory signals throughout the body. Every connection between cells, tissues, and organ systems will be restored to normal energetic status via the usage of low-level lasers, hence restoring normal physiological functioning of the organism (Karu, 2001; Oschman, 2000).

A laser causes activation of the cell, which in turn leads to an intensification of the biochemical processes. More recently, the work by Karu, Oschman, and others has enhanced our understanding of how low-level lasers work. According to Oschman, the current understanding of the cellular signaling cascade and amplification is that the receptors on the cell surface are the primary sites of action of low-frequency electromagnetic fields. It is at this receptor that cellular responses are triggered by hormones, growth factors, neurotransmitters, pheromones, antigens, or a single photon. Membrane signals closely associated with the receptors, such as adenylate cyclases and G proteins, are considered secondary messengers that couple a single molecular event at the cell surface to the influx of a huge number of calcium ions. Calcium ions entering the cell activate a variety of enzyme molecules and can produce a cascade of intracellular signals that initiate, accelerate, or inhibit biological processes (J. Oschman, 2000). The enzymes, in turn, are catalysts; and since catalysts are not consumed by reactions, they can continue to accelerate biochemical pathways until calcium levels drop to pre-stimulation values.

The work of Karu (1988) suggests that the mechanism of using a low-level laser at the cellular level is based on the electronic excitation of chromophores in cytochrome *c* oxidase that modulates a reduction-oxidation (redox) status of the molecule and enhances its functional activity. Oxidative metabolism is increased due to irradiation at all wavelengths used (Karu, 2001).

Two different viewpoints are considered: electromagnetic and thermodynamic (McMakin, 2004). From the electromagnetic point of view, living systems are mainly governed by the electromagnetic interaction of photons. Based on this concept, we can expect electromagnetic influences like that of a low-level laser of proper wavelength will have a strong impact on the living matrix (McMakin, 2004). From the thermodynamic point of view, living systems—in contrast to dead organisms—are open systems that need metabolism to maintain their highly ordered state of life. Such states can exist only far from thermodynamic equilibrium, thus dissipating heat so as to maintain their high order and complexity. Such nonequilibrium systems, called dissipative structures, have the ability to react on weak influences; for example, they are capable of amplifying very small stimuli (McMakin, 2004). The transition from a cell at rest to a rapidly dividing one will occur during a phase transition already influenced by the smallest fluctuations (J. Oschman, 1998). External stimuli can induce these phase transitions, which would otherwise not even take place. These phase transitions, induced by light, can be impressively illustrated by various chemical and physiological reactions as special kinds of dissipative systems. A vast amount of clinical and experimental research supports these two biophysical viewpoints concerning the interaction between life and laser light. Through the use of cytometric, photometric, and radiochemical methods, it is shown that the increase or decrease of cell growth depends on the applied wavelengths, on the irradiance, on the pulse sequence modulated to laser beams (constant, periodic, or random pulses), on the type of cells (leukocytes, lymphocytes, fibroblasts, normal and cancer cells) and on the density of the cells in tissue cultures (McMakin, 2004).

Low-level laser treatment confers numerous benefits, such as increased ATP at the cellular level via the stimulation of mitochondria, cellular enzymes, macrophage activation, collagen synthesis, significant increases in granulation tissue, increased permeability of cell membranes, and increased serotonin and endorphin with decreased C-fiber activity and bradykinin (Turner & Hode, 2002). See the flowchart in Figure 10-1 for more detailed explanation of how low-level laser works.

Clinical Application of Low-Level Laser

The therapeutic efficacy of low-level laser on healing wounds under suboptimal conditions has not gone unnoticed. An abundance of experimental studies supports a significant increase in fibroblast proliferation. It has been observed that the higher increase in proliferation occurs after irradiation at lower wavelengths (570 nm). Van Breugel et al. Every process creates a specific kind of vibrational frequency that travels through the tensegrity matrix. It has been postulated that low-level lasers can alter the resonant frequencies detected and hence stored by the living matrix. As a result, the new coherent vibrational frequency at the surface of a molecule, cell, or organism as a whole will likely trigger the integration of processes such as growth, injury repair, defense, and functioning of the organism as a whole (J. Oschman, 2000). The usage of low-level lasers by clinicians will enable them to manipulate and balance their patient's vibratory circuits and hence alter the body's systemic defense and repair mechanisms.

The mechanism of action of low-level lasers has not been fully elucidated, but current research tends focus on the following most encountered theories:

○ **Bioluminescence theory** is based on the observation that light emitted at a wavelength of 630 nm may accelerate DNA replication via photic stimulation. Laser irradiation at this frequency is said to be nonmutagenic, since

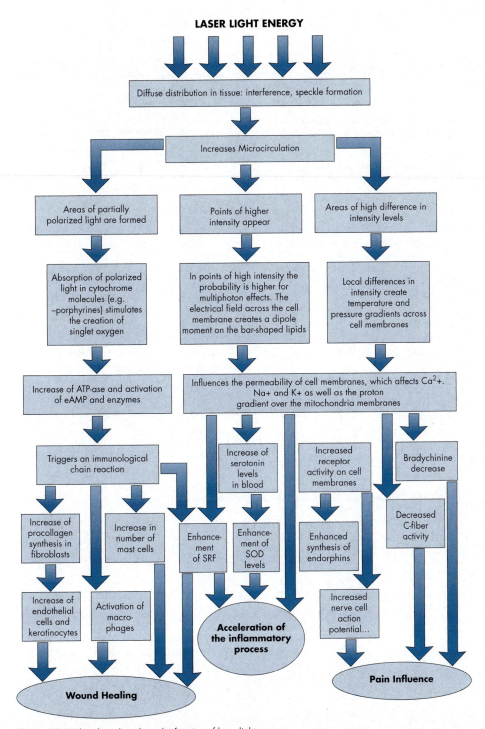

Figure 10-1 Flowchart describing the function of laser light energy.

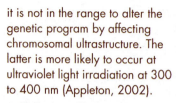

it is not in the range to alter the genetic program by affecting chromosomal ultrastructure. The latter is more likely to occur at ultraviolet light irradiation at 300 to 400 nm (Appleton, 2002).

○ **Cellular oscillation theory** is grounded on the notion that a low-level laser possesses characteristic resonant frequencies that are capable of altering the electromagnetic oscillations of single cells in tissues. This effect is thought to stimulate the biochemical processes that ultimately regulate the performance of various vital organs (Kleinkort).

○ **Biological field theory** observed a general decrease in absorption at longer wavelengths and concluded that several molecules in fibroblasts serve as photoacceptors, resulting in a range of absorption peaks (420, 445, 470, 560, 630, 690, and 730 nm; Turner & Hode, 2002; Van Breugel & Bar, 1992)

Karu also emphasizes that the use of the appropriate wavelength, namely, within the bandwidth of the absorption spectra of photoacceptor molecules (Karu, 2001), is an important factor to consider. It can be applied to the clinical use of low-level laser to aid in healing tears in the fascial sheath via several possible mechanisms, as shown earlier:

○ Increased procollagen synthesis in fibroblasts with resultant improved tissue strength values

○ Neovascularization of lymphatic and blood vessels, as well as vasodilation, improves microcirculation and lymphatic drainage (resorption of edema)

○ Larger quantity of granulation tissue and accelerated epithelization

○ Increase in number of mast cells around the area of injury

○ Increase of endothelial cells and keratinocytes

○ Activation of macrophages

○ Enhancement of Sarcoplasmic Reticulum Function (SRF)

○ Enhancement of superoxide dismutase (SOD) levels

○ Cytokine production

○ Increased DNA synthesis

○ Increased rate of cell proliferation

○ Increased ATP synthesis (Reddy, 2004)

○ Attenuates reactive oxygen species (ROS) production by neutrophils (Fujimaki, Shimoyama, Liu, Umeda, Nakaji, & Sugawara, 2003)

The goal of the soft tissue practitioner is to use a low-level laser to biomodulate the cells and tissues at the appropriate wavelength (target range) and enhance the cellular processes (just listed) in damaged tendons, ligaments, muscle (fascia), and epithelial tissue.

The clinician should use hand palpation to detect any fascial adhesions/restrictions, which are merely random arrangements of collagen fibers deposited in a cross-linked structure. The fascial adhesion/restriction will cause a global mechanical distortion throughout the body due to fascia tissue encompassing the whole body. In addition, an adhesion/restriction is a tear residing in the fascial tissue, and it will impede the transfer of information through the tissue; hence, the fascia will become a non-information-transferring tissue.

After detecting the site of fascial injury, the practitioner can set the frequency of low-level laser at the following levels to address the respective problem areas:

○ 3 Hz – inflammation

○ 25 Hz – fascia and muscle regeneration

○ 42 Hz – lymphatic regeneration

○ 125 Hz – reoxygenation

The low-level laser should be held at the area of focus no longer than 20 seconds at a time and then moved to surrounding areas of tenderness. The clinician should determine which fascial chain has been affected by the injury and from that point treat the respective anatomical areas. Additionally, the clinician may attempt to knead the tissue if it is accessible and may consider using renovator oil during the process. Two additional homeopathic preparations that can be used in conjunction with low-level laser and are worth mentioning are Inflamyar and Zellulisan. The application of both preparations involves a gentle massaging action of the ointments around and on the tender areas. Most users report enhanced flexibility and elasticity to muscles, tendons, and ligaments after routinely applying these homeopathic preparations.

Inflamyar is a homeopathic sports ointment that is designed to be used in conjunction with internal systemic therapy. Inflamyar treats arthritic and inflammatory conditions topically to greatly ease pain and bring quick relief to afflicted patients, all without the systemic side effects of conventional drug therapy. Other conditions effectively treated by Inflamyar include myalgia, contusion, hematoma, torticollis, tendovaginitis, epicondylitis, myogelosis, meniscopathia, neuralgia, lumbago, hip pain (sciatic pain), bursitis, and intercostal neuralgia. In addition to its use in treating chronic conditions, Inflamyar is now being used by athletes to treat various sports injuries such as sprains and bruises. It also can be used for fascial injuries with some degree of success.

Zellulisan ointment (a homeopathic formulation) is ideal in releasing toxin buildup due to lymphatic stasis caused by microtrauma to the fascia. Zellulisan combined with Inflamyar is ideal in treating inflammation of the connective tissue structures in addition to enhancing the excretion of metabolic, toxic by-products.

Some athletic trainers are currently attempting to improve the delivery of topical preparations such as Inflamyar, Traumeel, Diclofenac in Phlogel, and so on

across the stratum corneum of the skin. Lee, Shen, Lai, and Hu (2001) studied the influence of the yttrium aluminium garnet (YAG) laser on the transdermal delivery of drugs across the skin. The stratum corneum is a heterogeneous membrane consisting of a mosaic of cornified cells containing cross-linked keratin filaments and intercellular lipid-containing regions (Lee et al., 2001). Polar and nonpolar substances diffuse across the stratum corneum by different molecular mechanisms (Lee et al., 2001). In general, lipophilic drugs can relatively easily permeate the stratum corneum by the lipid-rich route (intercellular pathways), whereas hydrophilic drugs may predominantly diffuse across water-rich domains (intracellular pathways; Lee et al., 2001). It has been proposed that the YAG laser used by Lee et al. (2001) may predominantly interrupt the stratum corneum lipid bilayers to open intercellular pathways, resulting in a great increase in hydrophilic molecules across laser-treated skin (Lee et al., 2001). The most significant enhancement of drug permeation was observed for hydrophilic as opposed to lipophilic molecules (Lee et al., 2001). This is because the stratum corneum is a more important barrier to skin permeation of hydrophilic rather than lipophilic drugs, and the stratum corneum is ablated by laser irradiation. Enhanced absorption of topical preparations will allow practitioners to use smaller amounts, especially when treating areas of the body that are resistant to topical preparations.

Acupuncture Therapy

Acupuncture is a complex health therapy that has been practiced in China for more than 2,000 years. Its popularity has increased, and many North Americans now use acupuncture in treating pain resulting from a wide variety of chronic disorders. Despite considerable efforts to understand the anatomy and physiology of acupuncture points and meridians to connective tissue planes, knowledge of the principles behind this therapy has remained elusive for a long time. Many researchers have attempted to establish anatomical and functional connections between acupuncture points and a variety of body structures. These include receptors supplied by sensory nerves (Wang & Liu, 1989), tendon organs, encapsulated nerve endings, extensive neural terminals, vascular networks or superficial blood vessels (Gunn, 1976; Pan & Zhao, 1988), veins perforating fascia (Plummer, 1980), and mast cells (Zhai, 1988). However, it is only recently that Langevin, Churchill, and Cipolla (2001) have shown an intimate link with fascial anatomy that can still be better understood and have its effectiveness improved.

Traditional Chinese medicine contends that acupuncture points have specific therapeutic effects that are believed to occur at the site locally or at a distance via the system of acupuncture 'meridians'. More recently, Langevin and Yandow (2002) have formulated a model based on the notion that the biochemical effects derived from mechanical stimulation of connective tissue and potential spreading of these effects along connective tissue planes may explain acupuncture's therapeutic effects as well as traditional acupuncture theory does.

Langevin and colleagues (2001) proposed a mechanism of the therapeutic effects of acupuncture that takes into consideration the phenomenon of needle grasp. Their hypothesis coincides with the reaction to acupuncture needling known as 'di qi', which is widely viewed as essential to the therapeutic effects of acupuncture and may be the key to truly understanding its mechanism of action. Langevin and colleagues (2001) hypothesize first that needle grasp is due to mechanical coupling during needle rotation, and second that needle manipulation transmits mechanical signals to connective tissue cells via mechanotransduction.

Role of Connective Tissue Winding

During di qi, the needle is grasped due to the winding of connective tissue around the needle (Figure 10-2), which in turn results in a marked amplification of mechanical coupling between the inserted acupuncture

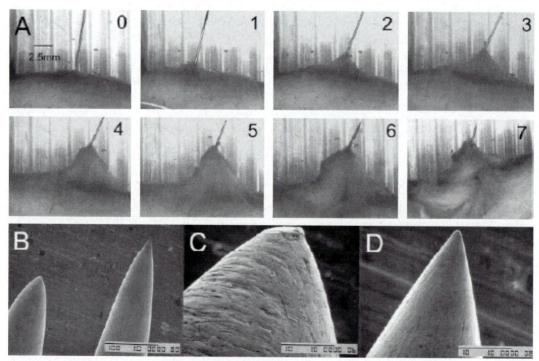

Figure 10-2 (A) "Whorls" of connective tissue from an acupuncture needle (inserted through tissue and rotated) and the number of rotations (numbered 1–7). (B) An electron microscopy of a gold (left) and stainless steel (right) needle magnified 350×. A 3,500× magnification of gold (C) and stainless steel (D) needles reveals different surface textures.
Source: Anatomical Record (New Anat.), 269 (2002): 257–265.

needle at the local connective tissue (Langevin et al., 2001). Langevin and colleagues (2001) believe that the initial grasp of the needle is due to electrical attractive forces between the needle and tissue, and that these forces can be accounted for by the extracellular matrix (ECM), which is made up of interwoven collagen and elastic fibers associated with glycoproteins and negatively charged proteoglycans (Aumailley & Gayraud, 1998). Once the acupuncture needle has been grasped by the connective tissue, movements of the needle (rotation and pistoning) may send a signal through connective tissue via deformation of the ECM to cells such as fibroblasts (Figure 10-3) and hence may contribute to the therapeutic effect of di qi (Langevin et al., 2001).

Mechanical Signal Transduction

Mechanical deformation of an integrin molecule via its attachment to the ECM can trigger the activation of a signaling cascade, resulting in a wide range of cellular responses. Some cells—such as fibroblasts, endothelial cells, and sensory neurons—are mechanically attached to the extracellular collagen matrix and intracellular cytoskeleton (Chicurel, Chen, & Ingber, 1998). The mechanism of mechanical load detection is thought to be due to the presence of an ECM–integrin–cytoskeleton-linked complex that is capable of activating a kinase cascade (Burridge,

Fath, Kelly, Nuckolis, & Turner, 1988; Giancotti & Ruoslahti, 1999). Any deformation of the connective tissue matrix, such as by inserting an acupuncture needle, will lead to transduction of the integrin molecules due to the presence of integrin-binding proteins (e.g., talin) that make up the matrix complex. One or more of these proteins can undergo a conformation change and initiate a series of phosphorylation and binding reactions in the protein complex (Banes, Tsuzaki, Yamamoto, Fischer, Brigman et al., 1995). Activation of a signaling cascade will lead to a wide range of cellular responses, for example, changes in the actin cytoskeleton with formation of stress fibers. Signal transduction caused by mechanical deformation of the fascia can lead to downstream cellular effects, including modification of the surrounding ECM (Figure 10-4; Brand, 1997).

Potential Downstream Effects of Needle Grasp

It is generally thought that cells exist in a dynamic state of balance that depends on the polymerization state of the cytoskeleton, the amount of extrinsic applied deformation, and the number and quality of focal adhesions (Wang, Yao, Xian, & Hou, 1985). Downstream effects of mechanical signal generated by acupuncture needle manipulation may include the synthesis and local release of

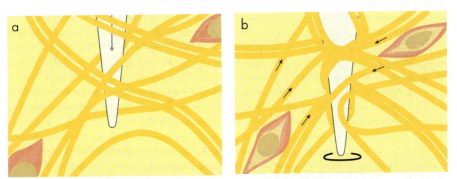

Figure 10-3 An illustration of needle insertion into connective tissue without rotation **(A)** and with rotation **(B)** as the needle pulls on collagen fibers (arrows). A mechanical signal is generated from rotating the needle, and energy is converted into local fibroblasts. Collagen fibers are seen as yellow lines and actin cytoskeleton as pink lines inside fibroblasts.

Source: *FASEB Journal, 15* (2002): 2275–2282.

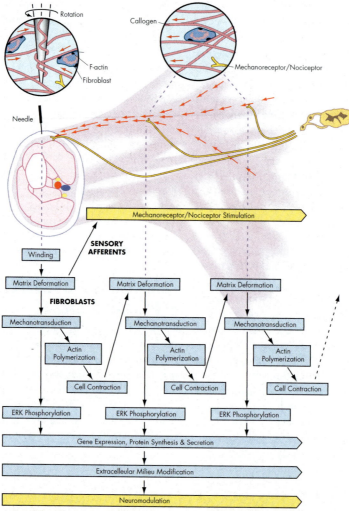

Figure 10-4 Mechanical Signal Transduction and Downstream Effects of Acupuncture Needle. The illustration represents a hypothetical summary at the microscopic level. The shaded gray area represents connective tissue of upper arm with a needle inserted into the biceps. During acupuncture needle manipulation, there is a pulling of connective tissue and deformation of the matrix (red arrows). Along the (lateral) border of the biceps is the "lung" acupuncture meridian, which may fall together with some planes of connective tissue. Source: *FASEB Journal, 15* (2001): 2275–2282.

growth factors, cytokines, vasoactive substances, degradative enzymes, and structural elements (Brand, 1997). Release of these substances can alter and hence influence the ECM and surrounding connective tissue cells, which can account for a change in the properties of fascia such as increased fluidity and fewer restrictions dispersed throughout the fascial web.

The effect of mechanical forces on mesenchymal tissues such as fascia can have important biomechanical, vasomotor, and neuromodulatory effects

(Duncan & Turner, 1995; Ryan, 1989; Stoltz, Dumas, Wang, Payan, Mainard et al., 2000). Contraction of fascia has been well documented during wound healing, tissue remodeling, and fibrotic processes. During acupuncture needle manipulation, pulling of collagen may cause reversible contraction of fibroblasts in the near vicinity of the acupuncture needle and will cause the fibroblast to change its phenotypic expression (Langevin et al., 2001). Contraction of the fibroblasts will cause further pulling of the collagen fibers, resulting in a deformation of the tissue matrix through the interstitial connective tissue. A proposed mechanism of action accounting for the influence of acupuncture needle manipulation on signal transduction and downstream effects can be seen in Figure 10-3.

Clinicians who are using acupuncture to relieve pain symptoms and release focal adhesions/restrictions in the fascia should be aware of some potential side effects that may be experienced by the patient. The list of symptoms is as follows: momentary discomfort where the needle is inserted, drowsiness and sleepiness, localized bruising, temporary worsening of symptoms, fainting, onset of a migraine headache, and feeling faint during or after treatment. A number of serious but rare conditions may occur following treatment: damage to an internal organ of the body from insertion of an acupuncture needle, infection in the area where the needle was inserted, infection spreading throughout the blood to infect previously damaged heart valves, premature onset of labor in a late stage of pregnancy, and other side effects.

Myofascial/Active Release Therapy

Both forms of soft tissue therapy decrease the tension in the fibrous bands of connective tissue, or fascia, that encases muscles throughout the body. Injury or adhesions to this network of fascia can be a major cause of pain and impede motion. Trauma and overuse of an affected body part causes adhesions in soft tissues and muscle. In myofascial therapy, the fascia is loaded with a constant force in a

specific direction until a release occurs, aiming to alleviate these problems by breaking up constrictions in the fascia (Kinakin, 2004). Active release therapy (ART) combines the use of a precisely directed tension with specific body movements to free restricted tissues and reduce the amount of scar tissue (Kinakin, 2004).

Various research models have been applied to deep connective tissue therapy, and this work has resulted in an applied format that directs clinicians on how to apply basic principles of engineering and biology to their soft tissue therapy approach. Table 10-1 (with some included modifications) has been adapted from Schleip (2003b) and can assist all practitioners interested in targeting adhesions established in fascia.

Fascial therapy focuses mainly on removing adhesions displaced throughout the connective tissue sheets. This in turn restores mobility and flexibility, opens the lines of communication throughout the body by erasing the tissue's somatic memory, clears the body of toxic substances that have been entrapped in a meshwork of fibers, and resolves soft tissue pain.

Discovery of the physiological basis of connective tissue therapy stems from discovery of the presence of mechanoreceptors, intrafascial smooth muscle cells, and autonomic nerves dispersed throughout the network of fascial tissue. Fascia is densely innervated by mechanoreceptors, which are responsive to manual pressure. Stimulation of these sensory receptors has been shown to lead to a lowering of sympathetic tonus as well as a change in local tissue viscosity (Schleip, 2003b). Additionally, smooth muscle cells that seem to be involved in active fascial contractility have been discovered in fascia. Fascia and the autonomic nervous system appear to be intimately connected (Schleip, 2003a).

Fascial manipulation causes a stimulation of intrafascial mechanoreceptors, which in turn alter the proprioceptive input entering the central nervous system. This effect results in a change in autonomic

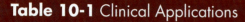

Table 10-1 Clinical Applications

Three key factors to effective treatment: knowing when, where, how

Time

- Only after water levels of patient have been assessed.
- Following rehydration period of the patient (close to full hydration).
- Following a thorough assessment after rehydration.
- As soon as possible.
- Heightened sympathetics: pay great attention to the state of the autonomic nervous system (which influences the body's overall tonus regulation).

Location

- Local area of concern (look for tightness in myofascia and antagonists).
- Assess and treat, if necessary, antagonists.
- Be aware of tissue physiology; areas containing large amounts of mechanoreceptors require much more attention (ligaments, myotendinous junctions).
- "Think outside the box": Give extra attention to myofascia of the face, hands, and feet; these tissues are always activated and might be the real cause of the patient's complaint.
- Abdomen and Pelvis: Deep pressure on visceral nerves as well as sustained pressure on the pelvis have been proven to increase vagal tone (increase parasympathetic state).

Method

- Timing: for example, for tonus decrease, use a slower type of treatment in order to avoid the myostatic stretch reflex.
- "Ruffini angle": Using lateral stretch is ideal to stimulate Ruffini organs and lower sympathetic tone.
- Use "unusual" sensations: create unusual body sensations that are most likely to be interpreted as "significant" by the filtering action of the reticular formation of the central nervous system; for example:
  - unusually strong stretch of fibers
  - unusually subtle stimulation ("whispering effect")
  - unusually specific stimulation
  - sensations that are always slightly changing/moving in a not precisely predictable manner
- Use a "feedback inclusion": As soon as you sense the beginning of a tonus change, mirror this with your touch in some way to the tissue. The more precise, immediate, and refined your "feedback inclusion" is, the more effective treatment will be.

(continued)

Table 10-1 Clinical Applications (continued)

Goal

- Engaging the patient in active micromovement participation (AMP); the slower, more demanding, and more refined the movements are, the more beneficial they will be for the patient.
- Ask and allow for a "deepening of proprioception."
- Relate body perceptions and movements to functional activities, and include the external space orientation as well as the social meaning aspects of altered body expressions.

Source: Adapted with permission from Schleip, R., Fascial plasticity—a new neurobiological explanation: Part 2. *Journal of Bodywork & Movement Therapies, 7*(2), 2003: 104–116.

tone via a change in gamma motor tone. Most of the fascial sensory nerve endings that are stimulated by fascial manipulation are interstitial receptors (type III and IV), which have been shown to induce a change in local vasodilation (Klingler, Schleip, & Zorn, 2004). The additional group of Pacinian receptors seem to be involved in high-velocity manipulation, while Ruffini endings are mostly stimulated by slow deep-pressure techniques, especially if they involve tangential forces—that is, lateral stretch (Klingler et al., 2004). Stimulation of fascial mechanoreceptors leads to changes in muscle tonus that come primarily from a resetting of the gamma motor system, rather than from the more volitional alpha motor coordination. Additionally, stimulation of Ruffini organs as well as many of the interstitial receptors affects the autonomic nervous system and can result in a lowering of sympathetic tone or changes in local vasodilation (Klingler et al., 2004).

In addition, the clinician attempts to restore the fibers to their original length while also working to restore the thixotropic properties of the matrix by attempting to depolymerize the matrix and achieve increased fluidity. According to Kruger, if the fascial interstitial fibers are strongly stimulated, there will be an extrusion of plasma from the blood vessels into the interstitial fluid matrix (Kruger, 1987). Such a change in local fluid dynamics means a change in the viscosity of the ECM. Unless irreversible fibrotic changes have occurred or other pathologies exist, the state of fascia can be transformed from that of a gel-like substance (which limits movement) to a more watery, flexible solute state via therapeutic interventions applied by the clinician. Therapies may include introduction of energy through muscular activity (active or passive movement provided by activity or stretching), soft tissue manipulation (provided by massage, skin rolling), heat (hydrotherapies, manual friction), vibration (manually or mechanically applied), and nutritional intervention (rehydration).

What Is Earthing™?

The earth's surface has a steady supply of electrons; hence, the earth acts as a global electron circuit (Chavalier, 2007). The human body's soft tissues (e.g., fascia) consist of a liquid crystal medium that has piezoelectric properties and allows the body to act as an excellent conductor of electricity (electrons). The free electrons on the earth's surface are easily transferred to the human body as long as there is direct contact (Chevalier, Mori & Oschman, 2006). Hence, earthing™ can be performed by an activity as simple as removing one's shoes and socks and standing on the ground. Standing barefoot allows a natural flow of electrons to and from our bodies and connects us to vital earth rhythms that set many of our biological clocks.

Unfortunately, synthetically soled shoes act as insulators and shield the body from direct contact with the ground, thus negating any benefits from the earth's electric field (Marchesi, 1985). When we are in homes and office buildings, we are also insulated and unable to receive the Earth's balancing energies. However, recent development of earthing™ technology has produced a conductive mattress pad that is connected by a wire to a rod that is placed into the earth (Earthing™ and EarthFx Products, 2006). Electrons and microcurrents from the earth instantaneously flow up the rod and wire and into the mattress pad (Earthing™ and EarthFx Products, 2006). The restorative influences of the earth are then transferred to the body, which is a good electrical conductor.

The Physiological Effects of Earthing™ (Grounding) in the Body

Earthing™ is poised to shake up the health field. Research on the patented earthing™ systems has produced immediate systemic and lasting health effects (Chevalier, Mori, & Oschman, 2006). Most recently, a number of researchers have observed the following benefits from earthing™: rapid reduction of pain and inflammation, relief from sleep disorders and reduction in the stress hormone cortisol, and so on (Amalu, Hobbins, Head, & Kolinsky, 2005; Ghaly & Teplitz, 2004).

Clinical Applications

People who sleep earthed report better rest, more energy, and waking more refreshed. They also experience less pain, stiffness, soreness, irritation, agitation, and fatigue; faster healing; the disappearance of chronic health problems; and more physical capacity and vitality (Earthing™ and EarthFx, 2006).

Athletic Recovery

Clinical applications of earthing™ have been used in the sports medicine field, most recently in the Tour de France by Dr. Jeff Spencer. Earthing™ involves connecting injured or painful areas of the body to the earth via conductive patches or bands placed on the skin. Infrared thermography was used to document the reduction in inflammation with earthing™ (Amalu). Research in several laboratories has shown rapid and permanent resolution of inflammation, pain, redness, swelling, and stiffness. The method works for acute injuries as well as

chronic problems—even in cases that have persisted for decades.

Normally, the inflammatory process is necessary to destroy pathogens and repair damaged tissues. But ongoing medical research is demonstrating that pathological diseases in the human body—such as osteoarthritis, rheumatoid arthritis, atherosclerosis, diabetes mellitus, neurodegenerative diseases, and a host of others—have been attributed to inflammation characterized by the buildup of reactive oxygen species (ROS; see Wulf, 2002). Unregulated overproduction of scavengers, free radicals and their derivatives, occurs in living tissues at low but measurable concentrations that are determined by the balance between the rates of radical production and their corresponding rates of clearance. Free radicals are positively charged molecules in search of negatively charged electrons (Earthing™ and EarthFx, 2006). As such, these free radicals can exist for only a nanosecond, because they are strongly attracted to sources of electrons. In a normal controlled inflammatory reaction, free radicals obtain the electrons they need by stripping them away from bacteria or damaged tissue (Earthing™ and EarthFx, 2006). This process in turn kills the bacteria or breaks down the damaged tissue cells for removal from the body.

Physiological Effects of Free Radicals in the Body

The most relevant radicals in biological regulation are superoxide and nitric oxide (NO). These radicals are formed by two groups of enzymes—the NAD(P)H oxidase and NOS isoforms, respectively. Many regulatory effects are mediated by hydrogen peroxide and other ROS that are chemically derived from superoxide. The term *redox signaling* is widely used to describe a regulatory process in which the signal is delivered through redox chemistry. Redox signaling is used by a wide range of organisms, including bacteria, to induce protective responses against oxidative damage and to reset the original state of "redox homeostasis" after temporary exposure to ROS.

Physiological Aspects of Redox Regulation

The radicals NO and superoxide anion (O_2) play an important role in biological regulation. Superoxide gives rise to other forms of ROS that serve as mediators in many regulatory processes. Most redox-responsive regulatory mechanisms in bacteria and mammalian cells serve to protect the cells against oxidative stress and to reestablish redox homeostasis (Wulf, 2002). Prominent examples are (1) oxidative induction of protective enzymes by the redox-sensitive bacterial OxyR and SoxR proteins and (2) the inhibition of nitric oxide synthase (NOS) by NO.

Molecular Aspects of Redox Regulation: Gain or Loss of Function, or Outright Destruction

The capacity of ROS to damage proteins and to hasten their proteolytic degradation has been employed as a regulatory mechanism in several cases; for example, in the degradation of the transcription factor subunit HIF-1a and the NF-kB inhibitor IkB (Wulf, 2002). Inhibition of protein tyrosine phosphatases is well defined on a molecular basis and provides an example of redox regulation by loss of function. In other cases, NO or ROS induce a gain of function in a signaling protein (Wulf, 2002). This mechanism is involved in the regulation of vascular tone and the functional activation of the bacterial OxyR and SoxR proteins (Wulf, 2002).

The oxidative enhancement of membrane receptor signaling and the corresponding downstream signaling pathways are not well characterized at the molecular level. However, they are likely to involve the simultaneous induction of several different redox-sensitive signaling proteins (Wulf, 2002).

Regulated versus Uncontrolled Free Radical Production: Increased ROS Levels in Old Age and Disease

There is evidence that ROS production may be substantially elevated in old age and certain disease conditions. Excessive stimulation of NAD(P)H oxidase by cytokines or other mediators is implicated in various disease conditions. Other sources of superoxide, such as the mitochondrial electron transport chain and xanthine oxidase, are not tightly regulated and may become increasingly relevant in old age, diabetes mellitus, and malignant diseases (Wulf, 2002). Regarding the free radical theory of aging, we are seeing a shift in paradigm. Changes in redox-responsive signaling cascades and in the expression of corresponding target genes may have a similar or even greater impact on senescence as the direct radical-inflicted damage of cellular constituents (Wulf, 2002). Receptor signaling was also found to be strongly influenced by the intracellular glutathione level in all cases where appropriate experiments were performed (Wulf, 2002). Many redox-sensitive signaling cascades respond equally well to ROS or to changes in the intracellular thiol/disulfide redox state (Wulf, 2002).

The massive oxidative shift in the human plasma thiol/disulfide redox state between the third and the tenth decade of life may, therefore, alter the set point of redox-sensitive signaling pathways in various somatic cells (Wulf, 2002). The pro-oxidative shift may account for age-related immunological dysfunctions and inflammatory processes as well as for the loss of the replicative capacity of fibroblasts.

Chances for Therapeutic Intervention—Earthing™

To ensure ordered redox-mediated signaling, life requires a delicately balanced intermediate level of free radicals and radical-derived ROS. There are some encouraging recent reports about the use of SOD/catalase mimetics in certain experimental systems. Dietary antioxidants are widely used to ameliorate excessive oxidative stress, but scientific proof of their efficacy is scarce. There is, nevertheless, a strong possibility that the process of senescence and disease-related wasting results, at least to some extent, from a progressive shift in biochemical conditions that may not be irreversible in principle.

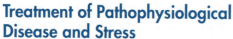

Treatment of Pathophysiological Disease and Stress

Oxidative stress plays a role in various clinical conditions such as malignant diseases, diabetes, atherosclerosis, chronic inflammation, human immunodeficiency virus (HIV) infection, ischemia reperfusion injury, and sleep apnea. These diseases fall into two major categories. In the first category, diabetes mellitus and cancer show commonly a pro-oxidative shift in the systemic thiol/disulfide redox state and impaired glucose clearance, suggesting that skeletal muscle mitochondria may be the major site of elevated ROS production (Wulf, 2002). These conditions may be referred to as mitochondrial oxidative stress. Without therapeutic intervention, these conditions lead to massive skeletal muscle wasting that is reminiscent of age-related wasting (Wulf, 2002). The second category may be referred to as inflammatory oxidative conditions because it is typically associated with an excessive stimulation of NAD(P)H oxidase activity by cytokines or other agents (Wulf, 2002). In this case, increased ROS levels or changes in intracellular glutathione levels are often associated with pathological changes indicative of a dysregulation of signal cascades and/or gene expression, exemplified by altered expression of cell adhesion molecules (Wulf, 2002). Earthing™ technology allows the flow of electrons from the earth back into the body, where they neutralize the positive charge of free radicals (Earthing™ and EarthFx, 2006). Once free radicals have been neutralized, they stop their destructive oxidative stress on the tissues, organs, and organ systems of the body (Earthing™ and EarthFx, 2006). Hence, scientists have extrapolated these observations and concluded that earthing™ acts as a natural anti-inflammatory that can result in a decreased incidence of chronic and debilitating diseases. EarthFx products represent a profound discovery that can affect the healing of many medical conditions and ailments that have plagued society. What we are learning from earthing™ is that dissociating ourselves from the electric field of our planet has had some serious long-term health consequences. These consequences are becoming more and more significant as people take on more and more stressful lifestyles. Disconnection from the earth has actually compromised the physiological systems that deal with stress and that permit recovery. The widespread incidence of both insomnia and chronic disease documents that our society in general is suffering serious consequences from the cycle of stress and lack of recovery.

Furthermore, there are some concerns regarding the possible biological effects of environmental fields. Living organisms and healing processes are extremely sensitive to environmental electric, magnetic, and electromagnetic fields. The Environmental Protection Agency recommends that consumers adopt "prudent avoidance" of extended exposure to 60 Hz and other electrical fields until science has determined whether such fields are harmful. Earthing™ causes an easily measurable decrease in the induced electrical field on the body, and at the same time has many positive health benefits.

Summary

Energy medicine involves electromagnetism, laser therapy, sound energy, and mechanical vibrations. Researchers have reported that healing can occur via tuning in the body to various energy fields. Various tissues and cells in the body respond to different frequencies of electrical current, and complementary medicine has focused on frequency-specific microcurrents (FSM), acupuncture, and therapeutic massage to enhance healing. Although energy medicine cannot be quantitatively assessed, there is enough anecdotal evidence to support claims of benefit over a placebo effect.

References

Amalu W., *Medical Thermography Case Studies.* Retrieved from http://www.earthfx.net/pdf/EFX_science_Amalu.pdf

Amalu, W., Hobbins, W., Head, J., & Kolinsky, D. (2005). Earth grounding and chronic inflammation: Alterations in plasma concentration levels of C-reactive protein. Project in progress.

Appleton, J. (2002). Arginine: Clinical potential of a semi-essential amino acid. *Alternative Medicine Review, 7*(6), 512–522.

Aumailley, M., & Gayraud, B. (1998). Structure and biological activity of the extracellular matrix. *Journal of Molecular Medicine, 76,* 253–265.

Ayala, A., Chung, C. S., Grutkoski, P. S., & Song, G. Y. (2003). Mechanisms of immune resolution. *Critical Care Medicine, 31*(8), S558–571.

Banes, A. J., Tsuzaki, M., Yamamoto, J., Fischer, T., Brigman, B., Brown, T., et al. (1995). Mechanoreception at the cellular level: The detection, interpretation and diversity of responses to mechanical signals. *Biochemistry & Cell Biology, 73,* 349–365.

Barros, E., Rodrigues, C. J., Rodrigues, N. R., Oliveira, R. P., Barros, T. P., & Rodrigues, Jr., A. J. (2002). Aging of the elastic and collagen fibers in the human cervical interspinous ligaments. *Spine Journal, 2,* 57–62.

Becker, R. (1967). The electrical control of growth processes. *Medical Times, 95,* 657–669.

Brand, R. A. (1997). What do tissues and cells know of mechanics? *Annals of Medicine, 29,* 267–269.

Burridge, K., Fath, K., Kelly, T., Nuckolls, G., & Turner, C. (1988). Focal adhesions: Transmembrane junctions between the extracellular matrix and the cytoskeleton. *Annual Review of Cell Biology, 4,* 487–525.

Chavalier, G. *The Earth's Electrical Surface Potential: A summary of present understanding.* Retrieved from http://www.earthfx.net/pdf/ EFX_science_Chevalier_EarthElecSurface.pdf.

Chevalier G., Mori K, and Oschman J. L., (2006). The effect of earthing™ (grounding) on human physiology. *European Biology and Bioelectromagnetics,* 600–621.

Chicurel, M. E., Chen, C. S., & Ingber. D. E. (1998). Cellular control lies in the balance of forces. *Current Opinion in Cell Biology, 10,* 232–239.

Duncan, R. L., & Turner, C. H. (1995). Mechanotransduction and the functional response of bone to mechanical strain. *Calcified Tissue International, 57,* 344–358.

Earthing™ and EarthFx Products. (2006). *A summary of research and development.* Retrieved from www.earthfx.net.

Fujimaki, Y., Shimoyama, T., Liu, Q., Umeda, T., Nakaji, S., & Sugawara, K. (2003). Low-level laser irradiation attenuates production of reactive oxygen species by human neutrophils. *Journal of Clinical Laser Medicine & Surgery, 21*(3), 165–170.

Ghaly, M., & Teplitz, D. (2004). The biologic effects of grounding the human body during sleep, measured by cortisol levels and subjective reporting of sleep, pain and stress. *Journal of Alternative & Complementary Medicine, 10*(5), 767–776.

Giancotti, F. G., & Ruoslahti, E. (1999). Integrin signaling. *Science, 285,* 1028–1032.

Gunn, C. C. (1976). Acupuncture loci: A proposal for their classification according to their relationship to known neural structures. *American Journal of Clinical Medicine, 4,* 183–195.

Ho, M. W. (1997). Quantum coherence and conscious experience. *Kybernetes, 26,* 265–276.

Ho, M. W., Popp, F. A., & Warnke, U. (1994). *Bioelectrodynamics and biocommunication.* Singapore: World Scientific.

Karu, T. (2001). Changes in absorbance of monolayer of living cells induced by laser radiation at 633, 670, and 820 nm. *Quantum Electronics, 7*(6): 982–988.

Kauffman, S. A. (1994). *The origins of order: Self-organization and selection in evolution.* Oxford: Oxford University Press.

Kinakin, K. (2004). *Optimal muscle training.* Windsor, ON: Human Kinetics.

Kleinkort, J. *The emerging paradigm of LLLT.* Retrieved October 15, 2007, from http://www.erchonia.com/pages/research_emerginparadigm.htm

Klingler, W., Schleip, R., & Zorn, A. (2004). European fascia research report. *Structural Integration (Journal of the Rolf Institute),*1–10.

Kruger, L. (1987). Cutaneous sensory system. In G. Adelman (Ed.), *Encyclopedia of Neuroscience,* Vol. 1 (p. 293). Cambridge, MA: Birkhauser, Boston.

Lamotte, M., Strulens, G., Niset, G., & Van de Borne, Ph. (2005). Influence of different resistive training modalities on blood pressure and heart rate responses of healthy subjects. *Isokinetics & Exercise Science, 13,* 273–277.

Langevin, H. M., Churchill, D. L., & Cipolla, M. J. (2001). Mechanical signaling through connective tissue: A mechanism for the therapeutic effect of acupuncture. *FASEB Journal, 15,* 2275–2282.

Langevin, H. M., & Yandow, J. A. (2002). Relationship of acupuncture points and meridians to connective tissue planes. *Anatomical Record, 269,* 257–265.

Lee, W. R., Shen, S. C., Lai, H. H., & Hu, C. H. (2001). Transdermal drug delivery enhanced and controlled by erbium: YAG laser—a comparative study of lipophilic and hydrophilic drugs. *Journal of Controlled Release, 75,* 155–166.

Lin, L. H., & Hopf, H. W. (2003). Paradigm of the injury-repair continuum during critical illness. *Critical Care Medicine, 31*(8), S493–495.

Marchesi, V. T. (1985). Inflammation and healing. In J. M. Kissans & W.A.D. Anderson (Eds.), *Anderson's pathology,* 8th ed. (Chapter 2, pp. 22–60). St. Louis, MO: CV Mosby.

McCraty, R., Atkinson, M., Tomasino, D., & Tiller, W. A. (1998). The electricity of touch: Detection and measurement of cardiac energy exchange between people. In K. H. Pribram (Ed.), *Brain and values: Is a biological science of values possible?* (pp. 359–379). Mahwah, NJ: Erlbaum.

McMakin, C. R. (2004). Microcurrent therapy: A novel treatment method for chronic low back myofascial pain. *Journal of Bodywork & Movement Therapies, 8,* 143–153.

Miyake, K., & McNeil, P. L. (1985). Mechanical injury and repair of cells. *Critical Care Medicine, 31*(8), S496–501.

Monnier, V. M., Mustata, G. T., Biemel, K. L., Reihl, O., Lederer, M. O., Zhenyu, D., et al. (2005). Cross-linking of the extracellular matrix by the Maillard reaction in aging and diabetes: An update on "a puzzle nearing resolution". *Annals of the New York Academy of Science, 1043,* 533–544.

Oschman, J. L. (1998). The cytoskeleton: Mechanical, physical, and biological interactions. *Biological Bulletin, 194*(3), 321–418.

Oschman, J. L. (2000). *Energy medicine.* London: Churchill Livingstone.

Oschman, J. L. (1997). What is healing energy? Part 3A: Silent pulses. *Journal of Bodywork & Movement Therapies, 1,* 185–186.

Oschman, J. L., & Oschman, N. H. (1994). Somatic recall, Parts I–II: Soft tissue memory/soft tissue holography, massage therapy. *American Journal of Massage Therapy Association, 34,* 36–45, 66–67, 101–167.

Plummer, J. P. (1980). Anatomical findings at acupuncture loci. *American Journal of Clinical Medicine, 8,* 170–180.

Reddy, K. G. (2004). Photobiological basis and clinical role of low-intensity lasers in biology and medicine. *Journal of Clinical Laser Medicine & Surgery, 22*(2): 141–150.

Rubin, C. T., McLeod, K. J., & Lanyon, L. E. (1989). Prevention of osteoporosis by pulsed electromagnetic fields. *Journal of Bone & Joint Surgery, 71-A*(3), 411–417.

Ryan, T. J. (1989). Biochemical consequences of mechanical forces generated by distention and distortion. *Journal of the American Academy of Dermatology, 21,* 115–130.

Schleip, R. (2003a). Fascial plasticity—a new neurobiological explanation: Part 1. *Journal of Bodywork & Movement Therapies, 7*(1), 11–19.

Schleip, R. (2003b). Fascial plasticity—a new neurobiological explanation: Part 2. *Journal of Bodywork & Movement Therapies, 7*(2), 104–116.

Siskin, B. F., & Walker, J. (1995). Therapeutic aspects of electromagnetic fields for soft-tissue healing. In M. Blank (Ed.), *Electromagnetic fields: Biological interactions and mechanisms.* (Advances in Chemistry Series 250, pp. 277–285). Washington, DC: American Chemical Society.

Stoltz, J. F., Dumas, D., Wang, X., Payan, E., Mainard, D., Paulus, F., et al. (2000). Influence of mechanical forces on cells and tissues. *Biorheology, 37,* 3–14.

Turner, J., & Hode, L. (2002). *Laser therapy.* Grangesberg, Sweden: Prima Books.

Van Breugel, H. H., & Bar, P. R. (1992). Power and density and exposure time of He–Ne laser irradiation are more important than total energy dose in photo-biomodulation of human fibroblasts in vitro. *Lasers in Surgery & Medicine, 12*(5), 528–537.

Wang K., & Liu, J. (1989). Needling sensation receptor of an acupoint supplied by the median nerve—studies of their electrophysiological characteristics. *American Journal of Chinese Medicine, 17,* 145–155.

Wang K., Yao S., Xian Y., & Hou Z. (1985). A study on the receptive field of acupoints and the relationship between characteristics of needling sensation and groups of afferent tissues. *Scientia Sinica, 28,* 963–971.

Weinberg, G. M. (2003). *An introduction to general systems thinking.* New York: Dorset House.

Werb, Z., & Gordon, S. (2005). Secretion of a specific collagenase by stimulated macrophages. *Journal of Experimental Medicine, 142,* 346–360.

Wulf, D. (2002). Free radicals in the physiological control of cell function. *Physiology Review, 82,* 47–95.

Zhai, N. (1988). Research on the histophysiological relation of mastocytes and meridians (Chinese). *Clinical Acupuncture Moxibust, 8,* 50–53.

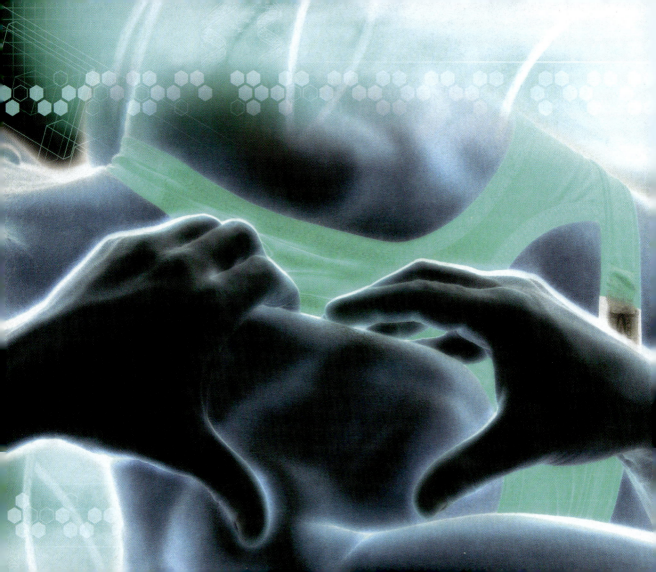

NUTRITION AND FASCIAL HEALTH

Fascia is a tough connective tissue that spreads throughout the body in a three-dimensional web from head to foot without interruption. The fascia surrounds every muscle, bone, nerve, blood vessel, and organ of the body, all the way down to the cellular level. Therefore, malfunction of the fascial system due to trauma, posture, or inflammation can create a "binding down" of the fascia, resulting in abnormal pressure on nerves, muscles, bones, or organs.

Fascial pathologies occur when fascial restrictions/distortions in the living matrix arise and need to be accurately diagnosed before proceeding with treatment. Most practitioners tend to limit their scope of treatment to physical therapy, such as trigger point therapy. Treating soft tissue should encompass treating causative factors such as the following:

o   Repetitive motions; excessive exercise; muscle strain due to overactivity

o   Lack of activity (leg or arm in a sling)

o   Nutritional deficiencies

o   Nervous tension or stress

o   Generalized fatigue

o   Sudden trauma to muscles, ligaments, or tendons

o   Hormonal changes (PMS or menopause)

A global approach to treatment must address the mechanical and biochemical modifications that trigger a microscopic structural change within tissues. Most practitioners address only the mechanical dysfunction of fascia. The purpose of this review is to introduce other treatment options that practitioners can employ in treating the fascial pathologies leading to physiological malfunction of tissues and organs that fascia encompasses.

NUTRITIONAL INTAKE AND ITS EFFECTS ON CONNECTIVE TISSUE HEALING

Nearly all knowledge gathered about the nutritional influences on human connective tissues is extrapolated from investigations with in vitro tissue and cell research, animal models, and clinical and surgical practice. Human in vivo investigations are costly and relatively difficult because serum levels of nutrients ordinarily inadequately reflect total body content. Measuring total body level of specific nutrients is complex and sometimes impossible. Measuring direct clinical effects on specific tissues resulting from individual nutrients in humans is equally complicated. Nearly all human measurements are indirect and from clinical studies.

Several studies have demonstrated that collagen production is sensitive to changes in short- and long-term food intake (Ruberg, 1984; Tinker & Rucker, 1985; Berg & Kerr, 1992). Within 24 hours of fasting, animal models have clearly shown a significant reduction of 50% in the rate of collagen synthesis in articular cartilage when compared to normal conditions. This reduction declines to 8–12% of control levels after 96 hours (Berg & Kerr, 1992). Most conditions are not as severe as starvation. However, energy restriction may reduce collagen synthesis, depending on duration and degree of food deprivation. Specific effects of malnutrition on connective tissue turnover depend on many factors, such as exercise activities, injuries, and disease. Nutrition restriction effects also may be age related. Youngsters who are still growing are more sensitive to nutritional changes (Tinker & Rucker, 1985). Replacement of tissue pools of macronutrients requires weeks to months and certainly affects turnover rates of tissue components.

Likewise, dietary deficiencies or excesses and physical activities influence turnover rates.

Caloric Intake

Calories provide the body with cellular energy for normal metabolism, building and repairing tissues, and stimulating hormonal responses. Individuals subjected to injuries to the fascia should avoid a reduction in caloric intake, even though their level of activity may have decreased overall. Instead they should focus on meeting a basic caloric intake equivalent to their maintenance level or slightly above, ensuring that the body's connective tissues are receiving adequate nutrients and energy for healing and repair of soft tissue.

Considering that fascia is created from all macronutrients, it is imperative to thoroughly understand the role of each macronutrient in the healing and maintenance of physiological function and anatomical structure.

Protein

Prolonged caloric restriction will generally result in a subsequent protein intake deficiency that in turn will be reflected by an increased rate of protein breakdown in the muscle tissue. This condition may be evident in elite athletes performing ultra-endurance activities and mountaineers whose energy consumption may be compromised; the result is loss of muscle protein and subsequent reduction in exercise performance (Friedlander, Braun, Pollack, MacDonald, Fulco, Musa, et al., 2005).

The two major sources of protein during times of bulk loss are muscle and connective tissue. Muscle tissue provides a steady source of amino acids, which serve numerous body functions such as those described in Table 11-1.

Table 11-1 Amino Acids and Their Function in the Body

Alanine An important source of energy for muscle tissue, the brain, and the central nervous system; strengthens the immune system by producing antibodies; helps in the metabolism of sugars and organic acids.

Arginine Significantly contributes to insulin production, muscle metabolism, and liver lipid metabolism; is a component of collagen. Arginine is a factor for maintaining the nitrogen balance in muscles and can enhance the body fat ratio of lean tissue to fat tissue (an important factor for weight management). Arginine also neutralizes ammonia, which helps in liver detoxification and regeneration. As a component of collagen, arginine can assist with wound healing, skin problems, arthritis, and connective tissue problems.

Asparagine Found mostly in meat sources, so vegetarians might need to consider supplementation. Asparagine balances the central nervous system and prevents excess nervousness and anxiety or excessive calmness and depression.

Aspartic acid Aids in the expulsion of harmful ammonia from the circulatory system. When ammonia enters the circulatory system, it acts as a highly toxic substance that can be harmful to the central nervous system and cause neural and brain disorders. Aspartic acid deficiency decreases cellular energy and may likely be a factor in chronic fatigue.

Carnitine Helps transport fat from adipose cells to the mitochondria of muscle cells so it can be utilized for energy. Carnitine is an important nutrient for diabetes prevention since poor fat metabolism is a causative factor for the development of type 2 diabetes. It is also used for heart disease prevention because it lowers triglycerides, improves organ muscle strength, and enhances the antioxidant effectiveness of vitamins C and E. Also, studies indicate that carnitine treatments can reduce the effects of cardiac surgery damage to the heart.

Citrulline Functions primarily in the liver. Like other amino acids, citrulline detoxifies ammonia, is involved in the energy cycle, and enhances the immune system.

Cysteine and Cystine These amino acids are structured very similarly and convert into each other as needed. They are involved in collagen production for skin elasticity and texture, and for alpha-keratin for fingernails, toenails, and hair. In fact, hair and skin are made up of 10–14% cystine. This makes supplemental cysteine great for burn and surgery recovery, and it is recommended in treating rheumatoid arthritis. Cysteine is a powerful free radical destroyer by itself, but it works best when vitamin E and selenium are present. It helps detoxify and protect the body from radiation damage, so it is often used in conjunction with chemotherapy and radiation cancer treatments. Cysteine is a precursor to the liver-detoxifying and antioxidant amino acid glutathione. This functionality has an antiaging effect on the body—even reducing the accumulation of age spots. Another impressive function is the breakdown of mucus in the respiratory tract, which can help in bronchitis, emphysema, and tuberculosis.

N-acetylcysteine The best form of cysteine supplementation; has been proven more effective at increasing glutathione levels than supplements of glutathione itself, or supplements of L-cysteine alone.

Dimethylglycine (DMG) Participates in formation of methionine, choline, DNA, and several neurotransmitters. DMG is good for the heart. It has been found to lower blood cholesterol and triglycerides, and its helps normalize blood pressure and blood glucose.

(continued)

Table 11-1 Amino Acids and Their Function in the Body (continued)

Gamma-aminobutyric acid (GABA) Functions in the central nervous system as a neurotransmitter; GABA occupies the nerve receptor sites for anxiety or stress-related messages so they are restrained from reaching the brain.

Glutamic acid The precursor of GABA, glutamic acid has somewhat the opposite function; it is an excitatory neurotransmitter. It is one of the few nutrients that crosses the blood–brain barrier and is the only means of detoxifying ammonia in the brain.

Glutamine Readily passes the blood–brain barrier and increases the amount of glutamic acid and GABA, thereby enhancing normal nervous system function. As amino acids chemically change, ammonia is released. Glutamine plays a role in removing this toxic ammonia from the brain. Because glutamine's role in the nervous system is so important, during times of stress, illness, or surgery, up to one-third of the muscle stores of glutamine are released for nervous system usage, causing extensive muscle deterioration and loss. The muscle glutamine release is much lower if glutamine levels are increased through supplemental L-glutamine. Supplemental L-glutamine is also used therapeutically in treating arthritis, autoimmune diseases, impotence, schizophrenia, and tissue damage from cancer radiation treatments.

Glutathione The liver produces glutathione from the amino acids cysteine, glutamic acid, and glycine. Glutathione deficiency results in early aging and in the loss of coordination, balance, tremors, and mental disorders. Glutathione levels decline with age; if not corrected, they will accelerate the aging process, so supplementation is important. But the assimilation of supplemental oral glutathione is questionable. Instead it is best to supplement with cysteine, glutamic acid, and glycine and have the body use those raw materials to manufacture needed glutathione.

Glycine Supplies additional creatine to muscles and is used to construct DNA and RNA. It functions in skin, connective tissues, the central nervous system, and the prostate.

Histidine Found abundantly in red and white blood cells; is a component of the myelin sheaths that protect nerve cells. Used in the treatment of arthritis, allergies, and ulcers.

Isoleucine One of three branched-chain amino acids (the others are leucine and valine) that enhance energy, increase endurance, and aid in muscle tissue recovery and repair. These amino acids also lower elevated blood sugar levels and increase growth hormone production. Supplemental isoleucine should always be combined with leucine and valine at a respective milligram ratio of 1:2:2.

Leucine One of three branched-chain amino acids (the others are isoleucine and valine) that enhance energy, increase endurance, and aid in muscle tissue recovery and repair. These amino acids also lower elevated blood sugar levels and increase growth hormone production. Supplemental leucine should always be combined with isoleucine and valine at a respective milligram ratio of 2:1:2.

Lysine Especially needed for adequate absorption of calcium and bone development in children. It aids in the production of antibodies, hormones, and enzymes.

Methionine A principal supplier of sulfur, which inactivates free radicals. Adequate methionine prevents disorders of the hair, skin, and nails; helps to lower cholesterol by increasing the liver's production of lecithin; reduces liver fat; and protects the kidneys.

(continued)

Table 11-1 Amino Acids and Their Function in the Body (continued)

Ornithine Participates in the release of growth hormone, which then prompts the metabolism of excess body fat. This process is enhanced by the presence of arginine and carnitine.

Phenylalanine Used by the brain to produce dopamine and norepinephrine, chemicals that promote alertness, elevate mood, decrease pain, aid in memory and learning, and reduce hunger and appetite.

Proline Obtained primarily from meat; aids in maintaining collagen (skin protein). Proline deficiency will cause an uncareful vegetarian to have early signs of skin aging. Proline also strengthens joints, tendons, connective tissue, and cartilage.

Serine A storage source of glucose by the liver and muscles; helps strengthen the immune system by providing antibodies; synthesizes fatty acid sheath around nerve fibers.

Taurine Helps stabilize the excitability of membranes, which is important in controlling epileptic seizures. Taurine and sulfur are considered to be factors necessary for the control of many biochemical changes that take place in the aging process; aids in the clearing of free radical wastes.

Threonine An important constituent of collagen, elastin, and enamel protein; helps prevent fat buildup in the liver; helps the digestive and intestinal tracts function more smoothly; assists metabolism and assimilation.

Tryptophan A natural relaxant; helps alleviate insomnia by inducing normal sleep; reduces anxiety and depression; helps in the treatment of migraine headaches; helps the immune system function; helps reduce the risk of artery and heart spasms; works with lysine in reducing cholesterol levels.

Tyrosine Promotes the healthy functioning of the thyroid, adrenal, and pituitary glands. Reduces appetite and helps to reduce body fat. Research indicates tyrosine may help chronic fatigue, narcolepsy, anxiety, depression, allergies, headaches, and Parkinson's disease.

Valine One of three branched-chain amino acids (the others are leucine and isoleucine) that enhance energy, increase endurance, and aid in muscle tissue recovery and repair. These amino acids also lower elevated blood sugar levels and increase growth hormone production. Supplemental valine should always be combined with isoleucine and leucine at a respective milligram ratio of 2:1:2.

Connective tissue is the second source of protein, which is reflective of the relative rate of turnover to muscle tissue (Tinker & Rucker, 1985). Many studies have demonstrated that a protein-deficient diet results in a reduction of growth and development of the organism as well as delay in wound healing and repairs (Ruberg, 1984).

All of the essential amino acids are necessary for synthesis of protein, growth factors, immune factors, and other components of the extracellular matrix (Tinker & Rucker, 1985). Some studies have shown that supplementing certain individual amino acids (methionine, lysine, arginine, and proline) to a protein-deficient diet may shorten the inflammation phase of connective tissue healing and aid in cross-linking of collagen fibers during the repair process of soft tissue healing (Ruberg, 1984). Countless studies demonstrate that protein malnutrition is significantly detrimental to normal turnover and healing of connective tissues, and most athletes are generally well nourished with protein intake. Unless an individual presents with severe trauma, surgery, or diabetes, a protein deficit that would negatively affect normal connective tissue metabolism should not be an issue.

Carbohydrates

Carbohydrates are a major component of an athlete's diet. They supply an efficient source of energy in the form of a monosaccharide known as glucose. Although little information exists on the direct effects of glucose deficiencies on connective tissues, it is well known that glucose is an energy source for several components and growth mediators. Phagocytes and other white cells that mediate the inflammatory process utilize glucose as an energy source. Activity by these cells during the acute and healing phases prepares tissue for repair after injury. Tissue cells such as fibroblasts and chondroblasts require glucose for synthesis of various macromolecules (Fisher, Mclennan, Tada, Heffernan, Yue, & Turtle, 1991). Glucose is a building block of glycosaminoglycans and glycoproteins in the ground substance of the matrix. Arguably, hypoglycemia (abnormally low level of plasma glucose) impairs normal cell function and delays wound healing (Ruberg, 1984). Production and release of several hormones, such as insulin and growth hormone, also decline with low levels of plasma glucose and further delay tissue growth and repair (Ruberg, 1984).

Conversely, high levels of plasma glucose may also be detrimental. Decreased insulin function may lead to hyperglycemia (abnormally high levels of plasma glucose), which also impairs wound healing (Ruberg, 1984). High levels of plasma glucose reportedly may inhibit the stimulatory action of ascorbic acid on proteoglycan and collagen production. Furthermore, recall that chronic high plasma and tissue glucose levels produce advanced glycation end products (AGE) that affect the physical, chemical, and mechanical properties of collagen and elastin protein (Serra, 1991). Although associated with aging, the AGE process is prematurely evident in diabetics. Proper glycemic control may delay the onset of complications related to excessive glycation and oxidation stress. For some type 2 diabetics, exogenous insulin may be necessary for glycemic control. Additionally, avoiding a diet with

excessive carbohydrate intake may prevent high accumulation of glycation and oxidative products.

Diets low in carbohydrates typically cause body water loss. For athletes, the resultant dehydration may compromise integrity of the connective tissues subject to mechanical loading. Considering that many connective tissues, such as in fascia, require relatively high water content for optimal functioning under stress, dehydration may increase incidence of injury and reduce the speed of healing and repair of injured fascia.

Fats

Fats are calorically dense and provide energy for the body. Both saturated and polyunsaturated fatty acids (PUFAs) act as precursors for hormones such as steroids and prostaglandins. PUFAs are essential constituents of the cell membrane, contributing to their structural and functional integrity. Saturated fats are commonly found in animal foods and in some vegetable plants and have little direct importance in the physiology of connective tissue. Hence there will be a greater focus (in this section) on the role of PUFAs on injured connective tissue.

PUFAs can be divided into two main subgroups: omega-3 and omega-6. The North American diet is particularly low in omega-6 fatty acids because diets are generally low in fish oils, which are the main source for this type of PUFA. Polyunsaturated fatty acids are precursors for a family of hormones, referred to as eicosanoids, that are released by macrophages and other cells. Eicosanoids have powerful autocrine (act on cell where released) and paracrine (act on nearby cell) actions. The major role of eicosanoids is in the inflammatory response; therefore, dietary PUFAs may moderate the length of the inflammatory phase (Serra, 1991).

Omega 6 gives rise to either series 1 or 2 eicosanoids. The preferred pathway is formation of series 1 eicosanoids but series 2 is formed predominantly. Omega-3 gives rise to series 3 eicosanoids. Series 2 eicosanoids are pro-inflammatory while series 1 and 3 are anti-inflammatory. Increasing the dietary ratio of omega-3 to omega-6 may decrease macrophage prostaglandin E_2 (PGE_2) and cytokine release and restore a balance between the eicosanoids, resulting in a reduction in inflammation and an enhanced healing and repair rate of connective tissue. Although increasing intake of n-3 PUFAs may not affect acute inflammation, such nutritional support quite possibly could moderate long-term inflammation related to excessive PGE_2 production and cytokine release from activated macrophages (Serra, 1991).

As we have seen, dietary macronutrient deficiencies and excesses influence metabolism of connective tissue components during growth, stress, and repair. Conceivably, nutrition may be used as adjunct therapy for tissue repair. However, most commonly, pharmaceuticals are used to moderate symptoms of inflammation resulting from injuries that may potentially interfere with normal turnover or repair of tissues (Bucci, 1995).

The following are additional dietary recommendations that will improve overall health:

○ Limit intake of stimulants (caffeine) and depressants (alcohol) because of their potential to disrupt neurological and metabolic function.

○ Limit intake of refined sugars to avoid fluctuation of blood sugar levels, mood swings, lowered energy, and lowered immunity.

○ Consume whole foods, such as fruits and vegetables, that contain phytochemicals and fiber. Fiber is helpful for maintaining digestive regularity. Eat more slowly, chewing food well.

○ Increase intake of cold-water fish, which supply essential fatty acid building blocks—gamma linolenic acid (GLA) and eicosapentaenoic acid (EPA)—that are needed for cell membrane maintenance and function.

○ Increase intake of probiotic cultures from food or supplements. (Probiotics are "health-promoting"

bacteria that normally reside in the gastrointestinal tract. Health-promoting bacteria aid the proper digestion of food and prevent the absorption of ingested toxins).

○ Drink plenty of water (preferably purified) to ensure adequate fluid levels.

SPECIFIC NUTRIENTS

Exercise has been linked to amino acid oxidation and increased muscle tissue loss if adequate protein is not available. Amino acid supplementation during exercise contributes to energy metabolism and increased protein synthesis.

Arginine

Injury significantly increases the need for the amino acid arginine, which is essential for a variety of metabolic functions. Animal studies have demonstrated that, following surgical trauma, dietary supplementation with arginine results in an increase in nitrogen retention and increased body weight, both of which are essential for successful recovery (Mane, Fernandez-Banares, Ojanguren, Castella, Bertran, Bartoli, et al., 2001). Supplementing arginine in patients who had major wounds significantly increased the amount of reparative collagen synthesized at the site of a "standard wound" (an incision 5 cm long and 1 mm in diameter, into which a catheter was inserted) made in healthy volunteers (Kirk, Hurson, Regan, Holt, Waserkrug, & Barbul, 1993). The same study found marked enhancement of the activity and efficacy of peripheral T-lymphocytes (white blood cells in the bloodstream).

Clinical studies have shown improved immune function in cancer patients fed arginine. Arginine's ability to improve wound healing and immune system function is thought to be related to its ability to stimulate the production of growth hormone. Growth hormone plays a critical role in modulating the immune system and is essential for muscle growth and development. That growth hormone secretion diminishes progressively with advancing age is one of the primary reasons for the decline in immune system function and muscular strength as we grow older. To accelerate wound healing, a supplemental dose of 10–22 grams of supplemental arginine daily is recommended.

Carnosine

Carnosine, a naturally occurring amino acid, was found to stimulate granulation and promote wound healing (Nagai & Suda, 1988). The breakdown product of carnosine, beta alanine, stimulates collagen and nucleic acid biosynthesis (Nagai, Suda, Kawasaki, & Mathuura, 1986). Typical dosing recommendations are 100 mg to 200 mg daily on an empty stomach. Possible side effects associated with a daily intake greater than 1,000 mg are muscle twitching, irritability, and insomnia.

Glutamine

The amino acid glutamine is an important substrate for rapidly proliferating cells, including lymphocytes (white blood cells). It is also the major amino acid lost during muscle protein catabolism in the initial response to injury. De-Souza and Greene (1998) documented the beneficial effects of supplementing burn victims with high doses of arginine and glutamine; this treatment significantly enhanced wound repair by stimulating an increased rate of collagen cross-linking.

Copper

Copper has been shown to play an important role in the healing of soft tissue injuries. The role of copper in the biosynthesis of bone and connective tissue has been well established, although its mechanism of action is only partially known (Tenaud, Leroy, Chebassier, & Dreno, 2000). Copper supplementation enhances bone healing. It works with vitamin C to create strong collagen, and it creates cross-links in collagen and elastin that strengthen the proteins that compose fascia. The typical dosing regimen requires a daily intake of 2 to 3 mg orally. At high doses (e.g., 1 gram), copper can cause numerous side effects and interactions such as the following: renal failure, gastrointestinal upset, and cardiovascular collapse. Vitamin C in doses of 1,500 mg daily reduces ceruloplasmin activity, resulting in high blood copper levels. Zinc in large doses can reduce copper absorption (*Natural Medicines Comprehensive Database*, 1999).

Zinc

Zinc plays a well-documented role in wound healing. Although zinc is present in the body in only a small quantity, it is found in many tissues, including bone, skin, muscle, and organs. It is a component of DNA, RNA, and numerous enzyme systems that participate in tissue growth and healing. Zinc appears to play little role in the initial inflammatory stages of wound repair but a greater role in the later stages of tissue repair and regeneration (Gray, 2003). Recommended daily intake is 15 mg daily for men and 12 mg daily for women. High doses of zinc are associated with gastrointestinal distress, and impairment of iron and copper absorption that may cause anemia (*Natural Medicines*, 1999).

Orthosilicic Acid

Orthosilicic acid is responsible for maintaining and building bone via the stimulation of type 1 collagen production by osteoblasts (Reffit, Ogston, Jugdaohsingh, Cheung, Evans, Thompson, et al., 2003; Calomme & Van den Berghe, 1997). Orthosilicic acid also plays a role in the formation of several components of the extracellular matrix comprising connective tissue. A recommended daily dose of stabilized orthosilicic acid ranges from 6 mg to 20 mg.

EPA

In vitro experiments done on ligament healing showed that the effect of omega-3 PUFAs (eicosapentaenoic acid–EPA) on collagen synthesis can be partially explained through its effect on PGE_2. When PGE_2 levels are low, the interleukin-6 (IL-6) level in tissues and collagen is increased. Only omega-3 PUFAs increase collagen production (through decreased PGE$_2$ production). In contrast, omega-6 PUFAs decrease collagen synthesis, resulting in a reduction in the rate of repair of fascia (Hankenson, Watkins, Schoenlein, Allen, & Turek, 2000). A recommended daily dose is 5 grams of fish oil containing EPA and docosahexanoic acid (DHA) twice daily (orally) with food. The most common side effects experienced while using EPA are an increased risk of bleeding due to its anticoagulant effects; use with caution in patients using heparin or warfarin. EPA can theoretically interfere with blood glucose control in diabetics; this effect can be potentiated with the use of antidiabetic drugs. Other side effects include loose stools and nosebleeds with high doses as well as belching and fishy taste (*Natural Medicines*, 1999).

Aloe Vera

Aloe vera is a plant well known for centuries to have healing properties. Aloe vera contains up to 200 different substances beneficial to the human body. These substances include enzymes, glycoproteins, growth factors, vitamins, and minerals. Long-chain sugars, or mucopolysaccharides (especially acemannan), have been of particular interest for their remarkable properties.

Aloe vera is commonly considered a general tonic for increasing well-being and longevity. It provides the micronutrients required for protein synthesis. Its many components work together to reduce inflammation and pain, promote healing, and stop infection. Some of these components cause cells to divide and multiply; some stimulate the growth of white blood cells. Aloe vera also enhances cell wall permeability, increasing cell access to nutrients and facilitating the removal of toxins from the cells. Aloe can be applied topically to wounds and taken internally for both skin wounds and gastrointestinal ulcers (Chithra, Sajithal, & Chandrakasan, 1998).

Aloe's mode of action may be through modulating macrophage function in the wound, enabling an immune response that ingests and destroys foreign pathogens (Zhang & Tizard, 1996). It has been sug-

gested that aloe works as a free radical scavenger and improves blood flow to the wound (Heggers, Elzaim, Garfield, Goodheart, Listengarten, Zhao, et al., 1997). A recommended daily oral dose of aloe vera is 50 to 200 mg daily of aloe gel (capsules). Aloe vera gel for internal use is obtained from the mucilaginous cells of the inner central zone of the leaf. Aloe juice is extracted from cells beneath the plant's skin and contains potent anthrone cathartics that have laxative and electrolyte-depleting effects. Some cross-contamination of extracted aloe gel with anthrones may occur. Theoretical interactions of anthrones may occur with digoxin, diuretics, and antiarrhythmic drugs. Oral aloe gel may increase the hypoglycemic effects of glyburide (diabetic medication; Jellin, Batz, & Hitchens, 1999).

Bromelain

Bromelain is found in pineapple and contains a proteolytic enzyme with the ability to break down, or dissolve, proteins. This mechanism of action can be helpful in chronic wounds or wounds having too much scar tissue. Bromelain speeds up healing time after surgical procedures and shows positive effects in the treatment of athletic injuries through reduction in inflammation and pain from injuries of the musculoskeletal system (Thorne Research, 1996).

Curcumin

Curcumin is an extract of the spice turmeric, known to have antioxidant properties and other health benefits. In Indian medicine, curcumin is used to reduce inflammation and treat wounds and skin ulcers. Researchers know that curcumin suppresses a factor that influences growth factors. This factor, nuclear factor kappa B (NF-κB), plays a prominent role in immunity and cell growth. Immediately after muscle injury, the immune system dispatches cells to the area. Their job is to destroy old tissue and begin new construction. NF-κB is one of the lines of communication used in immune cell function. By influencing NF-κB, curcumin modulates the repair process.

Muscle regeneration is a complex phenomenon. Curcumin works in part by changing the arrival time and status of chemical messengers known as cytokines. Cytokines appear at the scene early on, and they have a powerful effect on inflammation and cell growth. A cytokine known as interleukin-6 (IL-6), for example, makes muscle cells multiply. Another cytokine, called tumor necrosis factor (TNF), keeps cells from developing. By suppressing one, and enhancing the other, curcumin can speed up muscle regeneration.

Curcumin has a rapid effect on enhancing the healing rate of damaged muscle tissue. This implies that taking curcumin as soon as the injury occurs would be most beneficial. Curcumin may be useful not only for accidental injuries or sports but also to help repair surgical damage (Sidhu, Mani, Gaddipati, Singh, Seth, Banaudha, et al., 1999).

Typical recommended dosing involves oral dosages in the range of 0.5 to 3 grams (powdered root), taken daily in divided doses. Curcumin may cause gastrointestinal distress and is contraindicated in bile duct obstruction and peptic ulcer. Caution should be used in concomitant therapy with antiplatelet drugs due to theoretical additive blood-thinning effects (*Natural Medicines,* 1999).

Centella (Gotu Kola)

Centella has been found to induce levels of antioxidants in wounds and newly formed tissue, including superoxide dismutase, glutathione peroxidase, vitamin E, and vitamin C. Centella improves collagen formation and angiogenesis (Shukla, Rasik, Jain, Shankar, Kulshrestha, & Dhawan, 1999). A review article of centella noted that the most beneficial effects to date involved the stimulation and mutation of scar tissue by production of type I collagen and an inhibition of the inflammatory reaction. The ability of centella to aid in wound healing can be applied to connective tissue injuries involving fascia, and it can be used on a prophylactic basis.

Superoxide Dismutase (SOD)

During the initial phase of wound healing, immune cells are rushed to the wound site to protect against harmful invaders. They actually use free radicals to fight bacteria and to dispose of dead tissue. Once the free radicals have accomplished their job, however, they must be neutralized so the actual healing process can begin. SOD and other antioxidants such as vitamins C and D stop the free radical oxidation process and promote the healing and repair process itself. Soft tissue injuries can deplete SOD levels as well as those of other antioxidants (Ballmer, Reinhart, Jordan, Buhler, Moser, & Gey, 1994). SOD should be supplemented to encourage new tissue to grow, to enhance collagen, and to reduce swelling. Current research indicates that SOD taken orally is destroyed in the digestive tract. A lipid-encapsulated, injectable form of SOD (LIPSOD) and a sublingually administered form currently show the most promise for direct supplementation.

Vitamin A

Vitamin A enhances the early inflammatory stage and increases the number of monocytes and macrophages at the wound site. Animal studies have shown increased collagen cross-linking (MacKay & Miller, 2003). Dosing for connective tissue injuries is 25,000 IU orally daily. However, the recommended daily dose under normal conditions is in the range of 4,000 to 5,000 IU. Chronic use of large doses on the order of 50,000 to 100,000 IU from weeks to years can result in toxicity manifested as fatigue, malaise, lethargy, psychiatric changes, anorexia, nausea, vomiting, and joint and muscle pain. CNS symptoms include increased intracranial pressure, visual disturbance, and headache (*Natural Medicines,* 1999).

Vitamin C (Oral)

Vitamin C (ascorbic acid) is crucial for the proper function of the enzyme protocollagen hydroxylase, which produces collagen—the primary constituent of the granulation tissue that heals a wound and the key component in blood vessel walls. Vitamin C also has immune stimulating properties. A published review stated that vitamin C plays a variety of roles in the prevention and treatment of cancer, including stimulating the immune system and enhancing wound healing (Head, 1998). Wound healing requires more vitamin C than diet alone can easily provide. It must be replenished daily because it is water soluble. Suggested dosing guidelines are 100–120 mg daily to achieve cellular saturation and optimum risk reduction of heart diseases, stroke, and cancer in healthy individuals. For wound healing, 1,000–2,000 mg daily (in divided doses) to accelerate healing of fascia is recommended. Several interactions should be taken into consideration before supplementing a patient with vitamin C. Patients using oral contraceptives, estrogen, and salicylates require higher dosages of vitamin C. However, large oral doses can cause the following adverse side effects: diarrhea, heartburn, abdominal cramps, insomnia, and oxalate stones.

The dramatic positive effect of vitamin C on a wide array of infectious diseases has led to the pursuit of using this nutrient as an ideal nutrient to use in combating increased levels of oxidative stress accompanied by exercise stress. All toxic microtrauma to connective tissue can be repaired by a high enough dose of antioxidants. The timing and concentration of the administered dose are crucial; they must take effect before irreversible clinical consequences occur to the tissue. It is important to review how vitamin C works in the body and to understand the role of intravenous vitamin C for athletic purposes.

Vitamin C Intravenous

Szent-Gyorgyi, who discovered vitamin C, asserted that energy exchange in the body can only occur when there is an imbalance of electrons among different molecules, assuring that electron flow must take place (Szent-Gyorgyi, 1978). Vitamin C serves as one of the most important electron donors in the body and functions to maintain an ongoing supply of electrons to tissue. Damaged and necrotic connective tissue has a full complement of electrons that will prevent it from accepting any electrons; hence the tissue will not undergo an exchange of electrons, resulting in no energy flow.

When connective tissue is damaged by "loss of an electron" as in oxidation, an antioxidant counters this process by supplying electrons. Antioxidants do not function solely to donate electrons. Rather, many of them work to keep the more important antioxidant substances in the body in the reduced state, which allows the donation of electrons. For example, vitamin E is an antioxidant that is fat soluble; this characteristic is important in allowing it to be the primary antioxidant present in the lipid-rich cell membranes of the body. Vitamin C helps to restore oxidized vitamin E in the cell membranes to its electron-rich, reduced form. Even though vitamin C is not the primary antioxidant in the cell wall, it plays a vital role in maintaining optimal levels of the metabolically active antioxidant, vitamin E, at that site.

Local destruction of connective tissue through exercise-induced microtrauma or metabolic breakdown appears to be accounted for by the local loss of an electron (oxidation). An antioxidant can serve to immediately restore this loss of electrons, resulting in a prompt "repair" of the acutely oxidized tissue. Also, an antioxidant can often neutralize the oxidizing agent before it gets a chance to oxidize, or damage, the tissue.

Vigorous antioxidant therapy, such as intravenous vitamin C, goes a long way in reversing the clinical manifestations of such diseases as well. The dose administered must supply enough electrons on a daily basis to reverse the ongoing oxidative damage from the disease process.

In cases of severe burns and athletic injuries, an intravenous method of administering vitamin C (slow infusion) has been developed and used in conjunction with oxygen therapy. Typical dosing can range from 50 to 200 grams of intravenous vitamin C daily. Vitamin C is available in three sizes of ampules: 1 ml with 500 mg of vitamin C and 10 mg monothioglycerol; 10 ml with 1 g of sodium ascorbate and 0.5% monothioglycerol; and 25 ml with 25 grams sodium ascorbate. The pH of the solution is generally buffered with sodium hydroxide or calcium carbonate. Sodium hydrosulfite 0.5% is often used as an antioxidant. The pH is buffered from 5.5 to 7.0, and the 500 mg/ml solution has an osmolality exceeding 2,000 mOsm/kg. Avoid using a bolus dose of infusion in patients with renal insufficiency. Ascorbic acid gradually darkens on exposure to light. A slight color developed during storage does not impair the therapeutic activity. However, Abbott Laboratories recommends protecting the intact ampules from light by keeping them in the cartons until ready for use. High-performance liquid chromatography (HPLC) analysis showed that ascorbic acid was stable at room temperature (23°C) when protected from light and exhibited less than a 10% loss.

Cetylated Monounsaturated Fatty Acid

Cetylated monounsaturated fatty acid reduces inflammation and pain via the following possible mechanisms: (1) inhibition of 5-lipoxygenase enzyme, a potent mediator of inflammation; and (2) inhibition of pro-inflammatory cytokine release (e.g., tumor necrosis factor alpha, interleukin-1 beta). Reducing inflammation in the body is paramount in maintaining the pliability and integrity of fascia. Topical cream applied twice daily to the affected area, or oral dosing in the form of capsules or tablets at a strength of 1,050 mg (in divided doses) daily, should be used. The absorption from oral or topical formulation is similar (Hesslink, Armstrong, Nagendran, Sreevatsan, & Barathur, 2002; Kraemer, Ratamess, Maresh, Anderson, Volek, Tiberio, et al., 2005).

Vitamin B$_5$

Pantothenic acid (vitamin B$_5$) improves healing by encouraging the migration of cells into the wounded area, thus establishing epithelialization (Weimann & Hermann, 1999). At the same time that new cells are migrating into the wounded area, cell division is increased and protein synthesis is increased, improving the healing process in connective tissue. Vitamin B$_5$ also helps prevent an excess of inflammatory response in the wound and has been shown to improve surgical wound healing (Kapp & Zeck-Kapp, 1991).

Summary

Nutrition plays an important role in the metabolic functioning of the body. Blood vessels penetrate fascia, carrying nutrients and waste by-products of metabolism. Maintaining good nutrition becomes paramount when an injury occurs because certain nutrients can contribute to the overall healing process. Table 11-2 summarizes specific nutrients that can positively influence tissue health.

Table 11-2 Summary of Nutritional Supplements

Supplement	Function/Uses	Approximate Dose	Possible Side Effects
Arginine	Increases nitrogen retention Increases immune function Improves wound healing Increases growth hormone secretion	10 to 22 mg daily	Diarrhea, stomach cramps, bloating, exacerbation of cold sores
Carnosine	Promotes wound healing Stimulates collagen formation Antioxidant	100 to 1,000 mg daily	Muscle spasms at high dose Insomnia
Copper	Wound healing	2 to 3 mg daily	Acute: nausea, vomiting Chronic: diarrhea, jaundice, hemolytic anemia
Zinc	Wound healing	Adult male: 15 mg daily Adult female: 12 mg daily	Nausea, vomiting, GI irritation
Orthosilicic acid	Stimulates bone formation and collagen synthesis	Stabilized orthosilicic acid: 6 to 20 mg daily	None known

(continued)

Table 11-2 Summary of Nutritional Supplements (continued)

Supplement	Function/Uses	Approximate Dose	Possible Side Effects
EPA	Increases collagen production Brain development	100 to 3,000 mg EPA/DHA daily	Nausea, diarrhea, fishy taste, increased bleeding risk with anticoagulants
Aloe vera	Wound healing Reduces inflammation	50 to 200 mg daily	Diarrhea, abdominal pain and cramps, potassium loss, muscle weakness
Bromelain	Reduces inflammation Wound debridement Immune modulation	750 to 1000 mg daily	Allergic reaction Tachycardia in hypertensives
Curcumin	Anti-tumor Antioxidant Anti-inflammatory	0.5 to 3 g daily (root powder)	Gastrointestinal upset, stomach ulceration
Gotu kola	Anti-inflammatory Wound healing Venous insufficiency	600 mg 3 times daily (dried leaves)	Allergic itch, photosensitivity, contact dermatitis (topical use) Large doses: may increase blood pressure
Superoxide dismutase	Antioxidant Protects type I collagen (Petersen, et al., 2004) Anti-inflammatory (Hernandez-Saavedra, et al., 2005)	2,000 mg daily bound to wheat Gliadin	Wheat allergy
Vitamin A	Increases collagen cross-links Maintains healthy epithelial lining	25,000 IU daily × 10 days Usual dose: 4,000 to 5,000 IU daily	High doses: fatigue, malaise, nausea, vomiting, psychiatric changes, joint and muscle pain, liver abnormalities
Vitamin C	Fibroblast maturation Immune function Collagen synthesis	RDA: 100 mg daily Wound healing: 1,000 to 2,000 mg daily	Diarrhea, abdominal cramps, nausea, kidney stones
Cetylated monounsaturated fatty acid	Reduces inflammation and pain	Oral: 350 mg 3 times daily. Topical: Cream applied twice daily	None known
Vitamin B_5	Wound healing	5 to 10 mg daily	High doses: diarrhea

References

Ballmer, P. E., Reinhart, W. H., Jordan, P., Buhler, E., Moser, U. K., & Gey, K. F. (1994). Depletion of plasma vitamin C but not of vitamin E in response to cardiac operations. *Journal of Thoracic Cardiovascular Surgery, 108*(2), 311–320.

Berg, R. A., & Kerr, J. S. (1992). Nutritional aspects of collagen metabolism. *Annual Review of Nutrition, 12,* 369–390.

Bucci, L. R. (1995). *Nutrition applied to injury rehabilitation and sports medicine.* Human Kinetics Press: Boca Raton, FL.

Calomme, M. R., & Van den Berghe, D. A. (1997). Supplementation of calves with stabilized orthosilicic acid. Effect on the Si, Ca, Mg, and P concentrations in serum and the collagen concentration in skin and cartilage. *Biological Trace Element Research, 56*(2), 153–165.

Cerra, F. B. (1991). Nutrient modulation of inflammatory and immune function. *American Journal of Surgery, 161,* 230–234.

Chithra, P., Sajithal, G. B., & Chandrakasan, G. (1998). Influence of Aloe vera on collagen characteristics in healing dermal wounds in rats. *Molecular Cell Biochemistry, 181*(1–2), 71–76.

De-Souza, D. A., & Greene, L. J. (1998). Pharmacological nutrition after burn injury. *Journal of nutrition, 128*(5), 797–803.

Fisher, E., McLennan, S. V., Tada, H., Heffernan, S., Yue, D. K., & Turtle, J. R. (1991). Interaction of ascorbic acid and glucose on production of collagen and proteoglycan by fibroblasts. *Diabetes, 40,* 371–376.

Friedlander, A. L., Braun, B., Pollack, M., MacDonald, J. R., Fulco, C. S., Muza, S. R., et al. (2005). Three weeks of caloric restriction alters protein metabolism in normal-weight, young men. *American Journal of Physiology, Endocrinology, & Metabolism, 289,* E446–E455.

Gray, M. (2003). Does oral zinc supplementation promote healing of chronic wounds? *Journal of Wound, Ostomy, & Continence Nursing, 30*(6), 295–299.

Hankenson, K., Watkins, B., Schoenlein, I., Allen, K.G.D., & Turek, J. J. (2000). Omega-3 fatty acids enhance ligament fibroblast collagen formation in association with changes in interleukin-6 production. *Proceedings of the Society for Experimental Biology and Medicine, 223,* 88–95.

Head, K. A. (1998). Ascorbic acid in the prevention and treatment of cancer. *Alternative Medicine Review, 3*(3), 174–186.

Heggers, J. P., Elzaim, H., Garfield, R., Goodheart, R., Listengarten, D., Zhao, J., et al. (1997). Effect of the combination of Aloe vera, nitroglycerin and L-NAME on wound healing in the rat excisional model. *Journal of Alternative Medicine, 3*(2), 149–153.

Hernandez-Saavedra, D., Zhou, H., & McCord, J. M. (2005). Anti-inflammatory properties of a chimeric recombinant superoxide dismutase: SOD2/3. *Biomedicine & Pharmacotherapy, 59*(4), 204–208.

Hesslink, R., Jr., Armstrong, D., Nagendran, M. V., Sreevatsan, S., & Barathur, R. (2002). Cetylated fatty acids improve knee function in patients with osteoarthritis. *Journal of Rheumatology, 29(8)* 1708–1712.

Kapp, A., & Zeck-Kapp, G. (1991). Effect of Ca-pantothenate on human granulocyte oxidative metabolism. *Allergie et Immunologie (Paris), 37*(3–4), 145–150.

Kirk, S. J., Hurson, M., Regan, M. C., Holt, D. R., Waserkrug, H. L., & Barbul, A. (1993). Arginine stimulates wound healing and immune function in elderly human beings. *Surgery, 114*(2), 155–159.

Kraemer, W., Ratamess, N. A., Maresh, C. M., Anderson, J. A., Volek, J. S., Tiberio, D. P., et al. (2005). A cetylated fatty acid topical cream with menthol reduces pain and improves functional performance in patients with arthritis. *Journal of Strength & Conditioning Research*, 19(2), 475–480.

MacKay, D., & Miller, A. L. (2003). Nutritional support for wound healing. *Alternative Medicine Review, 8*(4), 359–377.

Mane, J., Fernandez-Banares, F., Ojanguren, I., Castella, E., Bertran, X., Bartoli, R., et al. (2001). The effect of L-arginine on the course of experimental colitis. *Clinical Nutrition, 20*(5), 415–422.

Nagai, K., & Suda, T. (1988). Realization of spontaneous healing function by carnosine. *Methods & Findings in Experimental & Clinical Pharmacology, 10*(8), 497–507.

Nagai, K., Suda, T., Kawasaki, K., & Mathuura, S. (1986). Action of carnosine and beta-alanine on wound healing, *Surgery, 100*(5), 815–821.

Natural Medicines Comprehensive Database, 2nd ed. (1999). Therapeutic Research Faculty. Stockton, CA

Petersen, S. V., Oury, T. D., Ostergaard, L., Valnickova, Z., Wegrzyn, J., Thogersen, I. B., et al. (2004). Extracellular superoxide dismutase (EC-SOD) binds to type I collagen and protects against oxidative fragmentation. *Journal of Biological Chemistry, 279*(14), 13705–13710.

Reffitt, D. M., Ogston, N., Jugdaohsingh, R., Cheung, H. F., Evans, B. A., Thompson, R. P., et al. (2003). Orthosilicic acid stimulates collagen type 1 synthesis and osteoblastic differentiation in human osteoblast-like cells in vitro. *Bone, 32*(2), 127–135.

Ruberg, R. L. (1984). Role of nutrition in wound healing. *Surgery Clinics of North America, 4,* 705–714.

Shukla, A., Rasik, A. M., Jain, G. K., Shankar, R., Kulshrestha, D. K., & Dhawan, B. N. (1999). In vitro and in vivo wound healing activity of asiaticoside isolated from *Centella asciatica*. *Journal of Ethnopharmacology, 65*(1), 1–11.

Sidhu, G. S., Mani, H., Gaddipati, J. P., Singh, A. K., Seth, P., Banaudha, K. K., et al. (1999). Curcumin enhances wound healing in streptozotocin induced diabetic rats and genetically diabetic mice. *Wound Repair Regeneration, 7*(5), 362–374.

Szent-Gyorgyi, A. (1978). How new understandings about the biological function of ascorbic acid may profoundly affect our lives. *Executive Health, 14*(8), 1–4.

Tenaud, I., Leroy, S., Chebassier, N., & Dreno, B. (2000). Zinc, copper and manganese enhanced keratinocyte migration through a functional modulation of keratinocyte integrins. *Experimental Dermatology, 9*(6), 407–416.

Kelly, G. (1996). Bromelain: a literature review and discussion of its therapeutic applications. *Alternative Medicine Review, 1*(4), 243–257.

Tinker, D., & Rucker, R. (1985). Role of selected nutrients in synthesis, accumulation, and chemical modification of connective tissue proteins. *Physiological Reviews, 65,* 607–657.

Weimann, B. I., & Hermann, D. (1999). Studies on wound healing: Effects of calcium D-pantothenate on the migration, proliferation and protein synthesis of human dermal fibroblasts in culture. *International Journal for Vitamin & Nutrition Research, 69*(2),113–119.

Zhang, L., & Tizard, I. R. (1996). Activation of a mouse macrophage cell line by acemannan: The major carbohydrate fraction from Aloe vera gel. *Immunopharmacology, 35*(2), 119–128.

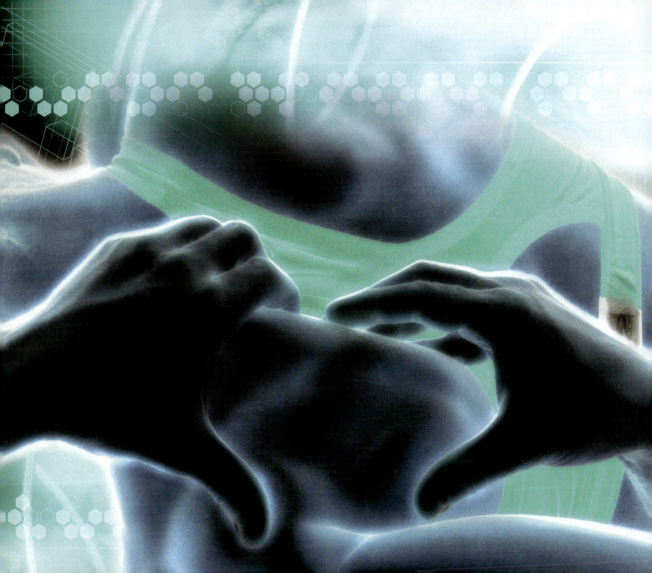

NUTRITIONAL SUPPORT FOR ISCHEMIC CONDITIONS

Ischemia is the reduction or absence of blood supply to an organ or tissue. The etiology of ischemia may be obstruction of blood supply by a blood clot, atherosclerotic plaque, traumatic disruption of the vascular supply, or hypoxemic vasoconstriction.

Nutrition has been used for a variety of health conditions, including ischemia. Antioxidants found in colorful fruits and vegetables quench reactive oxygen species (ROS) to reduce oxidative damage and inflammation.

EFFECTS OF ISCHEMIA ON ENERGY PRODUCTION

The cells of the body depend on an uninterrupted blood flow, which guarantees delivery of nutrients and oxygen for the continual production of cellular energy (ATP). Ischemia causes microcirculatory blockages, a change in tissue metabolism where the cells are no longer able to produce ATP by aerobic metabolism, and oxidative stress that damages multiple cellular components. When cellular oxygen levels fall due to failure of the circulatory system to deliver oxygen instead of oxygen-dependent aerobic metabolism, the cells switch to glycogenolysis and anaerobic glycolysis. These metabolic processes lead to the intracellular accumulation of nicotinamide-adenine dinucleotide (NADH), lactate, and H^+ ions and a reduction in intracellular levels of reduced glutathione. The accumulation of these substances and loss of reduced glutathione creates intracellular acidosis and a change in cellular reduction–oxidation (redox) status. If the ischemic process is prolonged, the accumulation of acids, lactate, and NADH inside of the cells eventually inhibits even anaerobic energy production (Opie, 1976; Stanley, Lopaschuk, Hall, & McCormack, 1997).

With loss of a continual supply of cellular energy, the energy-dependent metabolic functions of the cell grind to a halt. Within minutes, cell membrane disruption and organelle dysfunction occurs. Protein, fat, and carbohydrate catabolism and synthesis are also inhibited, as is control of intracellular mineral concentrations. Regulation of membrane mineral transport is lost, causing intracellular potassium and magnesium ions to leak out of the cells and extracellular sodium and calcium ions to leak into the cells' cytoplasm and mitochondria (Flatman & Lew, 1983). This redistribution of electrolytes creates osmotic changes and cellular edema (Carmeliet, 1999). When the energy supply is compromised to the point that it is inadequate to even meet survival needs, the cells die.

REPERFUSION INJURY

Restoration of blood flow and oxygen supply to previously ischemic tissues also contributes to the level of oxidative stress (McCord, 1985). This is called reperfusion injury. Ischemia and reperfusion activate an inflammatory response in the tissue, which can expand the area of injury and convert reversibly injured cells to irreversible injury (Maxwell & Lip, 1997).

One of the immediate effects of ischemia is direct damage to the vascular endothelium (Saeed, van Dijke, Mann, Wendland, Rosenau, Higgins, et al., 1998). The cell membranes of endothelial cells are disrupted, exposing the previously hidden inner leaflet of cell membranes and creating activation of coagulation. Subendothelial structures are also exposed, and collagenases are liberated. The exposure of cell membrane and subendothelial components as well as release of tissue factor (TF) trigger the extrinsic coagulation cascade and accelerate the production of thrombin (Esmon, 1998). In addition, the endothelial damage causes neutrophil activation, neutrophil–endothelial cell adhesion, neutrophil egress into the tissue, and production of inflammatory cytokines (Esmon, 1998).

The bloodstream's coagulation pathway is activated when blood comes into contact with subendothelial connective tissues or when the negatively charged surfaces of the cell membranes are exposed as a result of tissue damage. When cells are damaged, the bloodstream is exposed to the inner lining of cell membrane. In 1988 Feola and colleagues discovered that aminophospholipids of the inner wall of the cell membrane activates intravascular coagulation, causing a drop in the serum fibrinogen level and deposition of fibrin in the microcirculation (Feola, Simoni, & Canizaro, 1988).

The first step in the activation of coagulation is the binding of factors of the coagulation pathway to cell components that have been exposed by an injury. The end result is the production of thrombin, which subsequently converts soluble fibrinogen to fibrin.

The fibrin monomers produced are sticky and they aggregate with platelets, forming a deposit on the walls of the blood vessels that blocks or reduces blood flow through the blood vessel. These pathological processes compromise the microvascular system, resulting in decreased tissue perfusion and hypoxemia with resultant organ dysfunction and failure.

Plasmin is the principal effector of fibrinolysis. This enzyme is formed when tissue plasminogen activating factor (t-PA) triggers the conversion of plasminogen to plasmin. Once activated, plasmin breaks up (digests) fibrin deposits.

CELL INJURY DUE TO ISCHEMIA AND REPERFUSION

When muscles and associated fascia undergo ischemia, high-energy stores such as ATP decline, despite the attempt by large stores of muscle creatine phosphates to maintain ATP production. The muscle eventually undergoes necrosis unless blood flow and oxygen are restored by reperfusion, but this process is not without risk. Reperfusion can enhance cellular injury through induction of complement cascades, which attract neutrophils. These, in turn, release inflammatory cytokines that contribute to the production of reactive oxygen species that impair the microcirculation.

REACTIVE OXYGEN SPECIES

Free radicals are reactive substances containing one or more unpaired electrons. Once created in the body, these highly reactive compounds literally steal electrons from biological molecules and set up a chain reaction of destruction until they are neutralized. From the perspective of electronic nutrition, adequate availability of antioxidant nutrients and cell membrane factors that can neutralize and sponge up free radicals are necessary to combat free radical damage. Nutritionally, the key players are compounds that act as electron donors.

Excessive production of reactive oxygen species (ROS)—such as hydroxyl radicals, superoxide anions, hydrogen peroxide, and nitric oxide—lead to lipid peroxidation, which damages cell membranes and the oxidation of enzymes, proteins, and DNA, which in turn impairs the structures of these molecules and their functions (McCord, 1985). Normal cell defenses against ROS include a variety of antioxidant enzymes and dietary antioxidants (Meyers, Bolli, & Lekich, 1985).

When free radicals are produced in amounts that overwhelm the body's antioxidant systems, damage to the endothelial lining of the blood vessels takes place. This damage initiates a pathological process in the microvasculature, which causes the expression of inflammatory cytokines, activation of the complement cascade, platelet aggregation, fibrin deposition, and expression of neutrophil and endothelial cell surface adhesion molecules. These effects are followed by passage of neutrophils out of the bloodstream and into the tissues, resulting in neutrophil-mediated tissue destruction (Forman, Puett, & Virmani, 1989).

The endothelial cells play a critical protective function in maintaining blood flow by facilitating a state of relative vasodilation of the vessel wall; this state is mediated by the smooth muscle. Healthy endothelium limits the adherence of white blood cells and platelets to blood vessel walls, but this delicate balance quickly shifts to proadherence in cases of ischemia and injury to the blood vessel walls. The endothelium also both produces and responds to a multitude of chemical messengers to control the balance between anticoagulation and procoagulation. Endothelial disruption can result in vascular abnormalities, including vasospasm, coagulopathies, and microcirculatory dysfunctions (Hennig, Toborek, Cader, & Decker, 1994).

COAGULATIVE AND FIBRINOLYTIC PATHWAYS

The coagulative and fibrinolytic pathways are counterbalanced systems that are designed to maintain a steady flow of blood in the circulatory system and at the same time conserve blood in the event of trauma. Both of these systems are activated when their inactive precursors are converted into active components by the proteolytic activity of serine protease enzymes (Bachmann, 1987).

According to Ali, "Both systems involve intrinsic (plasma) and extrinsic (tissue) activation mechanisms that trigger a common pathway. In the coagulative system, the final common pathway involves polymerization of fibrinogen into fibrin, while that in the fibrinolytic system it involves activation of plasminogen" (M. Ali & O. Ali, 1997).

In the same paper, Ali also expounds on his belief that "the primary mechanisms underlying activation of both of these systems are related to oxidant phenomena," which affect circulating blood, cell membranes, and cytoplasmic components—particularly the mitochondria.

> Even though the coagulative and fibrinolytic systems are generally regarded as two discrete enzymatic pathways, in reality the intrinsic pathway of the fibrinolytic system is coupled to the intrinsic pathways of the coagulative, so that clot formation and resolution are initiated concurrently and perpetuated in tandem. We introduce the term clotting-unclotting equilibrium (CUE) in this article to integrate the oxidative nature of events that lead to the concurrent phenomena of clot formation and clot resolution. (M. Ali & O. Ali, 1997)

Hypercoagulation occurs within the circulatory system in a diverse group of conditions that are generally associated with inflammatory, infectious, traumatic, ischemic, allergic, and toxic processes (M. Ali, 1990).

Free radicals, particularly superoxide anions and hydroxyl radicals, are produced during and after ischemia and reperfusion events. "Superoxide anion is a relatively weak oxidant and owes most of its destructive potential to its ability to generate hydrogen peroxide by reacting with molecular oxygen. Hydrogen peroxide, in turn, generates highly toxic hydroxyl radicals in the presence of transition metals such as iron and copper" (Hennig et al., 1994).

Excessive free radical production in the circulatory system will initiate coagulation processes. Dr. Ali, in his excellent review article, notes that even healthy individuals will often exhibit platelet aggregates and microthrombi in their circulatory systems. He also discovered that these coagulation phenomena could be reversed by administration of antioxidants given both orally and as ascorbic acid infusions (M. Ali, 1990). The use of antioxidants provides an increased supply of electrons, which neutralizes these free-radical-mediated reactions. It will be interesting to find out whether equipment such as microcurrent units, pulsed electromagnetic fields, infrared devices, and phototherapy devices (lasers and LED)—which also increase the supply of electrons available to the bloodstream—exhibit similar effects. Coagulation phenomena such as platelet aggregation and microclots composed of fibrin deposits and neutrophil plugs can also be reversed by use of intravenous and oral proteolytic enzymes.

Research studies show that many septic, chronic fatigue, fibromyalgia, heart attack, stroke, diabetes, and osteonecrosis patients have hypercoagulable states evidenced by fibrin deposition in their small blood vessels.

Fibrin deposition is caused by excess thrombin generation. Hypercoagulable states associated with fibrin deposition in the microcirculation have a variety of causes, including genetic predisposition as well as activation of the clotting cascade by fragments from damaged cell membranes and by immune system IgG antibodies (Vermyeln, Hoylaerts, & Arnout, 1997).

Once the coagulation cascade is activated, clotting factors combine in a sequential manner to convert prothrombin (factor II) to thrombin (factor IIa).

Thrombin converts the soluble blood protein fibrinogen into fibrin. In healthy people a natural coagulation inhibitor called antithrombin, which is activated by heparin projections on the endothelial surface, maintains open flow of blood through the bloodstream. Once activated by heparin, the circulating antithrombin molecules combine with excess thrombin to form thrombin–antithrombin (TAT) complexes, which are then removed from the blood. The removal of active thrombin from the bloodstream stops production of fibrin.

When thrombin is generated in amounts greater than can be removed by antithrombin, the excess thrombin (IIa) then converts circulating fibrinogen into an intermediate protein called soluble fibrin monomer (SFM). SFM is a sticky protein that deposits on the capillary walls, creating a block that interferes with the passage of oxygen and nutrients from the bloodstream into the tissues.

When vascular endothelial cells are injured, fibrin deposition occurs and inactive tissue plasminogen activator (t-PA) is released. It then binds to fibrin and is consequently activated. The active t-PA converts the circulating inactive precursor protein, plasminogen, into a potent enzyme called plasmin. Plasmin's main job is to digest fibrin deposits and clots to keep the blood vessels open.

Another player in the mechanism of clot formation is the platelet. Platelets are cellular bloodstream elements that are inert until they encounter conditions that trigger their activation. Platelet activation causes the platelets to become sticky, providing a surface for clot formation. Platelets may be activated by thrombin, ischemia, trauma, or immunoglobulins. Once activated, platelets aggregate at the site of vascular injuries and bind to the damaged endothelial lining of vessels, where they will form a platelet plug and locally activate components of the coagulation cascade. The resulting activation of the complement cascade leads to production of a fibrin network that stabilizes the primary platelet plug.

Complement activation itself can occur via free radicals produced by neutrophil activation, by platelet activation, or by exposure of basement membranes and subcellular organelles. Activation of the complement pathway is a primary mediator in the pathogenesis of ischemia and reperfusion injuries. Complement activation results in the production of toxic metabolites. These toxic metabolites, along with the free radicals and enzymes released by the neutrophils, cause damage to the endothelial membrane, cell membranes, and subcellular structures. Structural membrane and organelle disturbances result in functional disturbances in which membrane signaling mechanisms, cellular energy production, and membrane control of cellular electrolytes and water content are disrupted.

Platelet-activating factor (PAF) is an inflammatory cytokine that stimulates the neutrophils to synthesize hydrogen peroxide, which initiates a PAF-dependent adherence of neutrophils to the vascular endothelium (Sundaresan, Yu, Ferrans, Irani, & Finkel, 1995). These processes facilitate the passage of circulating inflammatory cells (neutrophils and monocytes) from the bloodstream into the ischemic and reperfused tissues (Go, Murry, Richard, Weischedel, Jennings, & Reimer, 1988).

The white blood cells that leave the bloodstream create tissue-damaging inflammation (Dreyer, Michael, & West, 1991). These inflammatory cells generate oxygen-derived free radicals (respiratory burst) and release destructive lysosomal enzymes that can destroy cell structures and extracellular matrix (ECM) components. The enzymes released by activated neutrophils alter vascular permeability, disrupt the basement membrane of the vascular wall, and degrade collagen (collagenases), elastin (elastases), and ECM (gelatinase and heparinase).

When neutrophils have a respiratory burst, reactive oxygen products are released—such as superoxide anions, hypochlorous acid, hydrogen peroxide, and hydrogen anions (Freischlag & Hanna, 1991). These free radicals are usually controlled by enzyme antioxidants and nonenzyme antioxidants; but the antioxidant defenses can be exhausted, resulting in free-radical-mediated destruction of cellular structures, so it is important to maintain cellular antioxidant systems (Deveraj & Jialal, 2000).

Medical clinicians now recognize that oxidative injuries mediated by free radicals and the toxic metabolites arising from free radical damage to circulating low-density lipoproteins and cellular structures play key roles in the genesis of diabetes, atherosclerosis, and ischemia-induced tissue damage (Berliner, Territo, Sevanian, Ramin, Kim, Bamshad, et al., 1990; Steinberg, 1997; Steinberg, Parthasarathy, Carew, Khoo, & Witztum, 1989).

CHANGES IN THE MICROCIRCULATION IN ISCHEMIA

During the process of ischemia the activated complement pathway and the release of inflammatory cytokines by damaged tissues results in platelet aggregation, fibrin deposition, and vascular spasms that cause impaired blood flow—also called a no-flow phenomenon (El-Maraghi & Genton, 1980; Kiyak & Zerbino, 1996; Kloner, Ganote, & Jennings, 1974; Obrenovitch & Hallenbeck, 1985). Some tissue mechanisms may be involved in causing microcirculatory obstruction, including endothelial cell swelling, impaired nitric oxide release, vasospasms, and capillary occlusion with aggregated platelets and neutrophils (Forman, Puett, & Virmani, 1989; Kiyak & Zerbino, 1996).

ISCHEMIC EFFECTS ON HEART AND SKELETAL MUSCLE

When ischemia affects heart and skeletal muscle, the preferential efficient consumption of fatty acids decreases in favor of anaerobic glucose consumption (Chaundry, 1983). Intracellular acidosis is produced as well as alterations in cell membrane permeability and failure of the ATP-dependent mineral pumps. Failure of the membrane-bound ion pumps results in loss of the intracellular mineral potassium, magnesium, and zinc and elevates levels of free calcium in the cytoplasm. With ATP depletion the cellular concentrations of ADP and AMP increase and are soon catabolized to their waste products: adenosine, hypoxanthine, and xanthine (Swuartz, Cha, Clowes, & Randall, 1978).

The elevated cytosolic free calcium then produces activation of intracellular calcium-dependent proteases (Cheung, Bonventre, Malis, & Leaf, 1986; Lindsay, Liaw, Romaschin, & Walker, 1990). One of these proteases, calpaine, converts the enzyme xanthine dehydrogenase (XD) to xanthine oxidase (XO). The enzyme XD is in charge of converting xanthine into uric acid for renal excretion (McCord, 1985).

Normally, XD reduces nicotinamide-adenine dinucleotide (NAD) and cannot transfer electrons to molecular oxygen. On the other hand, the XO enzyme is capable of transferring electrons from hypoxanthine to oxygen. So upon reperfusion, this enzyme is responsible for formation of the destructive free radical superoxide anion. Normally the cells protect themselves against damage from superoxide anions by rapidly converting them via action of the enzyme superoxide dismutase (SOD) to the less destructive free radical, hydrogen peroxide.

The accumulation of oxygen-derived free radicals in ischemia and reperfusion leads to a situation of oxidative stress that can result in cellular death (Cochrane, 1991). When these free radicals attack the molecular components of the cell, they cause lipid peroxidation of cell membranes (Perry, 1990), protein oxidation, enzyme oxidation (White & Heckler, 1990), mitochondrial damage (Wolff, 1993), and DNA injury (Guyton & Kensleer, 1993).

The cells of our body normally contain enzymatic and nonenzymatic defenses against free radical attack. The enzymatic defenses include superoxide dismutase (SOD), catalase (CAT), and the enzymatic product glutathione (Zimmerman, 1991). SOD accelerates the conversion of superoxide anion to H_2O_2. CAT next metabolizes H_2O_2 to water and molecular oxygen. These enzymes have been found to be useful in preventing reperfusion injury in skeletal muscle (Walker, Lindsay, Labbe, Mickle, & Romaschin, 1987).

The endothelial cells of capillaries are the primary sites of injury in ischemia, since these cells are sensitive to hypoxia. During ischemia the XD conversion rate goes up in these cells (Punch, Rees, Cashmer, Wilkins, Smith, & Till, 1992) with increased generation of superoxide anions (Hardy, Homer-Vanniasinkam, & Gough, 1992). The superoxide and hydrogen peroxide free radicals act as chemotactic factors for polymorphonuclear leukocytes (PMN) by activating the alternate pathway of the complement cascade. An array of inflammatory components are created by damage to endothelial cells and leukocyte activation, including formyl peptides, tumor necrosis factor, interleukin-1 (Ward, Till, Kunkel, & Beauchamp, 1983), leukotriene B4, platelet-activating factor (PAF; Kirschner, Fyfe, Hoffman, Chiao, Davis, & Fantini, 1997), and thromboxane B2 (Patterson, Klausner, Goldman, Kobzik, Welbourn, Valeri, et al., 1989).

Because endothelial cell injury and complement activation occurs, the microcirculation becomes blocked by platelet microthrombi, fibrin deposition, and red blood cell and neutrophil plugs (Harstock, Seaber, & Urbaniak, 1989). Interstitial edema also occurs upon damage to the capillary cells (Kirschner et al., 1997). The activated neutrophils infiltrate the tissue and begin to release protease enzymes that further damage the ischemic tissue (Feng, Berger, Lysz, & Shaw, 1988; Weiss, 1989).

NUTRITIONAL TREATMENT OF ISCHEMIA

Free radicals are products of normal aerobic metabolism and by-products of inflammatory responses. Because uncontrolled production and activity of free radicals would disrupt the function and structure of cell membranes and subcellular organelles, living organisms rely on a protective antioxidant defense system (Arduini, Mezzetti, Porreca, Lapenna, Dejulia, Marzio et al., 1988). This antioxidant defense system includes both internally produced substances and dietary compounds. These antioxidants operate by in-

hibiting free radical formation, intercepting free radicals once they have formed, and repairing free-radical-induced injuries (Mutlu-Turkoglu, Erbil, Oztezcan, Olgac, Toker, & Uysai, 2000).

Minerals

The production and activity of the major intrinsic antioxidants (catalase, glutathione, and SOD) are controlled in part by the availability of key mineral cofactors. Magnesium, potassium, selenium, copper, chromium, zinc, and manganese are essential cofactors for enzymes involved in protecting tissues during ischemia, repairing damaged tissues, and reactivating disturbed metabolic pathways. Table 12-1 summarizes recommended intake for various minerals used in treating ischemia.

Table 12-1 Recommended Mineral Intake

Minerals	Daily Requirement (adult)
Manganese	2 to 5 mg
Selenium	50 to 200 mcg
Zinc aspartate	40 mg (12 mg elemental)
Zinc arginate	60 mg (9.45 mg elemental)
Chromium GTF	50 to 200 mcg
Potassium	1,560 to 3,120 mg
Magnesium	54 to 483 mg
Calcium	500 to 1,600 mg (elemental)
Vanadium	10 to 60 mcg
Copper	2 to 3 mg

Source: J. M. Jellin, F. Batz, & K. Hitchens, "Pharmacist's Letter/Prescriber's Letter," Natural Medicines Comprehensive Database. Stockton, CA: Therapeutic Research Faculty, 1999.

Some of these minerals are also involved with anti-oxidant activity—for example, selenium and magnesium in glutathione peroxidase, and copper, manganese, and zinc in SOD (Diplock, 1991; Evans & Henshaw, 2000).

Selenium is the essential mineral cofactor for the enzyme glutathione peroxidase, which maintains glutathione (Misso, Powers, Gillon, Stewart, & Thompson, 1996). Glutathione is required to control peroxides. When glutathione production and regeneration are compromised, uncontrolled peroxide radicals will damage the endothelium.

Zinc has a dual role; it is the cofactor for the antioxidant enzyme SOD as well as a cell membrane stabilizer. Zinc safeguards endothelial membrane integrity by protecting the endothelium against the inflammatory cytokine PAF. Copper and manganese are other essential mineral cofactors for SOD.

Enzymes

Clinically, it makes sense to use proteolytic enzymes to open up the circulation and magnesium to reduce vascular spasms. Magnesium, because of its multiple roles, has important anti-inflammatory properties that make it a useful mineral in ischemic conditions. Magnesium can inhibit neutrophil respiratory burst activity by blocking the entry of calcium into neutrophils (Cairns & Kraft, 1996). Magnesium can also decrease release of inflammatory mediators from mast cells and basophils, In addition, it can initiate smooth muscle relaxation and improve blood flow through spasmed blood vessels.

Clinicians have used high-potency oral enzyme supplements for decades to therapeutically address digestive difficulties, inflammation, infection, trauma, and other conditions. The following are possible applications of high-potency oral enzyme supplements:

- Inflammatory disorders
- Autoimmune disorders
- Hypercoagulation states
- Fibromyalgia

- Chronic fatigue syndrome
- Weight management
- Traumatic wounds
- Traumatic injuries such as auto accidents
- Athletic injuries
- High blood pressure
- Infections due to viruses, bacteria, and plasmodium
- Varicose veins
- Thrombophlebitis
- Atherosclerosis
- Ischemic conditions such as heart attacks and strokes
- Menstrual cramps
- Poor digestion
- Blood clots
- Cancer
- Blood sugar elevations
- Toxemia of pregnancy

Potential new uses include septic shock, traumatic shock, cavitations, adult respiratory distress syndrome, and toxin-induced injuries.

Proteolytic enzymes such as nattokinase, bromelain, papain, and serrapeptidase dissolve immune complexes and break down fibrin plugs in the microcirculation.

Bromelain

Bromelain is an enzyme extracted from pineapples. Bromelain is a mixture of sulfur-containing, protein-digesting enzymes known as proteolytic enzymes or proteases (Maurer, 2001). Papain, a proteolytic enzyme isolated from unripe papaya fruit, has effects similar to those of bromelain.

Bromelain was first introduced as a medicinal agent in 1957 and hundreds of scientific papers on its therapeutic applications have since appeared in the medical literature (Werbach & Murray, 1994).

Bromelain supplementation is useful in virtually any condition associated with inflammation, regardless of etiology. Hans Nieper found that bromelain and papain enzymes were effective in a diverse group of health conditions, including angina, cancer, indigestion, and upper respiratory tract infections. He used bromelain, serrapeptidase, and papain in his patients with angina because these enzymes inhibit platelet aggregation, reduce blood pressure, and break down atherosclerotic plaques (Nieper, 1978). When bromelain is given in excess of body tolerance, intestinal irritation with frequent urges to have a bowel movement may occur. Such symptoms indicate a need to lower the amount used.

Bromelain is a useful activator of fibrinolysis, especially in patients who have laboratory markers of impaired fibrinolysis such as high Lp(a) or high PAI-1 values. The recommended dosage of bromelain is 500 to 1,000 mg/day, between meals, three to four times per day.

Bromelain, papain, serrapeptidase, and nattokinase are oral alternatives to the use of injectable t-PA or urokinase as fibrinolysis activators in patients.

Nattokinase

Nattokinase is a powerful fibrinolytic enzyme extracted from a traditional Japanese food called natto. Natto is a cheese-like food produced by fermenting boiled soybeans with the beneficial bacteria *Bacillus subtilis* (Sumi, Hamada, Tsushima, Mihara, & Muraki, 1987). During the fermentation, various vitamins and enzymes, particularly nattokinase, are produced. People may receive the health benefits of nattokinase by either eating the fermented food or by using the purified nattokinase enzyme as a supplement.

The antithrombotic properties of nattokinase closely resemble the natural anticoagulation blood component plasmin. Besides acting like plasmin, nattokinase enhances the body's natural production of both plasmin and urokinase (Sumi, Banba, and Kishimoto, 1996.). Nattokinase has superior benefits for individuals with blood clots and hypercoagulable states—unlike the conventional clot-dissolving drugs (tissue plasminogen activators), which are effective only when taken intravenously, nattokinase is effective when taken orally even at doses as low as 100 mg/day (Sumi, Hamada, Nakanishi, & Hiratani, 1990). In addition, nattokinase's fibrinolytic activity lasts for more than eight hours after each oral dose.

After oral administration, nattokinase has a prolonged duration of fibrinolytic action in the bloodstream based on elevation of blood levels of euglobulin fibrinolytic activity (EFA) and fibrin degradation products (FDP). The levels of these substances in the bloodstream become elevated when fibrin is dissolved.

Nattokinase may useful in hypertension and in individuals with hypercoagulable states such as chronic fatigue syndrome, fibromyalgia, senile dementia, atherosclerosis, and neuralgia-inducing cavitational osteonecrosis. From the perspective of prevention, nattokinase may be a life-saving enzyme supplement for individuals at risk for heart attacks, strokes, and deep venous thrombosis.

Removal of Immune Complexes

Proteolytic plant enzyme supplements containing bromelain and papain can prevent the deposit of immune complexes in body tissues. When foreign substances (antigens) enter the bloodstream, the immune system generates antibodies to bind these foreign materials. When antigens and antibodies bind together, immune complexes are formed. Unless the body's internal enzymes rapidly remove them, these immune complexes will deposit in the circulatory system and initiate an inflammatory process. Researchers in Europe, Japan, and the United States have conducted studies, both in the test tube and in animals and humans, demonstrating the ability of plant and bacterial enzyme preparations to dissolve and clear these complexes.

Removal of Fibrin

Numerous conditions can create hypercoagulable states when fibrin deposition and platelet aggregation subsequently lead to the development of blood clots in the circulatory system. Proteolytic enzyme supplements are effective in removing these fibrin and platelet deposits. Proteolytic enzymes are often used therapeutically, treating a diverse group of inflammatory conditions. Bromelain decreases aggregation of blood platelets (Heinicke, Van der Wal, & Yokoyama, 1972) and increases fibrinolysis by activating the conversion of plasminogen to plasmin (Taussig & Batkin, 1988). Nattokinase works both directly and indirectly to remove fibrin deposits. Because it closely resembles plasmin, nattokinase acts directly on fibrin; indirectly, nattokinase increases the production of plasmin.

Inhibition of Pro-inflammatory Compounds

Bromelain (Werbach & Murray, 1994), papain, and nattokinase inhibit the production of pro-inflammatory compounds in ischemic tissues. These enzymes work by blocking the production of kinins, decreasing the synthesis of inflammatory prostaglandins of the 2 series, and increasing levels of anti-inflammatory PEG1 prostaglandins (Felton, 1980).

Hypercoagulability increases the risk of formation of fibrin deposits and large blood clots in blood vessels. This condition may be associated with an increased tendency to form thrombi (called thrombophilia) or by a reduced ability to remove thrombi once they form a condition called hypofibrinolysis.

Hypercoagulability can be predisposed by genetic factors or be initiated through physical stimulus to thrombosis, including viral and bacterial infection, medications (particularly estrogen and corticosteroids), and autoimmune diseases.

Summary

Sports injuries leading to ischemia can result in loss of function and death of the affected organ. Ischemia results in disruption of cellular energy production, and reperfusion causes further injury to tissues by the release of oxygen-free radicals. Nutritional support using minerals and enzymes reduces destructive free radicals, increases antioxidant defenses, dissolves blood clots, and reduces pro-inflammatory cytokines.

References

Ali, M. (1990). Ascorbic acid reverses abnormal erythrocyte morphology in chronic fatigue syndrome. *American Journal of Clinical Pathology, 94,* 515.

Ali, M., & Ali, O. (1997). AA Oxidopathy: The core pathogenetic mechanism of ischemic heart disease. *Journal of Integrative Medicine, 1,* 1–112.

Arduini, A., Mezzetti, A., Porreca, E., Lapenna, D., DeJulia, J., Marzio, L., Polidoro, G., & Cuccurullo, F.; (1988). Effect of ischemia and reperfusion on antioxidant enzymes and mitochondrial inner membrane proteins in perfused rat heart. *Biochimica et Biophysica Acta, 970,* 121–131.

Bachmann, F. (1987). Fibrinolysis. In M. Verstraeie, J. Vermylen, R. Lijnen, et al. (Eds.), *Thrombosis XIth Congress Hemostasis* (pp. 227–236). Leuven, Belgium: International Society on Thrombosis and Haemostasis and Leuven University Press.

Berliner, J. A., Territo, M. C., Sevanian, A., Ramin, S., Kim, J. A., Bamshad, B., et al. (1990). Minimally modified low-density lipoprotein stimulates monocyte endothelial interactions. *Journal of Clinical Investigation, 85,* 1260–1266.

Cairns, C. B., & Kraft, M. (1996). Magnesium attenuates the neutrophil respiratory burst in adult-asthmatic patients. *Academy of Emergency Medicine, 3,* 10931.

Carmeliet, E. (1999). Cardiac ionic currents and acute ischemia: From channels to arrhythmias. *Physiological Reviews, 79,* 917–1017.

Chaundry, I. H. (1983). Cellular mechanisms in shock and ischemia and their correction. *American Journal of Physiology, 245,* R117.

Cheung, J. Y., Bonventre, J. V., Malis, C. D., & Leaf, A. (1986). Calcium and ischemic injury. *New England Journal of Medicine, 314,* 1670.

Cochrane, Ch. G. (1991). Cellular injury by oxidants. *American Journal of Medicine, 91,* 23.

Deveraj, S., & Jialal, I. (2000). Low-density lipoprotein postsecretory modifications, monocyte function, and circulating adhesion molecules in type 2 diabetic patients with and without macrovascular complications: The effect of alphatocopherol supplementation. *Circulation, 102,* 191–196.

Diplock, A. T. (1991). Antioxidants nutrients and disease prevention: An overview. *American Journal of Clinical Nutrition, 53*(Suppl. 1), 189S–193S.

Dreyer, W., Michael, L., & West, M. (1991). Neutrophil accumulation in ischemic canine myocardium: Insights into the time course, distribution, and mechanism of localization during early reperfusion. *Circulation, 84,* 400–411.

El-Maraghi, N., & Genton, E. (1980). The relevance of platelet and fibrin thromboembolism of the coronary microcirculation, with special reference to sudden cardiac death. *Circulation, 62,* 936–944.

Esmon, C. T. (1998). Inflammation and thrombosis: Mutual regulation by protein C. *Immunologist, 6,* 84–89.

Evans, J. R., & Henshaw, K. (2000). Antioxidant vitamin and mineral supplementation for preventing age-associated macular degeneration. *Cochrane Database of Systematic Reviews, 2,* CD000253.

Felton, G. E. (1980). Fibrinolytic and antithrombotic action of bromelain may eliminate thrombosis in heart patients. *Medical Hypotheses, 6,* 1123–1133.

Feng, L. J., Berger, B. E., Lysz, T. W., & Shaw, W. W. (1988). Vasoactive prostaglandin in the impeding no-reflow state: Evidence for a primary disturbance in microvascular tone. *Plastic & Reconstructive Surgery, 81,* 755.

Feola, M., Simoni, J., Canizaro, P. C., Tran, R., Rashbaum, G., & Behal, F.J., (1988). Toxicity of polymerized hemoglobin solutions. *Surgery, Gynecology, & Obstetrics, 166,* 211–222.

Flatman, P. W., & Lew, V. L. (1983). Magnesium dependence of sodium pump mediated transport in intact human red cells. *Current Topics in Membrane Transport, 19,* 653–657.

Forman, M. B., Puett, D. W., & Virmani, R. (1989). Endothelial and myocardial injury during ischemia and reperfusion: Pathogenesis and therapeutic implications. *Journal of the American College of Cardiology, 13,* 450–459.

Freischlag, J. A., & Hanna, D. (1991). Superoxide anion release after ischemia and reperfusion. *Journal of Surgical Research, 50,* 565.

Go, L. O., Murry, C. E., Richard, V. J., Weischedel, G. R., Jennings, R. B., & Reimer, K. A. (1988). Myocardial neutrophil accumulation during reperfusion after reversible or irreversible ischemic injury. *American Journal of Physiology, 255,* H1188–H1198.

Guyton, K. Z., & Kensleer, T. W. (1993). Oxidative mechanisms in carcinogenesis. *British Medical Bulletin, 49,* 523.

Hardy, S. C., Homer-Vanniasinkam, S., & Gough, M. J. (1992). Effect of free radical scavenging on skeletal muscle blood flow during post-ischemic reperfusion. *British Journal of Surgery, 79,* 1289.

Harstock, L. A., Seaber, A. V., & Urbaniak, J. R. (1989). Intravascular thrombosis in skeletal muscle circulation after ischemia. *Microsurgery, 10,* 161.

Heinicke, R. M., Van der Wal, M., & Yokoyama, M. M. (1972). Effect of bromelain (Ananase) on human platelet aggregation. *Experientia, 28,* 844–845.

Hennig, B., Toborek M, Cader AA, Decker EA (1994). Nutrition, endothelial cell metabolism, and atherosclerosis. *Critical Reviews in Food Science & Nutrition, 34,* 253–282.

Kiyak, J. H., & Zerbino, D. D. (1996). Pathogenesis and morphogenesis of micro-circulatory

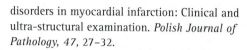
disorders in myocardial infarction: Clinical and ultra-structural examination. *Polish Journal of Pathology, 47,* 27–32.

Kirschner, R. E., Fyfe, B. S., Hoffman, L. A., Chiao, J. J., Davis, J. M., & Fantini, G. A. (1997). Ischemia-reperfusion injury in myocutaneous flaps: Role of leukocytes and leukotrienes. *Plastic & Reconstructive Surgery, 99,* 1485.

Kloner, R. A., Ganote, C. E., & Jennings, R. B. (1974). The "no-reflow" phenomenon after temporary occlusion in the dog. *Journal of Clinical Investigation, 54,* 1496–1508.

Lindsay, T. F., Liaw, S., Romaschin, A. D., & Walker, P. M. (1990). The effect of ischemia/reperfusion on adenine nucleotide metabolism and xanthine oxidase production in skeletal muscle. *Journal of Vascular Surgery, 12,* 8.

Maurer, H. R. (2001). Bromelain: Biochemistry, pharmacology and medical use. *Cellular & Molecular Life Sciences, 58*(9), 1234–1245.

Maxwell, S. R. J., & Lip, G. Y. H. (1997). Reperfusion injury: A review of the pathophysiology, clinical manifestations and therapeutic options. *International Journal of Cardiology, 58,* 95–117.

McCord, J. M. (1985). Oxygen-derived free radicals in postischemic tissue injury. *New England Journal of Medicine, 312,* 159–163.

Meyers, M., Bolli, R., & Lekich, R. (1985). Enhancement of recovery of myocardial function by oxygen free radical scavengers after reversible regional ischemia. *Circulation, 72,* 915–921.

Misso, N. L., Powers, K. A., Gillon, R. L., Stewart, G. A., & Thompson, P. J. (1996). Reduced platelet glutathione peroxidase activity and serum selenium concentrations in atopic asthmatic patients. *Clinical & Experimental Dermatology, 26,* 838–847.

Mutlu-Turkoglu, U., Erbil, Y., Oztezcan, S., Olgac, V., Toker, G., & Uysal, M. (2000). The effect of selenium and/or vitamin E treatments on radi-ation-induced intestinal injury. *Life Sciences, 66,* 1905–1913.

Nieper, H. A. (1978). Effect of bromelain on coronary heart disease and angina pectoris. *Acta Medica Empirica, 5,* 274–278.

Obrenovitch, T. P., & Hallenbeck, J. M. (1985). Platelet accumulation in regions of low blood flow during the postischemic period. *Stroke, 16,* 224–234.

Opie, L. H. (1976). Effects of regional ischemia on metabolism of glucose and fatty acids. *Circulation Research, 38*(Suppl. 1), 52–74.

Patterson, I. S., Klausner, J M., Goldman, G., Kobzik, L., Welbourn R., Valeri R., et al. (1989). Thromboxane mediates the ischemia-induced neutrophil oxidative burst. *Surgery, 106,* 224.

Perry, M. O. (1990). Postischemic cell membrane dysfunction. *Journal of Vascular Surgery, 10,* 179.

Punch, J., Rees, R., Cashmer, B., Wilkins, E., Smith, D. J., & Till, G. O. (1992). Xanthine oxidase: Its role in the no-reflow phenomenon. *Surgery, 111,* 169.

Saeed, M., van Dijke, C. F., Mann, J. S., Wendland, M. F., Rosenau, W., Higgins, et al. (1998). Histologic confirmation of microvascular hy-perpermeability to macromolecular contrast medium in reperfused myocardial infarction. *Journal of Magnetic Resonance Imaging, 8,* 561–567.

Stanley, W. C., Lopaschuk, G. D., Hall, J. L., & McCormack, J. G. (1997). Regulation of myocardial carbohydrate metabolism under normal and ischemic conditions. *Cardiovascular Research, 33,* 243–257.

Steinberg, D. (1997). Low-density lipoprotein oxidation and its pathobiological significance. *Journal of Biological Chemistry, 272,* 20963–20966.

Steinberg, D., Parthasarathy, S., Carew, T. E., Khoo, J. C., & Witztum, J. L. (1989). Beyond choles-terol: Modifications of low-density lipoprotein cholesterol that increases its atherogenicity. *New England Journal of Medicine, 320,* 915–924.

Sumi, H., Banba. T. and Kishimoto. N. (1996). Strong pro-urokinase activators proved in Japanese soybean cheese natto. [In Japanese] *Journal of the Japanese Society for Food Science and Technology, 43*(10), 1124–1127.

Sumi, H., Hamada, H., Nakanishi, K., & Hiratani, H. (1990). Enhancement of the fibrinolytic activity in plasma by oral administration of nattokinase. *Acta Haematologica, 84*(3), 139–143.

Sumi, H., Hamada, H., Tsushima, H., Mihara, H., & Muraki, H. (1987). A novel fibrinolytic enzyme 9 nattokinase in the vegetable cheese Natto; a typical and popular soybean food in the Japanese diet. *Experientia, 43*(10), 1110–1111.

Sundaresan, M., Yu, Z. X., Ferrans, V. J., Irani, K., & Finkel, T. (1995). Requirement for generation of H_2 and O_2 for platelet-derived-growth factor signal transduction. *Science, 270,* 296–299.

Swuartz, W. M., Cha, C. M., Clowes, G. H., & Randall, H. T. (1978). The effect of prolonged ischemia on high energy phosphate metabolism in skeletal muscle. *Surgery, Gynecology, & Obstetrics, 147,* 872.

Taussig, S. J., & Batkin, S. (1988). Bromelain, the enzyme complex of pineapple (*Ananas comosus*) and its clinical application: An update. *Journal of Ethnopharmacology, 22,* 199–203.

Vermyeln, J., Hoylaerts, M. F., & Arnout, J. (1997). Antibody-mediated thrombosis. *Journal of Thrombosis & Haemostasis, 78*(1), 420–426.

Walker, P. M., Lindsay, T. F., Labbe, R., Mickle, D. A., & Romaschin, A. D. (1987). Salvage of skeletal muscle with free radical scavengers. *Journal of Vascular Surgery, 5,* 68.

Ward, P. A., Till, G. O., Kunkel, R., & Beauchamp, C. (1983). Evidence of role of hydroxyl radical in complement and neutrophil-dependent tissue injury. *Journal of Clinical Investigation, 72,* 789.

Weiss, S. J. (1989). Tissue destruction by neutrophils. *New England Journal of Medicine, 320,* 365.

Werbach, M. R., & Murray, M. (1994). *Botanical influences on illness.* Tarzana, CA: Third Line Press.

White, M. J., & Heckler, F. R. (1990). Oxygen free radicals and wound healing. *Clinics in Plastic Surgery, 17,* 473.

Wolff, S. P. (1993). Diabetes mellitus and free radicals. *British Medical Bulletin, 49,* 642.

Zimmerman, J. J. (1991). Therapeutic application of oxygen radical scavengers. *Chest, 100,* 189S.

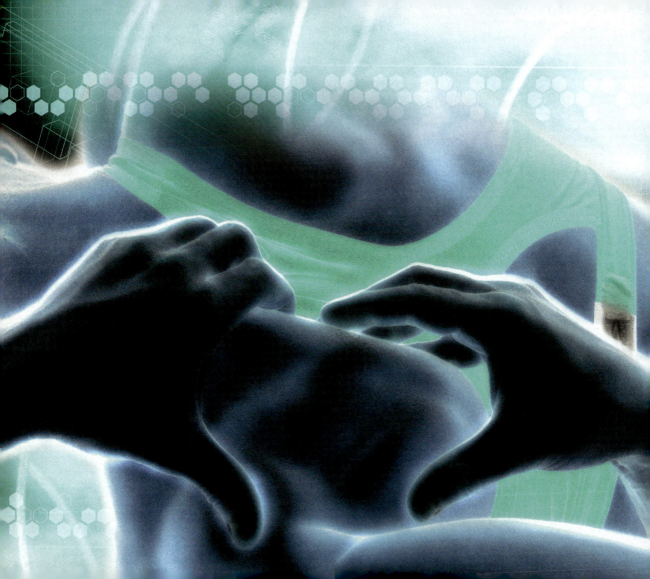

CHAPTER 13

NUTRITIONAL SUPPORT FOR INFLAMMATORY CONDITIONS

Inflammation is the response of the immune system or body tissues to infection, irritation, or injury (Feghali & Wright, 1997). The characteristic signs of inflammation present as redness, swelling, heat, pain, and dysfunction of the affected organ. This is commonly seen in connective tissue, muscle, tendons and fascia due to sports injuries, infections, and allergic reactions. Inflammation, which is mediated by various cytokines, can be categorized as acute (lasting a few days) or chronic (lasting several weeks or longer).

ACUTE INFLAMMATION

Acute inflammation results in the interaction of the immune system and inflammatory cells, which are mediated by proteins called interleukins (IL). Mobilization of various cytokines such as IL-1 and IL-6 activates neutrophils; this is followed by recruitment of macrophages to the injured site (Bedaira, Ho, Fua, & Huard, 2004). Neutrophils appear to have a phagocytic role in addition to releasing proteases to clean up cellular debris (Tidball, 2005). Neutrophils can also release cytotoxic and cytolytic molecules, which cause destruction through lysis of muscle cells, fascia, and surrounding tissues.

CHRONIC INFLAMMATION

Unresolved acute inflammation and overproduction of tumor necrosis factor alpha (TNF-alpha), IL-1, and IL-6 are implicated in chronic inflammation of prolonged duration. These are governed by cellular (cell mediated) and humoral (antibody mediated) immunity.

In the case where an injury to the fascia has not healed completely due to the release of transforming growth factor beta-1 (TGF-β1) during acute injury, fibrosis begins to take place (10–14 days post-injury) that interferes with regeneration of the perimysium, epimysium, and endomysium of muscle. Fibrous scar tissue may have long-lasting and damaging effects on the performance and recovery capability of an athlete's soft tissue. Some of the damaging effects attributed to scar tissue formation include the following:

○ Adhesions consisting of fibrous tissue that may limit movement, for example, between the layers of pleura, preventing inflation of the lungs; between loops of the bowel, interfering with peristalsis.

○ Fibrosis of infarcts. Blockage of an end-vessel by a thrombus or an embolus causes an infarct (area of dead tissue). Fibrosis of one large infarct or of numerous small infarcts may follow, leading to varying degrees of organ dysfunction, for example, in the heart, brain, kidneys, liver.

○ Tissue shrinkage occurs as fibrous tissue ages. The effects depend on the site and extent of the fibrosis.

There is interest in using nutritional supplements to mitigate the inflammatory reaction that occurs after exercise-induced or traumatic injury in order to minimize the impact of tissue damage and allow the body's immune system to begin the repair process. Evidence-based supplements are discussed below.

THE ROLE OF FLAVONOIDS

Flavonoids are polyphenolic compounds found extensively in fruits, vegetables, and drinks such as wine. They possess diverse functions in the body: anti-inflammatory, antioxidant, lipid lowering, antiviral, and anticancer; and they work through a variety of mechanisms (V. Stangl, Lorenz, & K. Stangl, 2006; Song, Lee, & Seong, 2005).

Flavonoids such as rutin, hesperidin, and quercetin reduce inflammation through their antioxidant effect on mast cells and by reducing phagocytosis and release of destructive lysozymes by neutrophils (Guardia, Rotelli, Juarez, & Pelzer, 2001). All three reduced inflammation (in the paw edema rat study) during the acute phase, with rutin being more effective during the chronic inflammatory stage. In general, rutin was more effective than the other two flavonoids, with quercetin possessing stronger activity than hesperidin.

Mast cells found in connective tissue do not circulate in the bloodstream. They participate in IgE-mediated reactions to release proinflammatory cytokines that act on connective tissue, smooth muscle, and the vasculature. Human umbilical cord blood-derived cultured mast cells (hCBMCs) were measured for their ability to secrete potent inflammatory mediators in the presence of certain flavonoids (quercetin, kaempferol, myricetin, and morin; Kempuraj et al., 2005). The effects of flavonoids on the release of tryptase, histamine, and inflammatory cytokines (IL-8, IL-6, and TNF-alpha) from hCBMCs showed an inhibitory effect; the greatest percent inhibition was by quercetin, followed by kaempferol, myricetin, and morin.

Phillips and colleagues conducted an experiment to see if markers of inflammation IL-6 and C-reactive protein (CRP) were attenuated after dietary supplements on postexercise muscle injury (Phillips, Childs, Dreon, Phinney, & Leeuwenburgh, 2003). CRP, an immune system molecule, is an inflammatory marker serving as a diagnostic tool for predicting various disease states associated with inflammation (Phillips et al., 2003). Forty men were randomized to receive either placebo (high oleic sunflower oil) or a dietary supplement consisting of 300 mg mixed tocopherols, 800 mg of docosahexaenoate, and 300 mg of flavonoids (100 mg hesperetin and 200 mg quercetin) on a daily basis for 14 days. Three days postexercise, the control group saw increases in CRP and IL-6, whereas this rise was minimal in the supplemented group. By day 14, both groups showed decreases in both inflammatory mediators with the supplemented group having a statistically significant difference ($P = 0.05$) in IL-6 and CRP ($P < 0.01$) over placebo. The researchers concluded that the anti-inflammatory properties of the dietary supplements attenuated the rise in inflammation associated with muscle damage due to eccentric exercise.

Quercetin

Quercetin is found in various concentrations in apples, onions, raspberries, red wine, citrus fruit, broccoli, and leafy greens. Its diverse effects on health include anticancer, cardiovascular, anti-inflammatory, and antiallergy properties that are due in part to quercetin's effect on quenching damaging reactive oxygen species (Nagata, Takekoshi, Takeyama,

Homma, & Osamura, 2004). Using the rat air pouch as a model to study acute inflammation, Morikawa and colleagues studied the mechanism by which quercetin reduces inflammation (Morikawa et al., 2003). The study demonstrated that quercetin-treated rats had reduced levels of certain inflammatory cytokines (TNF-alpha, Regulated upon Activation, Normal T-cell Expressed, and Secreted [RANTES], macrophage-inflammatory protein-2, and MIP-2) and prostaglandin E2 production resulting in less edema (Figure 13-1). Certain inflammatory cells that release destructive cytokines are inhibited by flavanols such as quercetin.

Boswellia

Boswellia and its main constituent, boswellic acid, are derived from the dried gum resin of *Boswellia carterii*. A study done on rats was designed to assess the efficacy of boswellia extract on reducing adjuvant-induced arthritis in rats (Fan et al., 2005). A single oral dose was administered daily for seven days, and edema and hyperalgesia were assessed and measured. At a dose of 0.45 g/kg/day, there was significant reduction in pain by day five, whereas a higher dose (0.9 g/kg/day) reduced pain at an early stage (5 to 24 hours) and on day five. The researchers speculate that the hyperalgesia effect is due to boswellia's anti-inflammatory properties brought about by immune modulation. Boswellic acids can reduce the production of leukotriene B4 by granulocytes and macrophages as well as slowing the movement of leukocytes to the site of inflammation.

Turmeric

Turmeric root contains volatile oil, diferuloyl methane (curcumin), demethoxycurcumin, and bisdemethoxycurcumin, all of which are known as curcuminoids (Jellin, Batz, & Hitchens, 1999). Curcumin, the lipid-soluble component in turmeric, possesses anti-inflammatory, anticarcinogenic, and antioxidant properties. Curcumin has been shown to consistently block the activity of the transcription factor nuclear factor kappa beta (NF-κβ) (a compound significant in the body's inflammatory response; Cohly, Taylor, Angle, & Salahudeen, 1998). Intraperitoneal injection

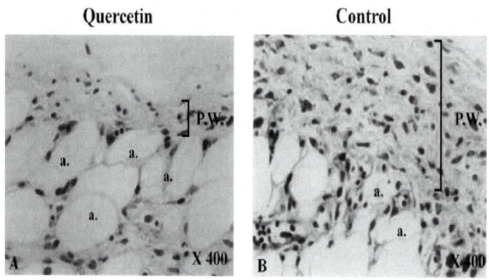

Figure 13-1 Quercetin-treated Rats Showing Histological Changes in Pouch Tissue. (A) Vehicle-treated rat showed tissue edema with a number of inflammatory cells (neutrophils, macrophages, and lymphocytes) and inflamed pouch walls (P.W.). Quercetin-treated rats (B) showed few inflammatory cells and less edema in P.W.

Source: Morikawa et al. (2003).

of mice with curcumin has been shown to stimulate muscle differentiation and enhance the regeneration process after injury through inhibition of NF-κβ expression on various inflammatory cytokines (Thaloor, Miller, Gephart, Mitchell, & Pavlath, 1999). Curcumin also mediates the metabolism of arachidonic acid (AA) by inhibition of cyclooxygenase-2. In addition, lipoxygenase, hyaluronidase, phospholipase, and collagenase enzymes, which also play a role in inflammation, are inhibited.

Resveratrol

Resveratrol is a naturally occurring polyphenolic compound produced by certain vines, pine trees, peanuts, grapes, and other plants. It has been studied for its antimicrobial, anti-inflammatory, anticancer, antioxidant, and beneficial cardiovascular properties. Resveratrol's vast anti-inflammatory properties have been elucidated by in vitro and in vivo studies: (1) inhibition of COX-1 and COX-2 enzymes; (2) antioxidant activity; (3) inhibition of 5-Lipoxygenase (5-Lox); (4) inhibition of mediators of inflammation from macrophage; (5) inhibition of TNF-alpha,

leukotrienes, histamines, and eicosanoids from mast cells; and (6) inhibition of protease and oxidant release from neutrophils (de la Lastra & Villegas, 2005; Figure 13-2).

Inflammation is a complex process that involves cytokine signaling and kinases such as mitogen-activated protein kinase (MAPKs), protein kinase C (PKC), phosphoinositide-3-kinase, and so on. MAPKs phosphorylates (adds a phosphate [PO_4] group to a protein or molecule) a variety of transcription factors, for example, NF-κβ and AP-1. Resveratrol inhibits the activation of these transcription factors and disrupts the signaling pathways required for initiation of the cascade toward inflammation. In addition, topical application of resveratrol can enhance wound healing by increasing connective tissue deposition and improving the overall integrity of the wound area.

Ginger

Ginger, a rhizome of the plant *Zingiber officinale*, has been used in traditional medicine for centuries as a

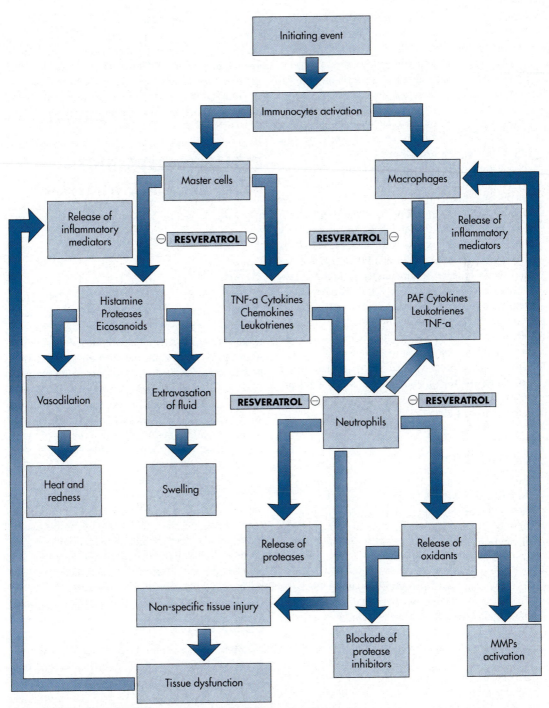

Figure 13-2 Resveratrol Inhibits All Phases of the Inflammatory Response.

*MMP: Matrix Metalloproteinase

Source: de la Lastra & Villegas (2005).

stimulant, diuretic, diaphoretic, and nausea. Today, interest in ginger lies in its antinausea and anti-inflammatory properties. The active components of ginger include phenolic compounds, sesquiterpenes, galanolactone, gingesulfonic acid, zingerone, monoacyldigalactosylglycerols, and gingerglycolipids.

Ginger is able to modulate inflammation through various pathways (Grzanna, Lindmark, & Frondoza, 2005). It does this by inhibiting COX-1 and COX-2 enzymes, thus lowering prostaglandin E2 production, inhibiting 5-Lox and thereby reducing leukotrienes and interfering with the induction of genes involved with inflammation. In addition to its anti-inflammatory property, ginger possesses analgesic effects. One of the active components [6]-gingerol, given in doses of 25 mg/kg and 50 mg/kg, was administered to mice intraperitoneally (Young, Luo, Cheng, Hsieh, Liao, & Peng, 2005). The results revealed a reduction in the acetic acid-induced writhing response (in the late phase) comparable to the nonsteroidal anti-inflammatory drug indomethacin. The acetic writhing test is used to study a drug's peripheral analgesic property, and since the late phase correlates with the inflammatory response and pain, it was concluded that [6]-gingerol acts peripherally rather than centrally.

Cat's Claw

Cat's claw is a tropical vine that grows in rain forest and jungle areas in South America and Asia. The bark and root contain active substances such as alkaloids, polyphenols, tannins, and several other phytochemicals that possess anti-inflammatory and antioxidant activity.

A study conducted by Aguilar and colleagues (Aguilar et al., 2002) compared a hydroalcoholic extract against an aqueous freeze-dried extract from the bark of cat's claw on carrageenan-induced paw edema model in mice (Sandoval et al., 2002). While both extracts significantly reduced edema, the hydroalcoholic extract (50 mg/kg) produced an anti-inflammatory effect at a much lower dose than the freeze-dried extract (200 mg/kg). Cat's claw mechanisms of action involve moderate to weak activity

against COX-1 and COX-2 in vitro, strong antioxidant properties of its proanthocyanidin content in scavenging various free radicals, and suppression of TNF-alpha production (Sandoval et al., 2002). But of the two cat's claw species, *Uncaria tomentosa* and *Uncaria guianensis*, the latter has the most potent antioxidant and anti-inflammatory properties.

OTHER NUTRIENTS AND INFLAMMATION

Other nutrients and compounds may play a role in inflammation.

Vitamin B_6

The active form of vitamin B_6, pyridoxal 5'-phosphate (P5P), is a water-soluble compound that may play a role in the etiology of inflammation. Kelly and colleagues found a direct dose response inverse relationship between CRP and P5P on subjects with new ischemic stroke when compared with matched controls (Kelly et al., 2004). Lower plasma P5P was associated with higher CRP levels. In another study, animals fed a B_6-deficient diet showed greater infiltration of inflammatory cells in the diaphragm, masseter, and heart muscles after infection with *T. Spiralis*, compared to mice fed a normal diet; B_6-deficient rats saw edema increase by 54% compared with weight-matched controls (Frydas et al., 1999; R. Lakshmi, A. Lakshmi, Divan, & Bamji, 1991). Thiobarbituric acid reactive substances (which indicate the extent of lipid peroxidation) increased by 30% and 43% in the edematous tissue of B_6-deficient mice. Collectively, the data show that pyridoxine deficiency enhances inflammation.

Lactoferrin

Lactoferrin, an iron-binding protein derived from milk and processed whey, possesses a host of biological activities such as antibacterial, antitumor, anti-inflammatory, antiviral, antifungal, and immune modulation (Brock, 2002). Neutrophils produce high levels of lactoferrin, which is stored in secondary granules and released during inflammation to contribute to its physiologic properties.

In vitro and in vivo studies have shown that lactoferrin can modulate the immune system and correct cytokine imbalance by inducing anti-inflammatory cytokines IL-4 and IL-10, inhibiting the proinflammatory cytokines TNF-alpha and IL-1 beta, and downregulating NF-κβ (Conneely, 2001; Togawa et al., 2001). Orally administered lactoferrin is broken down in the gut to form a new peptide, lactoferricin, with antibacterial activities similar to the parent compound. Mice fed lactoferrin have shown an increase in IgA and IgG in the intestinal fluid and induction of IL-18 secretion in the small intestine. (Tomita, Wakabayashi, Yamauchi, Teraguchi, & Hayasawa, 2002). IL-18 enhances activities of T helper-1 (Th-1) and natural killer (NK) cells.

Superoxide Dismutase

Superoxide dismutase (SOD) is a naturally occurring enzyme found in the cytosol and mitochondria. Manganese is required for the mitochondrial form, while copper and zinc are required for the cytosol form. SOD plays an important role in cellular antioxidant defenses.

SOD possess potent free radical scavenging activity, and this is thought to be one mechanism by which it interrupts the inflammatory cascade (Riedl et al., 2005). Another mechanism, shown in vitro, involves reduced movement of leukocytes, suggesting a reduction in infiltration of inflammatory cells (Michelson, 1987).

Fish Oil

Docosahexaenoic acid (DHA) and eicosapentaenoic acid (EPA) are omega-3 polyunsaturated fatty acids (PUFAs) capable of regulating the inflammatory process (Simopoulos, 2002). Human studies have shown that fatty acid metabolism is linked to the immune system through effects on eicosanoids (prostaglandins, leukotrienes, and thromboxanes). Prostaglandins are regulators of the immune response, and their formation is influenced by fatty acids that affect arachidonic acid (AA) metabolism. EPA and DHA compete with AA to reduce prostaglandin E2 and leukotriene B4 formation. In addition, these PUFAs have the ability to reduce the capacity of monocytes to produce IL-1 and TNF-alpha.

By reducing the amount of saturated fat in the diet and incorporating omega-3 PUFAs, studies have shown that the immune and inflammatory processes in the body can be regulated through modification of cytokines, ecosanoids, and gene expression. But consumption of PUFAs beyond three to four grams daily may impair immunity and result in increased lipid peroxidation and resultant oxidative species, causing a reduction in T-cell directed function, NK cell function, and macrophage activity (Meydani, 1996). Therefore, consumption of other antioxidants may be required to reduce the overall rise in oxidant by-products.

Cetylated Monounsaturated Fatty Acid

Cetylated monounsaturated fatty acid reduces inflammation and pain via the following possible mechanisms: (1) inhibition of 5-lipoxygenase enzyme, a potent mediator of inflammation; and (2) inhibition of pro-inflammatory cytokine release (e.g., tumor necrosis factor-alpha, interleukin-1 beta), which mediates inflammation. Reducing inflammation in the body is paramount in maintaining the pliability and integrity of fascia. Topical cream applied twice daily to affected area or oral dosing in the form of capsules/tablets at a strength of 1,050 mg three times daily should be used. The absorption from oral or topical formulations is similar (Hesslink, Armstrong, Nagendran, Sreevatsan, & Barathur, 2002; Kraemer et al., 2005).

Summary

Nutritional intervention in sports-related trauma can have a dramatic impact on the recovery of the affected organ. The link between the immune system and inflammation increases our understanding of how supplements can confer benefits without the gastrointestinal adverse effects associated with conventional drug therapy. Acute inflammation, while beneficial to some extent in the healing phase, can lead to chronic inflammation; and the use of nutritional supplements is gaining popularity as a means of mitigating the destructive effect of the inflammatory response.

References

Aguilar, J. L., Rojas, P., Marcelo, A., Plaza, A., Bauer, A., Reininger, E., et al. (2002). Anti-inflammatory activity of two different extracts of *Uncaria tomentosa* (Rubiaceae). *Journal of Ethnopharmacology, 81,* 271–276.

Bedaira, H. S., Ho, A. M., Fua, F. H., & Huard, J. (2004). Skeletal muscle regeneration: An update on recent findings. *Current Opinion in Orthopaedics, 15:* 360–363.

Brock, J. H. (2002). The physiology of lactoferrin. *Biochemistry & Cell Biology, 80,* 1–6.

Cohly, H. H., Taylor, M. F., Angel, A., & Salahudeen, A. K. (1998). Effect of turmeric, turmerin and curcumin on H_2O_2-induced renal epithelial (LLC-PK1) cell injury. *Free Radical Biology & Medicine, 24,* 49–54.

Conneely, O. M. (2001). Anti-inflammatory activities of lactoferrin. *Journal of the American College of Nutrition, 20*(5), 389S–395S.

de la Lastra, C. A., & Villegas, I. (2005). Resveratrol as an anti-inflammatory and anti-aging agent: Mechanisms and clinical implications. *Molecular Nutrition & Food Research, 49,* 405–430.

Fan, A. Y., Lao, L., Zhang, R. X., Zhou, A. N., Wang, L. B., Moudgil, K. D., Lee, D. Y., et al. (2005). Effects of an acetone extract of *Boswellia carterii Birdw.* (Burseraceae) gum resin on adjuvant-induced arthritis in Lewis rats. *Journal of Alternative and Complementary Medicine.* 11(2), 323–31 .

Feghali, C. A., & Wright, T. M. (1997). Cytokines in acute and chronic inflammation. *Frontiers in Bioscience, 2,* d12–26.

Frydas, S., Papaioanou, N., Vlemmas, I., Theodoridis, I., Anogiannakis, G., Vacalis, D., et al. (1999). Vitamin B_6-deficient diet plus 4-deoxypyridoxine (4-DPD) reduces the inflammatory response induced by *T. spiralis* in diaphragm, masseter and heart muscle tissue of mice. *Molecular Cell Biochemistry, 197*(1–2), 79–85.

Grzanna, R., Lindmark, L., & Frondoza, C. G. (2005). Ginger—a herbal medicinal product with broad anti-inflammatory actions. *Journal of Medicinal Food, 8*(2), 125–132.

Guardia, T., Rotelli, A. E., Juarez, A. O., & Pelzer, L. E. (2001). Anti-inflammatory properties of plant flavonoids. Effects of rutin, quercetin and hesperidin on adjuvant arthritis in rat. *Il Farmaco, 56,* 683–687.

Hesslink, R., Jr., Armstrong, D., Nagendran, M. V., Sreevatsan, S., & Barathur, R. (2002). Cetylated fatty acids improve knee function in patients with osteoarthritis. *Journal of Rheumatology, 29,* 1708–1712.

Jellin, J. M., Batz, F., & Hitchens, K. (1999). *Pharmacist's Letter/Prescriber's Letter, Natural medicines comprehensive database,* 2nd ed. Stockton, CA: Therapeutic Research Faculty.

Kelly, P., Kistler, J. P., Shih, V. E., Mandell, R., Atassi, N., Barron, M., et al. (2004). Inflammation, homocysteine, and vitamin B_6 status after ischemic stroke. *Stroke, 35,* 12.

Kempuraj, D., Madhappan, B., Christodoulou, S., Boucher, W., Cao, J., Papadopoulou, N., et al. (2005). Flavonols inhibit proinflammatory mediator release, intracellular calcium ion levels and protein kinase C theta phosphorylation in human mast cells. *British Journal of Pharmacology, 145,* 934–944.

Kraemer, W., Ratamess, N. A., Maresh, C. M., Anderson, J. A., Volek, J., Tiberio, D., et al. (2005). A cetylated fatty acid topical cream with menthol reduces pain and improves functional performance in patients with arthritis. *Journal of Strength & Conditioning Research 19*(1), 115–121.

Lakshmi, R., Lakshmi, A. V., Divan, P. V., & Bamji, M. S. (1991). Effect of riboflavin or pyridoxine deficiency on inflammatory response. *Indian Journal of Biochemistry & Biophysics, 28*(5–6), 481–484.

Meydani, S. N. (1996). Effect of (n-3) polyunsaturated fatty acids on cytokine production and their biologic function. *Nutrition, 12*(Suppl.1), S8–S14.

Michelson, A. M. (1987). Medical aspects of superoxide dismutase. *Life Chemistry Reports, 6,* 141–142.

Morikawa, K., Nonaka, M., Narahara, M., Torii, I., Kawaguchi, K., Yoshikawa, T., et al. (2003). Inhibitory effect of quercetin on carrageenan-induced inflammation in rats. *Life Sciences, 74,* 709–7217.

Nagata, H., Takekoshi, S., Takeyama, R., Homma, T., & Osamura, Y. (2004). Quercetin enhances melanogenesis by increasing the activity and synthesis of tyrosinase in human melanoma cells and in normal human melanocytes. *Pigment Cell Research, 17,* 66–73.

Phillips, T., Childs, A. C., Dreon, D. M., Phinney, S., & Leeuwenburgh, C. (2003). A dietary supplement attenuates IL-6 and CRP after eccentric exercise in untrained males. *Medicine & Science in Sports & Exercise,* 35 (12) , 2032–2037.

Riedl, C. R., Sternig, P., Gallé, G., Langmann, F., Vcelar, B., Vorauer, K., et al. (2005). Liposomal recombinant human superoxide dismutase for the treatment of Peyronie's disease: A randomized placebo-controlled double-blind prospective clinical study. *European Urology,* 48, 656–661.

Sandoval, M., Okuhama, N. N., Zhang, X. J., Condezo, L. A., Lao, J., Angeles, F. M., et al. (2002). Anti-inflammatory and antioxidant activities of cat's claw (*Uncaria tomentosa* and *Uncaria guianensis*) are independent of their alkaloid content. *Phytomedicine, 9,* 325–337.

Simopoulos, A. P. (2002). Omega-3 fatty acids in inflammation and autoimmune diseases. *Journal of the American College of Nutrition, 21*(6), 495–505.

Song, J. M., Lee, K. H., & Seong, B. L. (2005). Antiviral effect of catechins in green tea on influenza virus. *Antiviral Research, 68*(2), 66–74.

Stangl, V., Lorenz, M., & Stangl, K. (2006). The role of tea and tea flavonoids in cardiovascular health. *Molecular Nutrition & Food Research, 50*(2), 218–228.

Thaloor, D., Miller, K. J., Gephart, J., Mitchell, P. O., & Pavlath, G. K. (1999). Systemic administration of the NF-κβ inhibitor curcumin stimulates muscle regeneration after traumatic injury. *American Journal of Physiology, 277*(2 Pt 1), C320–329.

Tidball, J. G. (2005). Inflammatory processes in muscle injury and repair. *American Journal of Physiology Regulatory, Integrative & Comparative Physiology, 288,* 345–353.

Togawa, J., Nagase, H., Tanaka, K., Inamori, M., Umezawa, T., Nakajima, A., et al. (2001). Lactoferrin reduces colitis in rats via modulation of the immune system and correction of cytokine imbalance. *Advances in Nutritional Research, 10,* 247–269.

Tomita, M., Wakabayashi, H., Yamauchi, K., Teraguchi, S., & Hayasawa, H. (2002). Bovine lactoferrin and lactoferricin derived from milk: Production and applications. *Biochemistry & Cell Biology, 80,* 109–112.

Young, H. Y., Luo, Y. L., Cheng, H. Y., Hsieh, W. C., Liao, J. C., & Peng, W. H. (2005). Analgesic and anti-inflammatory activities of [6]-gingerol. *Journal of Ethnopharmacology, 96,* 207–210.

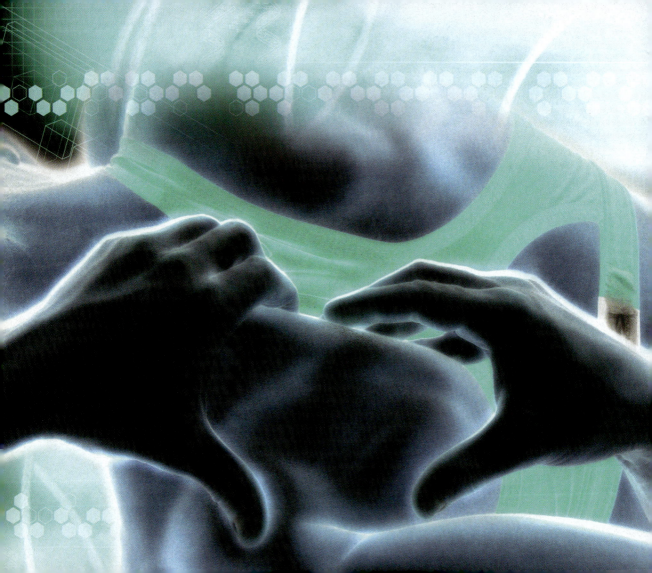

PHARMACOLOGICAL MANAGEMENT OF FASCIAL PATHOLOGIES

Pharmacology is defined as the interaction between chemical agents and biological systems. In regards to muscle and its associated fascia, growth factors regulate the protein metabolism of muscles. In conditions of inflammation and overzealous response of TGF-1 beta, antifibrotics can play a role in reducing scarring and enhance functional recovery of muscles. Nonsteroidal anti-inflammatory medications, on the other hand, while effective for reduction of pain and inflammation, have adverse effects that can impair muscle healing. Local injection therapy is also discussed.

GROWTH FACTORS AND IMMUNE RESPONSE

Research involving growth factors in connective tissue care management is very intriguing from the standpoint of its potential role as a therapeutic alternative in the treatment of tissue fascia injuries. Growth factors are biological factors that cause cellular growth and proliferation of new tissue.

The major growth factor families (Komarcevic, 2000) are epidermal growth factor (EGF), transforming growth factor-beta (TGF-beta), insulin-like growth factor 1 (IGF-1), interleukins (ILs), platelet-derived growth factor (PDGF), fibroblast growth factor (FGF), vascular endothelial growth factor (VEGF), and colony-stimulating factors (CSF). The growth factors described in this section have been used in research and are currently being assessed clinically.

Epidermal Growth Factor (EGF)

Epidermal growth factor (EGF) promotes epidermal growth and is commonly found in tears. The concentration of EGF in an individual's tears has been found to be a positive determinant for healing following eye surgery (Fagerholm, 2000). When EGF is applied to injured skin, such as burns, ulcers (skin or GI tract), and surgical corneal (eye) wounds, it does promote healing. Therefore, EGF has been used for diabetic leg ulcers and venous stasis ulcers as a topical application. Hence, EGF can enhance healing time in suspected cases of fascial tears overlying the muscle.

Insulin-like Growth Factor (IGF-1 and other IGFs)

Many tissues in the body (including muscle, GI tract, and skin, as well as many others) have receptors for IGF-1. IGF-1, and IGF-2 and are important in skeletal muscle repair and regeneration (MacGregor & Parkhouse, 1996). IGF-1 is available usually at

medical research institutions or in medical trials. Nutrients such as dihydroepiandrosterone (DHEA), which increase IGF-1, may also have a clinical role in accelerating the repair of connective tissue injuries.

Human Growth Hormone (HGH)

Human growth hormone (HGH) is secreted abundantly in children to enable them to achieve normal growth. In young adults, still-high levels of HGH help keep them physically healthy and youthful looking. With aging, growth hormone secretion and IGF-1 production decline, contributing to a variety of biochemical and physical degenerative changes, including delayed skeletal muscle healing. Synthetically produced HGH is taken intravenously by some individuals under the supervision of a physician specialist to slow or in some cases even reverse the effects of aging. HGH is much more readily available than IGF-1 and has been used in a variety of clinical studies to improve body composition and effect healing (Chen et al., 1999).

Antiaging physicians who treat their aging patients with HGH are accustomed to the accelerated healing time these patients have compared with age-matched individuals with very low IGF-1 levels. In general, individuals taking proper dosing of HGH have adequate levels of IGF-1, so they heal faster.

HGH works by increasing levels of IGF-1, and as a result promotes anabolism and the healing of fractures due to receptors for IGF-1 being found in fibroblasts, chondrocytes, and osteoblasts (Bail et al., 2002; Raschke et al., 2001). Most common side effects experienced by HGH users are hypoglycemia (low blood sugar level) and inadequate thyroid function. A huge misconception, brought on by the mass media, is that giantism is a common side effect of using GH in the normal human body. This is true only if GH is used during the prepubescent period in one's life. It is very important that a person be fully grown and mature before using GH. Other rare side effects include diabetes, heart enlargement, high blood pressure, and enlargement of the kidneys.

Fibroblast Growth Factor-10 (FGF-10)

Application of fibroblast growth factor-10 (FGF-10) improves wound strength, collagen content, and epidermal thickness (Jimenez & Rampy, 1999). The parameters for wound strength involve fibroblast cells that produce connective tissue and scarring. At present, FGF-10 is used in research investigations only. Fibroblast growth factor is also known as keratinocyte growth factor-2 (KGF-2).

Vascular Endothelial Growth Factor (VEGF)

Vascular endothelial factor (VEGF) promotes the development of new blood vessels, including the smooth muscle cells found in the walls of blood vessels. New blood vessels must form and reconnect to each other in order for fascia to be reperfused with oxygen and nutrients, and thus form new tissue. VEGF is produced by neutrophils during the inflammatory process of a soft tissue injury and as a result promotes the revascularization of fascia (McCourt, Wang, Sookhai, & Redmond, 1999).

Modulating the Immune Response During Healing

Interleukin (IL) refers to non-antibody proteins called cytokines that act as cellular mediators in generating an immune response. An appropriate immune response depends upon the proper balance of cytokines, some that induce antibody action and others that inhibit the action when no longer needed for healing. IL-6 is a cytokine that stimulates a number of immune system reactions that promote the healing action of antibodies at the wound site (Gallucci et al., 2001). However, in cases of excessive inflammation where the IL-6 concentration is too high, there are negative consequences. In rehabilitation of injured tendons and ligaments, oversecretion of IL-6 during the rehabilitation exercise phase may cause exaggerated proliferation of fibroblast cells, leading to scarring and scar contraction. Conversely, in

ligament injuries such as the medial collateral ligament (MCL) of the knee, a certain level of fibrous tissue must form in order for the ligament to heal. The release of IL-6 promotes MCL collagen synthesis, leading to fibrous tissue formation (Hankenson, Watkins, Schoenlein, Allen, & Turek, 2000). It has been suggested that IL-6 levels should be monitored in skeletal joints, aiming for a certain optimal level that promotes enough influx of inflammatory cells to encourage healing, but not so much as to damage healing tissue with excessive scarring. This suggestion also applies to body workers who are assessing and treating injuries to fascia (Skutek, Van Griensven, Zeichen, Brauer, & Bosch, 2001).

ANTIFIBROTICS

Although administering exogenous growth factors (e.g., IGF-1, bFGF, or NGF) can enhance muscle regeneration, it does not prevent fibrosis in injured muscle. Preliminary results strongly suggest that researchers should focus their efforts on eliminating fibrosis to enhance healing within injured skeletal muscle. TGF-beta 1 plays a crucial role in fibrosis, and by inhibiting its signaling pathway the formation of fibrotic scar tissue can be minimized (Bedair, Ho, Fu, & Huard, 2004).

Researchers have looked at a number of antifibrosis agents with the goal of blocking fibrosis and promoting improved functional recovery of injured skeletal muscle. Using different animal models of muscle injury, the antifibrotics decorin, suramin, and interferon-gamma (IFN-g) can antagonize the effect of TGF-β1 in different ways. Decorin works by directly inhibiting TGF-β1 suramin competes with TGF-β1 receptors, and IFN-g interferes with TGF-β1 signal transduction (Chan, Li, Foster, Horaguchi, Somogyi, et al., 2003; Foster, Li, Usas, Somogyi, Huard, 2003; Fukushima et al., 2001; Li, Foster, Deasy, Chan, Prisk, et al., 2004; Sato, Li, Foster, Fukushima, Badlani, et al., 2003). All these antifibrosis agents block the action of TGF-β1, inhibit skeletal muscle fibrosis induced by traumatic injury, enhance muscle regeneration, and improve the functional recovery of injured muscle. See Figure 14-1 for a summary of antifibrosis therapy.

Relaxin, a hormone produced during pregnancy that facilitates the birth process, belongs to the insulin-like growth factors family. Negishi and colleagues used an animal model of fibrosis in skeletal muscle after injury and found that relaxin increased muscle regeneration and strength in addition to reducing fibrotic scar tissue development by inhibiting collagen production caused by TGF-β1 and interleukin-1 beta (Negishi, Li, Usas, Fu, & Huard, 2005). Like superoxide dismutase (SOD), relaxin can increase the expression of myogenic proteins like desmin.

Timing of relaxin administration is important in controlling fibrosis and maintaining a balance between muscle fiber regeneration and growth of connective tissue. The researchers found that relaxin injected into muscle three days after injury, during the inflammatory phase, produced the best results in the functional recovery of injured muscle and reduced fibrosis. The optimal timing for decorin administration to maximize antifibrosis and enhance muscle regeneration and strength is 10 to 15 days after injury (Fukushima et al., 2001). Fukushima and colleagues have demonstrated that 50 mcg of decorin post-injury results in a greater number of regenerating myofibers than do lower concentrations (Figure 14-2).

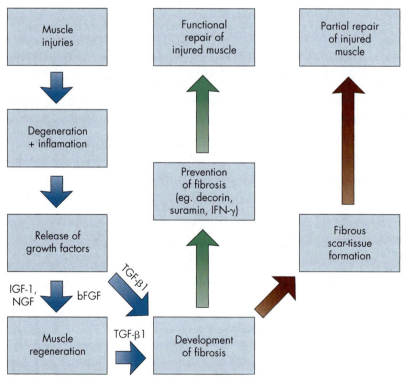

Figure 14-1 Pathway Showing Development of Fibrosis by TGF-beta-1 and Its Prevention Using Antifibrotic Therapy (decorin, suramin, interferon-gamma).
Igf-1 = insulin-like growth factor, bfGf = basic fibroblast growth factor, NGF = nerve growth factor, **TGF-**β1 = transforming growth factor, IFN-gamma = interferon gamma.
Source: Yong, et al., 2005.

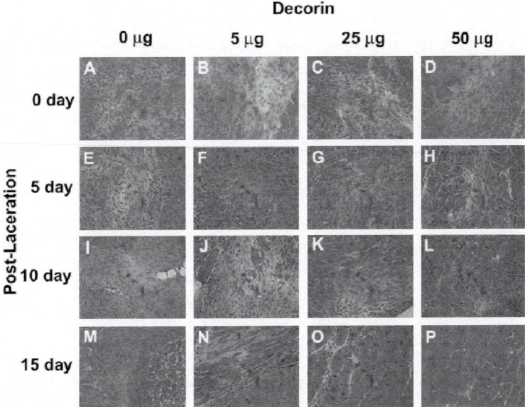

Figure 14-2 Panels A, B, C, and D Show Lacerated Muscle Injected with 0, 5, 25, and 50 mcg of Decorin Immediately Post-injury. The same concentrations of decorin were used for the following: panels E, F, G, and H showing decorin injected 5 days after injury; panels I, J, K, and L showing muscle injected with decorin 10 days after laceration; and panels M, N, O, and P showing decorin injected 15 days after muscle laceration.

Source: Fukushima et al. (2001).

NONSTEROIDAL ANTI-INFLAMMATORY DRUGS (NSAIDS)

Nonsteroidal anti-inflammatory drugs (NSAIDs) are commonly prescribed for injuries involving inflammation. NSAIDs work by blocking the activity of the cyclooxygenase (COX) enzyme. There are two types of COX enzymes (COX-1 and COX-2), and they differ in their physiological function. COX-1 has a protective role on the gastric mucosa and renal blood flow, whereas COX-2 is implicated in inflammatory reactions (Cordero, Camacho, Obach, Domenech, & Vila, 2001). These two enzymes catalyze the formation of ecosanoids from arachidonic acid (Figure 14-3), and these metabolites are involved in acute inflammation (de Leval et al., 2000). Another property by which certain NSAIDs (diclofenac, indomethacin, piroxicam, and tenoxicam) are able to reduce inflammation involves their inhibition of reactive oxygen species (ROS) generation by neutrophils (Paino et al., 2005). Upon injury, neutrophils generate ROS at the affected area as a line of defense to reduce bacterial infection (Paino et al., 205). However, these highly reactive substances damage tissue, leading to chronic inflammation.

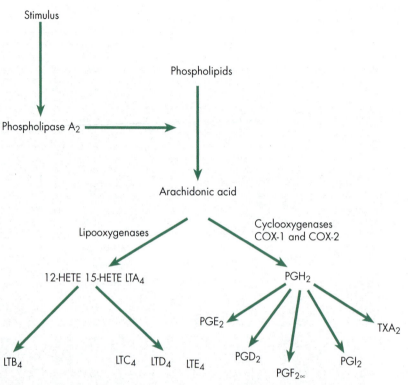

Stimulus

Phospholipids

Phospholipase A$_2$

Arachidonic acid

Lipooxygenases

Cyclooxygenases
COX-1 and COX-2

12-HETE 15-HETE LTA$_4$

PGH$_2$

PGE$_2$

TXA$_2$

LTB$_4$

LTC$_4$ LTD$_4$ LTE$_4$

PGD$_2$

PGF$_{2\infty}$

PGI$_2$

Figure 14-3 **Formation of Various Eicosanoids (prostaglandins and leukotrienes) That Are Pro-Inflammatory Compounds.**
Source: de Leval et al. (2000).

Problems with NSAIDs

The nonspecific NSAIDs (e.g., indomethacin, ibuprofen, naproxen, piroxicam) inhibit both COX-1 and COX-2 enzymes. The COX-1 enzyme is expressed in a variety of organs such as the gastrointestinal tract, kidney, fetal cells, and neurons of the brain. Due to the nonspecific nature of COX enzyme inhibition, these NSAIDs are implicated in producing harmful side effects. For example, common adverse events stemming from a reduction in prostaglandin (PG) derived from COX-1 results in loss of protective barrier of the gastric mucosa and reduction in renal blood flow. Studies have shown that concomitant use of two or more NSAIDs increases gastrointestinal, hepatic, and renal injury by two times over single drug use (Clinard et al., 2004).

Specific COX-2 inhibitors

COX-2 inhibitors were designed to reduce the adverse effects of COX-1 inhibition from nonspecific NSAIDs, but studies have shown that this newer class of drugs possesses other undesirable side effects resulting from COX-2 enyzme blockade.

The COX-2 enzyme is considered to be an inducible enzyme that can contribute to chronic inflammation with prolonged use (Doux, Bazar, Lee, & Yun, 2005). NSAIDS that block COX-2 enzyme activity can increase the production of this enzyme and contribute to high levels of latent COX-2. When NSAIDs are withdrawn or blood levels fall below therapeutic values due to noncompliance, the high levels of COX-2 can increase synthesis of PG, leading to an increase in inflammation.

The growth of muscle myofibers is dependent on COX-2 activity. Using a mouse model for muscle atrophy, Bondesen and colleagues demonstrated that multiple mechanisms of muscle growth are regulated by the COX-2 pathway (Bondesen, Mills, Kegley, & Pavlath, 2004). Prostaglandins, for example, play a crucial role in various stages of myogenesis; and inflammation enhances muscle repair soon after injury. PG derived from COX-2 but not COX-1 is important for muscle regeneration after trauma, and specifically blocking the activity of COX-2 can delay muscle regeneration.

Topical NSAIDs

Diclofenac is an NSAID that is used to treat arthritis or pain originating in soft tissues. As with other NSAIDs, it can produce gastric irritation or ulceration, fluid retention, and other systemic side effects. When diclofenac is delivered transdermally, it can be selectively concentrated in the joints or soft tissues, thereby minimizing the gastric side effects. A study by Cordero and colleagues has shown that not all NSAIDs applied topically are effective at mitigating inflammation derived from COX-2 (Cordero et al., 2001). In vitro study has revealed that indomethacin, ketorolac, ketoprofen, and diclofenac showed the strongest activity against COX-2 when applied topically; however, penetration enhancers are required to increase efficacy (Cordero et al., 2001).

The ability of diclofenac to be efficiently absorbed depends on its formulation base. Absorption enhancers such as oleic acid and d-limonene increase permeation of the drug (Escribano, Calpena, Queralt, Obach, & Domenech, 2003). Other studies have used microemulsion formulations of water, lauryl alcohol, and Labrasol (surfactant)/ethanol (cosurfactant) (1:2) (Kweon, Chi, & Park, 2004) and mixed micelle formulas of lecithin with cholate or deoxycholate in an attempt to increase absorption while minimizing skin irritation (Hendradi, Obata, Isowa, Nagai, & Takayama, 2003).

While NSAIDs work through various mechanisms to mitigate inflammation, judicious use of these agents has been implicated in adverse reactions ranging from gastrointestinal intolerance to drug interactions and impaired wound healing. Because of these untoward side effects, nutritional therapies appear more favorable as healing agents in sports injuries involving inflammation.

LOCAL INJECTION THERAPY

Local injection therapies are used in the management of a number of soft tissue disorders and include the local infiltration of substances like methylprednisolone or triamcinolone with or without lignocaine (Neer, 1983) More recently Actovegin (Wright-Carpenter, Klein, Schaferhoff, Appell, & Mir, 2004) injections into the fascial adhesions were used in an attempt to increase glucose and oxygen delivery.

Local Anesthetic Injections and Dry Needling

The local injection of an anesthetic such as methylprednisolone into the fascial adhesion aims to reduce symptoms of pain. Dry needling may be equally effective, although the use of local anesthetic may reduce postinjection soreness. According to Fricton (1994) and Jaeger and colleagues (1987), the main action of anesthetic injections and dry needling rests with the mechanical disruption of the trigger point; and in the case where a local anesthetic is used, desensitization of the area will occur (Fricton, 1994; Jaeger & Skootsky, 1987).

It is important that a properly trained and certified clinician localize the adhesions/restrictions in the fascia using careful manual palpation and/or percussion with a tendon hammer. Prior to injection it is important to stretch the area locally, followed by insertion of the needle parallel to the muscle fibers. Upon inserting the needle, the clinician may experience resistance by the taut band of muscle fibers, while the patient may report a feeling of a dull ache along a referred zone.

Some physicians have experimented with using a low dose paraben-free Celestone Soluspan injectable suspension coadministered with a local anesthetic, such as 1% or 2% lidocaine hydrochloride, for adhesive capsulitis. Adhesive capsulitis, or frozen shoulder, is characterized by marked fibrosis and adhesions. The initial dosage of Celestone Soluspan injectable suspension can vary from 0.5 to 9.0 mg/daily, depending on the type of fascial pathology being treated. In situations of less severity, lower doses will generally suffice; in selected patients, higher initial doses may be required.

The Celestone Soluspan injectable serves a number of purposes. Corticosteroids are useful in suppressing inflammation in the short term—and in the long term, dissolving scar tissue, stabilizing the body's defenses, and speeding the healing process—and are very effective in causing certain cysts to disappear. In addition, cortiscosteroids may have a weakening effect on fascial restrictions, making it easier for the clinician to break down the scar tissue. Besides the local anesthetic, compressed air is injected in conjunction with the Celestone Soluspan injection. If the air is injected at a high enough pressure, a breakage of the collagen cross-links spreads throughout the web of fascia, hence restoring full range of motion.

Many users and treating clinicians report significant increases in range of motion within a single treatment! The only downfall with this type of treatment is the short duration of pain caused by the establishment of inflammation attributed to microtrauma to various soft tissue structures.

Local Administration of Actovegin

For years, a standard German practice for the treatment of muscle strain injuries has been a local injection of Actovegin, a deproteinized dialysate from bovine blood which contains electrolytes and essential trace elements and 30% of organic components as amino acids, oligopeptides, nucleosides, intermediary products of the carbohydrate and of the fat metabolism, and components of the cellular membranes such as glycosphingolipids (Nycomed, 2007). One of the physiologic components of Actovegin is inositol phospho-oligosaccharides (IPOs; Nycomed, 2007). These compounds are thought to possess central and peripheral insulin-like effects (Fricton, 1994).

The active components in Actovegin promote glucose uptake by cerebral and skeletal muscle and other cells and stimulate intrinsic glucose transport by regulating glucose carrier GluT1; Actovegin activates pyruvate dehydrogenase (PDH), resulting in increased cellular utilization of glucose and formation of energy-rich substances (Jaeger & Skootsky, 1987). Actovegin also increases uptake and utilization of oxygen by hypoxic tissues and cells. It does this by promoting mitochondrial function and decreased lactate formation to protect hypoxic tissue (Nelson et al., 1989). Actovegin is commonly combined with Traumeel, a homeopathic anti-inflammatory drug, along with extracts of arnica, calendula, and camomile, among others.

Actovegin works by generally increasing the amount of cellular energy available for a tissue or organ system to use by increasing the uptake and utilization of glucose and oxygen (Nycomed, 2007). These two effects are coupled and give rise to increased levels of ATP and thus a greater availability of energy for the cell (Nycomed, 2007). Actovegin is indicated for cases where the body is in a state of increased energy requirement—during wound healing, soft tissue injuries, and in states where the body is experiencing an impairment of normal physiological functioning such as during hypoxia, which can occur during soft tissue injuries or substrate deficiency (Nycomed, 2007).

As one can see, a number of injection therapies are available for the management of soft tissue injuries such as fascial adhesions and fascial tears. Although an increasing number of techniques and injectables are available, such as Actovegin, the current evidence for connective tissue injury use is scant.

Summary

Growth factors are necessary for cell differentiation and proliferation. During wound healing, various growth factors are released at different stages in the repair process to stimulate angiogenesis, fibroblast formation, and wound contraction.

To enhance wound healing and reduce symptoms from injury, some people resort to pharmacologic therapy such as NSAIDs (oral, topical) and local injection therapy. Each has its own advantages and disadvantages. NSAIDs are easy to administer and contribute to immediate pain relief, but not without adverse gastrointestinal side effects. Local injection is more site specific and provides dramatic relief from pain. The caution with corticosteroid injection is its damaging effect on joint cartilage if overused.

References

Bail, H. J., Kolbeck, S., Krummrey, G., Schmidmaier, G., Haas, N. P., & Raschke, M. J. (2002). Systemic application of growth hormone for enhancement of secondary and intramembranous fracture healing. *Hormone Research, 58*(Suppl. 3), 39–42.

Bedair, H. S., Ho, A. M., Fu, F. H., & Huard, J. (2004). Skeletal muscle regeneration: An update on recent findings. *Current Opinion in Orthopaedics, 15,* 360–363.

Bondesen, B. A., Mills, S. T., Kegley, K. M., & Pavlath, G. K. (2004). The COX-2 pathway is essential during early stages of skeletal muscle regeneration. *American Journal of Physiology Cell Physiology, 287,* 475–483.

Chan, Y. S., Li, Y., Foster, W., Horaguchi, T., Somogyi, G., Fu, F.H., & Huard, J (2003). Antifibrotic effects of suramin in injured skeletal muscle after laceration. *Journal of Applied Physiology, 95*(2), 771–780.

Chen, K., Nezu, R., Wasa, M., Sando, K., Kamata, S., Takagi, Y., et al. (1999). Insulin-like growth factor-1 modulation of intestine epithelial cell restitution. *Journal of Parenteral and Enteral Nutrition, 23*(5 Suppl), S89–S92.

Clinard, F., Sgro, C., Bardou, M., Hillon, P., Dumas, M., Kreft-Jais, C., et al. (2004). Association between concomitant use of several systemic NSAIDs and an excess risk of adverse drug reaction. A case/non-case study from the French Pharmacovigilance system database. *European Journal of Pharmacology, 60,* 279–283.

Cordero, J., Camacho, M., Obach, R., Domenech, J., & Vila, L. (2001). In vitro based index of topical anti-inflammatory activity to compare a series of NSAIDs. *European Journal of Pharmaceutics and Biopharmaceutics, 51,* 135–142.

de Leval, X., Delarge, J., Somers, F., de Tullio, P., Henrotin, Y., Pirotte, B., et al. (2000). Recent advances in inducible cyclooxygenase (COX-2) inhibition. *Current Medicinal Chemistry, 7,* 1041–1062.

Doux, J. D., Bazar, K. A., Lee, P. Y., & Yun, A. Y. (2005). Can chronic use of anti-inflammatory agents paradoxically promote chronic inflammation through compensatory host response? *Medical Hypotheses, 65,* 389–391.

Escribano, E., Calpena, A. C., Queralt, J., Obach, R., & Domenech, J. (2003). Assessment of diclofenac permeation with different formulations: Anti-inflammatory study of a selected formula. *European Journal of Pharmaceutical Sciences, 19*(4), 203–210.

Fagerholm, P. (2000). Wound healing after photorefractive keratectomy. *Journal of Cataract Refractory Surgery, 26*(3), 432–447.

Foster, W., Li, Y., Usas, A., Somogyi G, Huard J. (2003). Gamma interferon as an antifibrosis agent in skeletal muscle. *Journal of Orthopaedic Research, 21*(5), 798–804.

Fricton, J. R. (1994). Myofascial pain. *Baillieres Best Practice & Research. Clinical Rheumatology, 8,* 857–880.

Skutek, M., Van Griensven, M., Zeichen, J., Brauer, N., & Bosch, U. (2001). Cyclic mechanical stretching enhances secretion of Interleukin-6 in human tendon fibroblasts. *Knee Surgery, Sports Traumatology, Arthroscopy, 9*(5), 322–326.

Wright-Carpenter, T., Klein, P., Schaferhoff, P., Appell, H. J., Mir, L. M., & Wehling, P. (2004). Treatment of muscle injuries by local administration of autologous conditioned serum: A pilot study on sportsmen with muscle strains. *International Journal of Sports Medicine, 25,* 588–593.

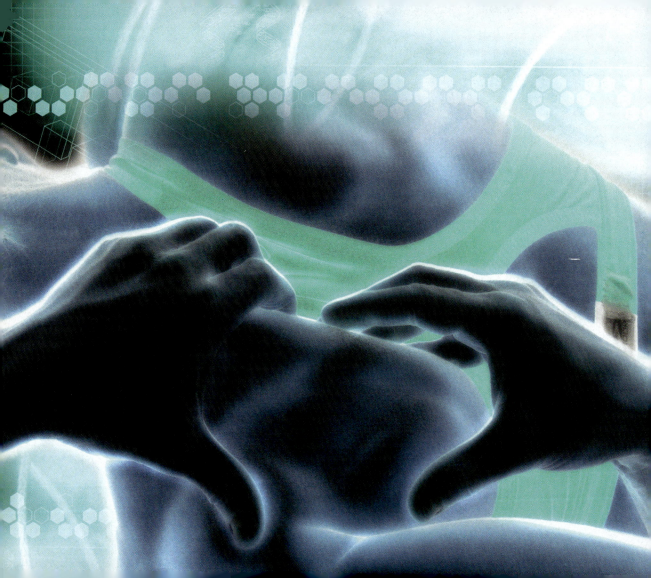

CHAPTER 5

MANAGEMENT OF MYOFASCIAL INJURIES IN THE ATHLETE—CASE STUDIES

Injuries to fascia inevitably will cause myofascial pain and musculoskeletal dysfunction that can result in residual tightness, weakness, decreased endurance, and a loss of full range of motion and flexibility. As a result, there occurs an imbalance in the agonist/antagonist muscle function, with resultant loss of efficient functioning of the myotatic unit. This leads to premature fatigue and break-down of the normal smooth reciprocal pattern of contraction and relaxation that occurs with activity, as well as to the subsequent development of clinical symptoms. Both speed and load (resistance) pro-mote earlier breakdown of the myotatic unit by primarily affecting the activity of the antagonist mus-cles or the stabilizers. The antagonistic muscles are necessary for the timed dynamic breaking forces and for protecting the agonist against overload injury. At high rates of speed, recruitment of antagonistic function is impaired and predisposes the agonist to breakdown.

One of the most common causes for recurring myofascial pain and dysfunction is the incomplete or inadequate rehabilitation of a previously painful process that had presumably resolved without the patient having achieved a full range of motion or normal strength. This generally occurs because the focus of treatment was on pain relief rather than on correction of the underlying tissue dysfunction.

In all cases of myofascial dysfunction, treatment must be individualized, comprehensive, and goal directed. Formal treatment programs are mainly for pain relief rather than focusing on restoring func-tion and promoting a speedy return to functioning activity. In the case studies presented in this chap-ter, the therapist's goal in all cases is not only to provide pain relief but also to restore the myofascial capacity of the athlete exceeding that prior to injury in the shortest time frame possible. These case studies will highlight the usage of a variety of highly developed techniques such as physical therapy (e.g., articular pumping, segmental reinforcement, proprioception exercises, ELDOA), injection therapy, acupuncture, low-level laser, and supplementation and nutrition.

Because sport is inherently not a healthy endeavor, the goal of every trainer or strength and conditioning coach should be first and foremost to put a healthy athlete on the field. The coach of tomorrow will work synergistically with technical coaches, team doctors, therapists, and the athlete to optimize the athlete's performance capabilities when needed.

TREATING AT A GLOBAL LEVEL

In treating a myofascial dysfunction, it is important to look at the individual on a global, or holistic, level. Focusing on just the area of complaint will usually not be as effective, if at all effective, as identifying all areas or regions that an injury might affect. Consequently, treatment of the fascial/meridian system should consider addressing a variety of factors.

The clinician should assess the area of complaint (area of pain presentation). However, it is important not to overly focus one's attention on the area of complaint, but move on to a more global treatment pain reduction program. The assessment should carefully determine which fascial planes, trains, chains, and meridians are affected using both hand palpation and observation skills. The therapist needs to perform these skills at a velocity consistent with the thixotropic properties of the tissue. To complete a thorough assessment, the clinician should use palpation in conjunction with orthopedic and muscle testing. At this point, the clinician should focus attention on actively working the fascial tissue at the appropriate depth and direction depending upon whether superficial or deep fascia is injured and on the respective plane and/or chain of the injured fascia. However, it should be pointed out that when working deeper fascia, it is important not to engage the fascia deeply or too quickly before loosening the overlying layers, because doing so can result in driving already existing structural abnormalities deeper into the fascia. Fascial connective tissue therapy will consist of using both active and passive movements to provide tension along the fascial planes, trains, chains, and meridians being treated.

In addition to the above-mentioned goals, here are some other treatment objectives: complete body image, skeletal alignment and support, tensegrity, connective tissue length and resilience, ability to hold and release a somato-emotional charge, establishment of full range of motion, and reduction of pain.

Treatment of Fascia

Bednar and colleagues have noted that degenerative changes to fascia are consistently due to bundles of collagen with the formation of a hardened, granular tissue that is infiltrated by lymphocytes and plasma cells (Bednar, Orr, & Simon, 1995). Vascular proliferation "capillarization" with certain patients is dependent on anomaly changes to the capillary's external basal lamina, while in other patients there is the presence of microcalcifications (Bednar et al. 1995).

The release of tissue from tension and spasm, which allows for a correction in posture, is very important for maintenance of good hemodynamics. If the hemodynamics within tissue is not disturbed, the tissue exchange will be normal. Tissue that is well vascularized will receive all its necessary elements (hormones, proteins, growth factors, electrolytes, etc.) and appropriate removal of its waste products, thus avoiding local irritation and dysfunction due to a buildup of metabolic by-products. The neurological system is able to influence the exchange and transport signals that are required to maintain body homeostasis. We as clinicians should carefully make sure that the body and its tissues are free of any constraints that serve as a source of soft tissue dysfunction, which can eventually result in degeneration. One of the most important goals for any bodyworker is the prevention and release of fascial adhesions, throughout the fascial web, that can alter both the body's biomechanics and physiological function.

CASE STUDY 1: TREATMENT OF PROXIMAL HAMSTRING PAIN USING ACTIVE RELEASE TECHNIQUE® APPLIED TO THE MYOFASCIAL MERIDIANS

This case report involves a 38-year-old triathlete competitor presenting with chronic pain in the proximal hamstring tendon. Treatment of this condition included the use of Active Release Techniques® along the "superficial back line" myofascial meridian, resulting in complete resolution of symptoms.

Many manual medicine therapists direct soft tissue treatment to individual muscle groups. However, due to the recent publication of literature regarding continuums between various structures by way of connective tissues (i.e., myofascial meridians), manual therapists should consider revising the way they identify and deal with tension and strain development within the body.

Background

Hamstring injuries are among the most, if not the most, common soft tissue injuries in athletes (Jonhagen, Nemeth, & Eriksson, 1994; Kujala, Orava, & Jarvinen, 1997; Turi & George, 1998). The high rate of reinjury and persistence of the complaint make the management of hamstring conditions difficult, and often frustrating, for attending physicians, trainers, and the athletes themselves (Croisier, Forthomme, Namurois, Vanderthommen, & Crielaard, 2002; Jonhagen et al., 1994; Kujala et al., 1997; Turi & George, 1998; Hennessy & Watson, 1993; Verrall, Slavotinek, Barnes, & Fon, 2003). Furthermore, the lack of consensus as to the proper treatment and rehabilitation of this condition serves to increase the aggravation (Kujala et al., 1997). Factors causing hamstring injuries have been studied for many years, and various suggestions have surfaced as to the underlying cause of the problems. Some of the more commonly noted etiologic factors include muscle weakness, strength imbalance, lack of flexibility, fatigue, inadequate warm-up, and aberrant posture (Bednar et al., 1995; Croisier et al., 2002; Jonhagen et al., 1994; Kujala et al., 1997; McHugh et al., 1999; Puranen & Orava, 1988; Stanton & Purdam, 1989; Turi & George, 1998; Hennessy & Watson, 1993; Verrall et al., 2003; Worrell, 1994). Traditionally, these etiological factors have been thought to be independent of one another. However, a theoretical model for hamstring injury proposed by Worrell and Perrin considered the interaction between these etiological factors as being most important; and as such, treatment and rehabilitation should specifically assess and correct deficits in all of these areas (Leahy, 1996; Puranen & Orava, 1988).

Hamstring conditions usually result from noncontact injuries that present in two forms: (1) sudden onset

with immediate incapacitating pain; and (2) slow, insidious onset with muscle tightness. Often the slow onset of hamstring strain will develop into a sudden onset (Worrell, 1994). This concept leads one to believe that an underlying presence of increased myofascial tension may precipitate hamstring conditions, as well as being a cause for the high rate of recurrence and chronicity of the problem. Literature has suggested (Blankenbaker & De Smet, 2004; Kaplan et al., 2001) that passive muscle stiffness primarily reflects the lack of extensibility of the connective tissue elements in parallel with the muscle fibers (parallel elastic component). McHugh and colleagues looked at the role of passive muscle stiffness in symptoms of exercise-induced muscle damage (McHugh et al., 1999). They proposed that strain imposed by active lengthening of stiff muscle is transferred from the rigid tendon–aponeurosis complex to the muscle fibers, resulting in myofibrillar strain (McHugh et al., 1999).

Correction of the underlying causes of hamstring injuries has been approached in a variety of ways. Following the usual progression of treatment rendered, passive therapy is usually performed first, followed by a more active rehabilitation protocol. The final phase of therapy often includes more detailed sport-specific rehabilitation protocols. Many methods of passive therapy are presently being utilized by practitioners with the intention of affecting changes in soft tissue structures; these methods include massage, Graston technique®, and proprioceptive neuromuscular facilitation/ post-isometric relaxation (PNF/PIR) stretching. Another common treatment method utilized by therapists in managing soft tissue complaints is Active Release Technique (ART®), developed by Michael Leahy.

Leahy proposed a mechanism to explain increased tissue stiffness, or tension, that he called the cumulative injury cycle (Leahy, 1996). In this cycle, repetitive microinjury in tight muscles leads to an increase in the friction and tension within the myofascial structures. This tension leads either to decreased circulation to the tissue in what is termed the "chronic cycle," or it leads to the "inflammation cycle," whereby a tear or crush injury ensues, followed by inflammation. Both of these cycles lead to the same result: an accumulation of adhesions and fibrosis within the tissue. This in turn increases the tightness of the tissue. As such, the cumulative injury cycle is self-perpetuating, and as this downward spiral continues, the symptoms and syndromes of cumulative injury disorder are produced. It is the goal of ART®, as with other soft tissue techniques, to remove these "adhesions," thereby decreasing tissue tension and thus stopping the cumulative injury cycle. In the case of ART®, the involved tissue is taken from a shortened position to a fully lengthened position while the contact hand holds tension longitudinally along the soft tissue fibers and the lesion (Kruger, 1987). The effectiveness of this treatment method has been described in a variety of case reports and is utilized by many practitioners for the treatment of a variety of conditions involving soft tissue dysfunction (Agrios & Crawford, 1999; Baer, 1999; Buchberger, 1999; Buchberger, Rizzoto, & McAdam, 1996; Drover, Forand, & Herzog, 2004; Kazemi, 2000; Pajaczkowski, 2004). However, as with any treatment method, effectiveness is subject to proper diagnosis as well as to anatomical and biomechanical considerations.

The hamstring muscle group occupies the posterior compartment of the thigh and consists of three muscles: (1) semitendinosus, (2) semimembranosus, and (3) biceps femoris. These hamstring muscles, spanning the hip and knee joints, arise from the ischial tuberosity deep to the gluteus maximus. They are innervated by the tibial division of the sciatic nerve—except for the short head of biceps femoris, which is innervated by the peroneal division (all via spinal segments L5, S1, and S2; Moore & Dally, 1999). Both of the "semi" muscles, as well as the long head of biceps femoris, attach proximally to the ischial tuberosity. Semitendinosus inserts distally to the medial surface of the superior part of the tibia, while semimembranosus attaches to the posterior part of the medial condyle of the tibia. The long head of biceps femoris joins the short head arising from the linea aspera to insert onto the side of the head of the fibula.

This description of the origin and insertions of muscles is somewhat misleading when considering how strain and tension are distributed throughout the body. The muscle–bone concept presented in standard anatomical descriptions gives a purely mechanical model of movement. It separates movement into independent muscular functions, failing to give a picture of the seamless integration in a living body. Functionally, the tissue that provides this integration is the myofascia. The word *myofascia* denotes the inseparable nature of muscle tissue (*myo*) and its accompanying connective tissue (*fascia*). The myofascial units communicate and extend across lines and broad planes within the body. These myofascial connections, termed "myofascial meridians" by Myers, transmit strain and tension throughout connections within the body (Myers, 2001). As stated by Myers, muscles never attach to bone. Their movement pulls on the fascia, the fascia is attached to the periosteum, and the periosteum pulls on the bone. In other words, muscles and fascia are continuous with each other, transmitting tension, strain, and lines of pull from one structure to the next. Therefore, if one of the structures within a meridian develops tension, it will be distributed along the entire myofascial continuum. With this in mind, theoretically there is "only one muscle; it just hangs around in 600 or more fascial pockets" (Myers, 2001). In his text *The Anatomy Trains*, Myers describes seven myofascial lines or "meridians." Two of these meridians, the "superficial back line" (SBL) and the "superficial front line" (SFL), are directly related to the present case.

The purpose of this case report is to describe the use of ART®, applied to the myofascial meridians, as a method of relieving pain and tissue tension present in a case of a chronic hamstring injury. The case also outlines the importance of the myofascial sling system (myofascial connections), which plays an important role in the force and tension distribution throughout the body as well as in the complete management of soft tissue dysfunction.

Case History

A 38-year-old competitive triathlete presented to the clinic with a complaint of chronic proximal hamstring pain and tightness in the right leg.

The pain was described as constant and exacerbated by running. The patient's complaint stemmed from a running injury that she had suffered two years prior in which she developed what was diagnosed as an acute tendinopathy of the proximal hamstring that caused her to withdraw from her training regimen. At that time, the patient was treated using the rest, ice, compression, and elevation (RICE) principle of acute injury management that served to greatly decrease the pain intensity. Since then, a residual subjective feeling of "discomfort/pain" and "tightness" remained that she felt greatly decreased her running performance. The patient decided to stop running altogether, which subsequently forced her to stop participating in the Ironman Competition, in which she had competed for many years. Shortly after the resolution of the acute phase of the injury, the patient then sought out chiropractic care for her complaint. The practitioner managed the condition using electro-acupuncture and home stretching, as well as Active Release Technique® directed solely on the hamstring muscle group. This treatment protocol, which lasted approximately six months, served to lessen the symptoms for short periods of time (one–two days); however, it failed to resolve the complaint and allow the patient to return to running.

Upon presenting to our clinic approximately two years after the initial incident, the patient's symptoms had not lessened, nor had she returned to any running activities. Postural examination revealed moderate anterior head carriage, internally rotated shoulders, and anterior pelvic tilt causing an increased lumbar lordosis. During lateral postural examination it was noted that during weight bearing, dorsiflexion of the ankles was present. This gave the impression that the patient was leaning forward (i.e., there was approximation of the dorsal surface of the foot to the anterior leg when standing). It should be noted that according to Meyers, these findings are consistent with a "tight" superficial front line (Myers, 2001). Muscle length testing resulted in mild discomfort as well as a mildly decreased range of motion in the right hamstring relative the left (approximately 15°). Also, the right rectus femoris and both the right and left pectoralis major muscles demonstrated a decreased range of

motion. Palpatory findings revealed tenderness in the proximal hamstring myotendinous junction and hamstring insertion, as well as tightness and fibrosis in the ipsilateral plantar fascia, gastrocnemius, sacrotuberous ligament, long dorsal sacral ligament, and the midthoracic longissimus thoracis. Nonpainful dyskinesis (decreased joint play) was noted in the right subtalar joint with joint palpation. Gait analysis revealed a "hunched forward posture," while running resulting in excessive dorsiflexion of both ankles. No other gait abnormalities were observed. Manual muscle testing of the lower limb musculature was unremarkable and was graded as 5/5 bilaterally. Sensory testing of the lower extremities was bilaterally symmetrical, and all deep tendon reflexes were graded as 2+. Systems review did not reveal any concurrent illness or disease processes.

A diagnosis of chronic proximal hamstring tendinopathy was given. Treatment frequency was three times a week for the first two weeks, followed by twice per week for the next three weeks. Treatment included ART® applied to the right superficial back line (see discussion) including the plantar fascia, gastrocnemius, hamstrings group (including the proximal tendon), sacrotuberous ligament, long dorsal sacral ligament, and the ipsilateral erector spinae. Drop piece manipulation was performed for a total of three visits until the subtalar dyskinesis was resolved. Home stretches for the hamstring muscle group and the superficial front line (see discussion) were also prescribed at a frequency of two times per day, holding each stretch for 40 to 60 seconds per repetition. Postural advice was also administered to relieve stress placed on tissues when using the computer, driving, talking on the phone, and so on.

The patient reported a subjective decrease of 60–70% in pain intensity and tightness after only two treatments. By the fifth visit, the pain was felt only during testing of the end range of motion. At this time the patient began running again. She was also started on eccentric hamstring exercises. This included eccentrics on the hamstring curl machine, which involves first performing the concentric portion with both legs and then doing the eccentric portion only with the symptomatic leg. Repetitive eccentric hamstring catches were also prescribed (Verrall et al., 2003). In addition, proprioceptive training was added to the treatment. This consisted of proprioceptive leg drops (patient is prone, practitioner lifts up the leg, then drops it at random times as the patient is instructed to "catch" the leg before it hits the table) and rocker/wobble board training. By the eighth visit, the patient had progressed to 8- to 10-km runs with no restrictions or pain caused by the hamstring group. The only factor interfering with the patient's run lengths at this point was cardiovascular deconditioning stemming from her lack of training. Simultaneously, during visit eight, end ROM testing was unremarkable. At this point, the patient progressed to more extensive rehabilitative protocols such as plyometrics to improve running economy and kinesthetic awareness of the joints (Swanik, 2002; Turner, Owings, & Schwane, 2003).

Discussion

As mentioned earlier, hamstring conditions are usually the result of either a sudden onset of tissue injury with immediate incapacitating pain or a slow, insidious onset preceded by muscle tightness that may later develop into an acute strain of the tissue (Worrell, 1994). Consequently, this concept leads one to believe that an underlying presence of increased myofascial tension or stiffness may precipitate hamstring conditions. ART® is a widely used method of soft tissue therapy aimed directly at relieving tissue tension and restoring normal biomechanical function. Various clinical case reports have cited the benefits of this technique in managing a variety of musculoskeletal conditions (Agrios & Crawford, 1999; Baer, 1999; Buchberger, 1999; Buchberger et al., 1996; Drover et al., 2004; Kazemi, 2000; Pajaczkowski, 2004).

The reader may now be wondering why this technique failed to provide the desired results when applied by the previous treating practitioner in this particular case. The answer may lie in the anatomy of the hamstrings muscle group, as well as in the concept of the myofascial continuum referred to earlier.

Recall that of the seven myofascial meridians described in Meyers's text, two meridians—the SBL and the SFL—are of direct relevance in this case (Myers, 2001). Theoretically, the SBL extends from the plantar fascia, around the calcaneous, and into the Achilles tendon, and the SBL continues with the gastrocnemius. Interestingly, Meyers postulates that tightness in these structures will create a compressive force in the subtalar joint by forcing the calcaneous into the tallus (Myers, 2001). This will create dyskinesis, or "fixation," of the subtalar joint. This was one of the findings identified and subsequently used as treatment in the current case report. From the gastrocnemius, the line continues up the hamstrings, into the sacrotuberous ligament, to the long dorsal sacral ligament, and up the ipsilateral erectors all the way to the galea aponeurotica. Part of this meridian, or "myofascial sling" as it is often termed, has in part been demonstrated by the work of Vleeming, Pool-Goudzwaard, Stoeckart, and Snijders (Pool-Goudzwaard, Vleeming, Snijders, & Mens, 1998; Van Wingerden, Vleeming, Snijders, Pool, & Stoeckart, 1993; Vleeming et al., 1989; Vleeming et al., 1996; Vleeming, Stoeckart, & Snijders, 1989). These authors used buckle transducers in embalmed cadaveric specimens to demonstrate force translation between the biceps femoris (the most commonly injured hamstring muscle), the sacrotuberous ligament, the long dorsal sacral ligament, and the thoracolumbar fascia. In these studies, tension was applied to individual structures along this chain while tension readings were collected from the hypothesized connected structures. Results demonstrated that tension applied to these structures transferred into the adjacent tissues along this fascial chain.

In the running athlete, the hamstring is subject to eccentric force loading as the leg is propelled forward just prior to heel strike. It is this required increase in eccentric muscle activity that appears to be related to hamstring injuries occurring in the late swing phase of gait as the foot strikes the ground (Stanton & Purdam, 1989). Thus, if there is increased tension in any part of the SBL, it will cause increased tension in the hamstring, which is already subject to microinjury and tears via running mechanics during eccentric loading. Hence the hamstring becomes the "weakest link" in the myofascial sling, which may explain why it becomes the symptomatic tissue in running athletes.

The other myofascial meridian that may have been involved in the present case was the SFL. According to Myers (2001), this sling represents the myofascial connection running from the anterior crural compartment, to the subpatellar tendon, and up the rectus femoris to the anterior inferior iliac spine (AIIS). From the AIIS, tension is transferred via the bony pelvis to the rectus abdominus, up the sternalis muscle or sternochondral fascia, to the sternocleidomastoid. The patient's static posture helped to identify the SFL as being involved in the current case. Tension in the SFL may have resulted in the anterior head carriage with rolled-forward shoulders via the upper component of the sling, as well as the anterior pelvic tilt of the lower trunk via the pull of the rectus femoris. Interestingly, the anterior pelvic tilt serves to increase lumbar lordosis, which has been identified as a postural contributor to hamstring injury (Turl & George, 1998).

The SBL and SFL are thought to have a reciprocal relationship, such that contracture, or shortening, of one will draw tension via lengthening and/or stretching of the other (Myers, 2001). Following the works of Janda, anterior head carriage and anterior pelvic tilt are common postural compensations (Hammer, 1996). This follows the theory and observation by Myers (2001) that it is very common for the SFL to be pulled down, and thus "locked short," while the SBL hikes up the back, thus drawing tension into it ("locked long"). This pattern is encouraged by improper posture, such as that of individuals slumping forward while at the computer screen or driving their cars.

Returning to the original question of why ART® to the hamstrings alone was insufficient in dealing with this case, the meridian concept may provide the answer. By treating the entire SBL with ART® and stretching, while simultaneously stretching the SFL, the lines of pull and/or strain within the patient were balanced. Thus, any tension that was

causing persistence of the symptoms was relieved, and the myofascial mechanics were returned to normal.

The concept of adverse neural tension has also been identified as a possible cause for repetitive hamstring strain (Kujala et al., 1997). Turl and George (1998) noted that 57% of their study population suffering from grade I repetitive hamstring strain were diagnosed with adverse neural tension using the slump test. Their theory describes how repeated injury to the hamstrings can produce inflammation and possible scarring that interferes with normal mobility and nutritional well-being of the sciatic nerve. The slump test procedure has the patient sit at the edge of the table with the plinth in contact with the popliteal fossa at the back of the knee. The patient is instructed to flex the neck and slump the shoulders forward as the practitioner applies overpressure. The patient is then instructed to extend the knee as much as possible. For the test to be positive, the patient's original hamstring pain must be reproduced and then decreased on cervical extension. This combination of movements draws tension directly into the SBL. Therefore, Turl and George's diagnosis of adverse neural tension using the slump test would be positive in patients with tension in the superficial back line—such as the patient in the current case (Danto, 2003).

By dealing with the affected tissues, the locked-short SFL and the locked-long SBL, symptoms in this patient were effectively relieved. However, other predisposing factors of this type of pattern (example: aberrant posture) must also be addressed in order to sustain the soft tissue alterations. This includes postural retraining by way of patient instruction, postural reminders (e.g., a note placed on the top of the computer screen reminding the patient to correct his or her posture), as well as home stretching to sustain the corrected posture.

In addition to postural corrections, rehabilitative efforts are essential to aid with tissue healing and to correct other predisposing factors such as muscle weakness, strength imbalance, lack of flexibility, and fatigue.

Conclusion

The focus of this case report was to describe how treating an entire myofascial meridian may be effective in resolving chronic or recurring hamstring problems. If focused soft tissue treatment protocols directed solely at the hamstring muscle group fail to resolve the symptoms, it may be because all of the lines of tension are not adequately addressed. Methods of soft tissue treatment, in our case Active Release Techniques®, while anecdotally effective, are limited to the practitioner's knowledge of the involved anatomy and soft tissue mechanics. Many manual medicine therapists direct such treatment protocols in isolation. Due to the recent publication of literature regarding continuums between various structures by way of connective tissue, manual therapists may want to consider revising the way they identify and deal with tension and strain development within the body. More research is needed to demonstrate the presence of these lines of pull, since many of them are currently only theoretical constructs.

Now that applying the knowledge learned so far into clinical practice has been discussed, attention can be turned to specific techniques, as well as the treatment of specific patient populations and specific conditions.

The goal of the next three case studies is to briefly introduce the concept of globality of training in the rehab model with respect to the fascial systems and their importance to an athlete in rehabilitation.

Three common injuries seen in sport will be presented along with a general protocol of rehabilitation performance-oriented training to expedite the recovery phase and get the athlete back on the field and ready to perform optimally as soon as possible. The phrase "rehabilitation performance-oriented training" is used here with a purpose. Nearly all North American models of physical therapy are geared toward the average Mr. and Mrs. Smith and not toward the athlete who needs to perform at a high level.

Strength and conditioning coaches are faced with numerous difficult situations of having an athlete who has a limited time to get ready for sport but has not yet been adequately prepared to train at a high level. The area between recovery and therapy from injury training is an area that is not well defined, and a good trainer and/or coach must be able to bridge the gap.

The trainer/coach should walk away after reading this chapter and know that his or her protocol must be approached with respect to the globality of all the systems of the body. The importance of the fascial systems with regard to rehabilitation and performance must be recognized and always addressed. These concepts and methods are thoroughly discussed and taught by Guy Voyer, who put together a system of advanced somato-therapy (training of the body).

CASE STUDY 2: GLOBAL TREATMENT OF A SURGICALLY REPAIRED TORN SUPRASPINATUS IN AN OVERHAND-THROWING PITCHER

The first case study is that of a 21-year-old right-handed relief pitcher who is recovering from a surgically repaired torn supraspinatus muscle on his throwing arm. Please keep in mind that his is a hypothetical case study and that literally hundreds of different subjective factors would or could change the recommended protocol. Having said that, here is an outline to demonstrate a possible approach this patient's treatment.

The first task would be to get the athlete to a competent and experienced therapist trained in the necessary systems to help speed up the rehabilitation period. If possible, the patient should have Dr. Guy Voyer, Dr. Keith Pyne, or Ming Chew P.T. see the athlete immediately post surgery and as often as humanly possible. The goal for the first 21 days post surgery would be to pump the area and use various treatment modalities to expedite the healing process.

One of the initial treatment modalities would be the use of pompage. Dr. Voyer recommends pumping be performed immediately post surgery to allow the fascia to be released, hydrate the area, and speed the healing process up. The therapist in this particular case could pump the shoulder joints and liquid pump the scapula even though it is the origin of the supraspinatus muscle. Some examples might be pumping of the movement of the scapula and pumping of the movement of the clavicle.

Post 21 days, according to Dr. Guy Voyer, is sufficient time to allow for proper healing of the repaired tissue. At this point the trainer/coach can begin the rehabilitation performance-oriented training process. In this particular case, the trainer/coach must know the anatomy of the total shoulder and the relationship of the supraspinatus muscle to all of the five joints that comprise the shoulder in its entirety.

The trainer/coach cannot address a problem in one joint of the shoulder without looking at its effects on the other joints of the shoulder. A problem in one joint of the shoulder may affect function of other joints. For the dynamic explosive athlete such as a baseball pitcher, this situation will spell potential injury down the road.

The focus should be on the proper pumping, myofascial stretching, reinforcement (strengthening), proprioception, and ELDOA (*Etierement Longitudinaux avec Decoaptation OsteoArticulaire*, which means "longitudinal stretching with osteoarticular decoaptation") of the repaired shoulder with respect to the globality of the system. The first protocol may proceed as described in the following paragraphs.

First, a general warm-up should be performed. An example might be 10–12 minutes on a stationary bike. Secondly, the trainer performs some general pumping techniques of the shoulder joints.

Since the primary function of the supraspinatus muscle is lateral abduction of the arm, any joint relationship to this function should be done last. A good flow might be:

- Sternoclavicular joint
- Acromioclavicular joint
- Scapular/thoracic joint
- Glenohumeral joint
- Mobility of the "false" subdeltoid joint (including pumping of the supraspinatus bursa)

Finally, the pumping of the supraspinatus bursa should be performed.

As a side note, it should be clarified that in the initial stages of rehabilitation, myofascial stretching is performed before the segmental strengthening (reinforcement), and reinforcement is performed before the proprioception.

As the recovery progresses and the range of motion and strength increase, the myofascial stretching should be performed after the reinforcement; the proprioception will eventually be performed before the reinforcement. After the pumping of the shoulder joints, myofascial stretching can be performed for the following:

- Pectoralis major (deep fibers), serratus anterior, and latissimus dorsi
- Long and short head of biceps, coracobrachialis, and the three triceps heads
- Anterior and posterior deltoid
- Rotator cuff muscles including teres minor and major, subscapularis, infraspinatus, and supraspinatus

Once again, the repaired area is stretched last.

An understanding of the fascial chains with relation to the shoulder will allow the trainer/coach to put together the best protocol for the repaired area. Once the correct myofascial tension is obtained, performing 3 sets of 30 seconds for each structure is fine. Segmental reinforcement means the strengthening of the individual muscles with respect to the laws of their biomechanical functions, ranges, and fiber placement. Sequential reinforcement of the following muscles would be prescribed in this first phase:

1. Rhomboids—external range, intermediate fibers
2. Upper trapezius—total range
3. Posterior deltoid—external range, intermediate fibers
4. Medial deltoid—internal range only, intermediate fibers

Perform 3–5 sets of 50 repetitions at a moderate tempo for each exercise.

Proprioception for the shoulder joint can now be performed in the following order:

1. Posterior glenohumeral
2. Anterior glenohumeral
3. Medial glenohumeral (performed last)

Once the proper position is obtained, from 45 seconds to 1 minute of these drills can be performed while respecting the laws of joint placement and progression (with support/eyes open, without support/eyes open, without support/eyes closed).

As another side note, it is important to understand as a coach/trainer the neurological value of proprioception to the athlete. Proprioception is the ability to reflexively adapt and coordinate the ligaments, capsules, and tendons to adapt to the correct posture of the joint. The Somato-therapy course previously mentioned provides the trainer/coach with the knowledge and practical application of this invaluable tool.

ELDOA is a system that instructs the athlete how to use various postures which will allow decoaptation of the functional units that may have been compressed or coapted as a result of his/her sport, position, injury or compensation caused by the injury. Hence, ELDOA postures can be prescribed for the following anatomical structures in the pitcher in this case study:

○ Coxofemoral (both sides) sacrum
○ T8/T9 (if range of motion permits)
○ T6/T7 (if range of motion permits)
○ C4/C5
○ L5/L7 (if range of motion permits)

It is recommended that the contralateral uninjured arm be trained as well during this phase to take advantage of the neurological benefits of the injured side. The player is put through this segment of rehabilitation as many times as possible until the trainer/coach determines that the player can progress into the next phase and ultimately into a more global, dynamic, rehab/training performance-oriented protocol.

CASE STUDY 3: GLOBAL TREATMENT OF A SURGICALLY REPAIRED LEFT ANTERIOR CRUCIATE LIGAMENT IN A SOCCER PLAYER

Our next case is a 30-year-old male soccer player recovering from a postsurgical repair of the left anterior cruciate ligament (ACL). As with the previous case, pumping should be performed by a trained therapist immediately following surgery. The therapist can perform liquid pumping of the knee, the ankle, and the hip, and fascial treatment of the lower limb.

Post 21 days, the trainer/coach can step up and begin the training process. First, have the patient do a general warm-up of 10–12 minutes (bicycling if possible, or exercising in a warm pool if the surgeon permits). Physical therapist Bill Knowles prefers to use the warm pool and various drills.

According to Guy Voyer, D.O. and Sport M.D., if the athlete is able to perform rehabilitation training in water, then he or she should do so as much as possible. The water provides a safe environment and allows for the fascial system to relax, hydrate, and communicate more efficiently.

The proper pumping will follow post warm-up:

1. Pumping of knee in lateral translation
2. Pumping of knee in medial translation
3. Pumping of knee in flexion and external rotation
4. Pumping of knee in flexion and internal rotation
5. Pumping of knee in extension and external rotation
6. Pumping of knee in extension and internal rotation. (Last one done because of direct effect on ACL.)

The myofascial stretching of the following should follow:

1. Biceps femoris
2. Semimembranosus
3. Farabeuf's deltoid (superficial gluteus maximus, gluteus medius, tensor fascia lata)
4. Gracilis
5. Quadriceps (each portion as range permits), excepting the vastus medialis
6. Gastrocnemius (medial and lateral)

Segmental reinforcement of the following muscles could be done:

1. Gluteus medius—total range, neutral fibers
2. Gluteus maximus—total range, medial to lateral fibers
3. Gastrocnemius—total range, medial to lateral fibers
4. Quadriceps—static wall squat with support—all positions up to 1-minute holds, medialis to lateralis

Segmental proprioception of the following joints should occur in this order and once again respecting the laws of progression:

1. Patellofemoral joint
2. Medial and lateral tibiofemoral joints
3. Fibulofemoral joint
4. Medial tibiofemoral joint

It should be noted that at some point during this phase, this running athlete should begin a periodized water and running protocol as part of his rehabilitative training. As long as the surgeon believes there is no risk of infection, the athlete may begin water work and running to train those muscles globally within those neural patterns, thereby providing more information to the nervous system.

CASE STUDY 4: GLOBAL TREATMENT OF SURGICALLY REPAIRED ACHILLES TENDON IN A VOLLEYBALL PLAYER

This case involves a 26-year-old female volleyball player recovering from a postsurgical Achilles tendon repair. The volleyball player is a front-line player whose role is primarily spiking and blocking. This athlete requires and will have to be able to sustain very high eccentric loading on the repaired tissue in order to compete again at a high level. Immediately post surgery, the trained therapist can begin pumping the area. Treatment may include the following:

1. Pumping of the sinus tarsus
2. Pumping of the naviculocuboid junction
3. Pumping of the anterior gliding of the talus

Post 21 days, the rehabilitation performance-oriented training phase begins. General warm-up (15-minute warm-water pool drills recommended) and pumping of the following:

1. The knee in anterior and posterior translations
2. The sinus tarsus
3. The cuboid
4. Posterior gliding of the talus
5. The calcaneus
6. The navicular
7. The cuneiforms

Myofascial stretching of the following:

1. Biceps femoris, semitendinosus, semimembranosus
2. Extensor hallusis longus, extensor digitorum
3. Tibialis anterior
4. Lateral and medial gastrocnemius muscles, soleus

Reinforcement (segmental strengthening) of the following:

1. Tibialis anterior, total range
2. Lateral gastrocnemius—external range
3. Medial gastrocnemius—external range
4. Soleus—total range (last performed)

Finally, the proprioception of the following should be performed, again while respecting the laws of progression:

1. Knee in medial and lateral rotation
2. Talus and medial part of the tibia
3. Tibial/calcaneum joint
4. Fibular/calcaneum joint
5. Rotation movement of the navicular

6. Rotation movement of the cuboid
7. Second cuneiform

Discussion

If there is a lesion in a peripheral joint, there will subsequently be a compensation with the spine between the pelvis and the skull. During all the rehabilitation protocols, the therapist must continuously assess the spine and pelvis so that they choose the appropriate ELDOA to correct this compensatory posture and augment the rapidity of the rehabilitation.

Conclusion

Together, these systems of training and rehabilitation will allow the trainer/coach to deliver the greatest amount of information to the functional units and nervous system in the least amount of time. If this goal can be accomplished, the athlete has the greatest chance of recovering fully by not allowing compensation to set in within the functional unit, the global physiological system, and the nervous system as a whole.

Further information on the training and treatment methods of Guy Voyer, D.O. can be found at www.guyvoyer.com.

CASE STUDY 5: QUANTIFYING PREFUNCTIONAL AND FUNCTIONAL REHABILITATION IN AN INJURED SOCCER PLAYER

Groin pain is an increasing symptom seen in certain athletes over the last few years. In fact, research shows that 2.5% of all sports injuries suffered are groin injuries (Morelli & Smith, 2001). These injuries tend to occur more commonly in sports that require repetitive use of the proximal musculature of the thigh and lower abdominal muscles, particularly when the motion involves hip abduction and violent external rotation (K. E. LeBlanc & K. A. LeBlanc, 2003). It can also be seen in individuals who run for prolonged periods and those who do speed interval sports/training. Some of these sports include hockey, soccer, football, basketball, and tennis. Two of the most common groin injuries in sport have to do with adductor strains and osteitis pubis (Morelli & Smith, 2001).

This case study deals with a 17-year-old soccer player diagnosed with osteitis pubis. Osteitis pubis was first described in athletes in 1924 by Beer, and later in 1932 by Spinelli (Holt, Keene, Graf, & Helwig, 1995; Rodriguez, Miguel, Lima, & Heinrichs, 2001). Osteitis pubis is a painful, noninfectious, inflammatory condition that affects the pubic bone, pubic symphysis, adductor muscles, abdominal muscles, and surrounding fascia. The abdominal fascia and adductor fascia and muscles attach to the pubic bone and symphysis, causing antagonistic tension forces to be placed on the pubic symphysis. The result is "mechanical traction microtrauma" and consequently an inflammatory response or osteitis pubis (Holt et al., 1995; Rodriguez et al., 2001). Other factors such as limitation of internal rotation of the femoral-acetabular (hip) joint, or fixation of the sacroiliac joint, also place excessive stress on the joint (Morelli & Smith, 2001; Rodriguez et al., 2001).

Clinical presentation of osteitis pubis falls into three categories: (1) mechanical (sports related), (2) obstetric, and (3) inflammatory reaction of the symphysis (Grzanna, Lindmark, & Frondoza, 2005; Young et al., 2005). Full recovery for this condition is slow and is estimated to be seven to nine months from the beginning of symptomatology (Grzanna et al., 2005; Young et al., 2005). Often the athlete or patient is misdiagnosed and/or mismanaged, resulting in prolonged symptoms and increased frustration by the health practitioner, athlete, and coach.

Therefore, one of the most important steps in managing patients with osteitis pubis is an accurate diagnosis. The health-care practitioner has to take an appropriate and thorough history in order to reach a differential diagnosis. Onset of injury, location of complaint, and mechanism of injury, as well as palliative and/or provocative activities, will assist in creating a differential diagnosis list. Pain that becomes worse with activity may suggest bursitis, myofascial strain, or even a tear. Nevertheless, intra-abdominal pathologies, genitourinary abnormalities, referred lumbosacral pain, and/or hip joint disorders must also be considered (Morelli & Smith, 2001). Once these conditions have been ruled out (usually following physical examination and imaging techniques), a diagnosis of osteitis pubis can be established. A differential diagnosis should be performed to rule out some other related conditions prior to establishing a definitive diagnosis (Morelli & Smith, 2001).

Table 15-1 Differential Diagnosis for Osteitis Pubis

Pathological diseases and/or soft tissue injuries
Inflammatory bowel disease (IBS)
Diverticulosis
Urinary tract infection
Nerve entrapment (femoral, inguinal, obturator)
Stress fracture
Sports hernia
Iliopsoas strain
Referred lumbosacral pain
Acetabular labral tear
Osteomyelitis
Abdominal/inguinal hernia
Scrotal/testicular abnormality

Case History

A 17-year-old soccer player presented with groin pain of 10 months duration. The patient is a defenseman and noted groin pain following a soccer game in which he did not recollect any traumatic impact. The patient had been treated at another facility for the previous few months using electrical stimulation, anti-inflammatories, and recommendation of rest. In fact, the athlete had not played soccer, nor was he involved in any physical activity over this 10-month period. The diagnosis at the time was adductor strain. The athlete complained of pain with walking, running, stair climbing, and changing from a sitting to a standing position. He also reported pain with coughing, sneezing, and bowel movements. The patient indicated pain in his abdominal and inguinal areas bilaterally as well. Previous medical history was unremarkable, and he did not report any noticeable increases in temperature. The patient denied any numbness, tingling, or feeling of "pins and needles." The pain described was sharp in nature and grew worse with activity. Rest did not seem to elicit any symptoms.

Physical Examination

Physical examination involved each region of the groin that has the potential to produce groin pain. This included the adductor muscles, abdominal muscles, the pelvic bones, the hip joints, the hip flexors, and the lumbopelvic joints.

First, the patient was observed standing. Postural assessment revealed forward head carriage, elevated left shoulder, an anterior pelvic tilt bilaterally, and medial knee rotation on the left. Observation of the athlete walking revealed little hip movement, a short stride length, and adduction of the left lower extremity during swing phase. Active movement of the hip joint was limited in extension and external rotation, bilaterally producing pain. Active lumbar spine movement was within normal limits. Active abdominal flexion and iliopsoas flexion both produced pain above the pubic symphysis and in the inguinal area respectively. Passive movements of the hips, lumbar spine, and sacroiliac joints revealed restriction in the left sacroiliac joint. Resist[ed] movements of hip flexion, hip adduction, ab[dominal] flexion, and iliopsoas contraction all produced pain in the pubic bone and groin region (specifically adductor insertion and above the pubic symphysis). Palpation of the adductor tendons (adductor brevis, longus), and rectus abdominus insertion (pubic symphysis) revealed they were tender to touch.

Functional movement testing—such as sit-ups, hopping, lunges, and zigzag running—all produced groin pain. Sit-up testing also produced pain just above the pubic symphysis. Pelvic symmetry testing revealed a higher iliac crest on the left and a left leg length inequality (consistent with previous sacroiliac joint fixation). The Thomas test (for psoas length) revealed shortened hip flexors bilaterally. Cough impulse testing was positive for groin pain, while Valsalva testing was negative. Finally, the squeeze test was performed on this patient as a diagnostic for osteitis pubis. During this test, the examiner places one fist between the patient's knees and instructs the patient to "squeeze." In this case study, the squeeze test was positive for pubic symphysis pain indicative of osteitis pubis.

Imaging

X-ray imaging of athletes with osteitis pubis may show widening of the pubic symphysis, irregular contour of the articular surfaces, and/or periarticular sclerosis (Morelli & Smith, 2001). The chronic stage of this condition usually shows a "moth eaten" appearance along the margins of the pubic symphysis.

Radionucleide bone scan may show increased uptake in the area (pubic symphysis). However, this is not diagnostic for osteitis pubis but just adds it to the differential diagnosis list.

CT scan and MRI (most preferred) are the two imaging techniques most sensitive to diagnosing osteitis pubis (Kjaer, 2004). Bone marrow edema can be detected early on with MRI; however, chronic bony changes associated with osteitis pubis are not as easily seen on MR imaging (Fricker, Taunton, & Ammann, 1991; Machlum & Bahr, 2004; Morelli & Smith, 2001).

Blood Testing for the Athlete

When assessing a patient's blood test results, the physician's main concern is that a particular result should not fall outside a normal "reference range." The problem with applying normal reference ranges to athletes is that these ranges usually represent the average population, rather than the optimal level required to maintain the superior physiological functioning required for an athlete to perform at a high level of competition. Hence it appears that the most standard reference ranges are too broad to adequately detect health problems or prescribe appropriate therapy on an individual basis.

Conventional medicine tends to neglect hormone imbalances that develop in both men and women as they get older or when athletes partake of pharmaceutical enhancement (e.g., anabolic and androgenic steroids, human growth hormone, thyroid hormone, insulin). As a result, many athletes who use drugs that exhibit toxic side effects are at risk of suffering a variety of discomforts and lethal diseases that are correctable and preventable if simple hormonal adjustments are made.

When it comes to assessing hormone status, the use of standard reference ranges will fail aging people and athletes. This occurs because standard laboratory reference ranges are not flagging dangerously high levels of estrogen and insulin or deficient levels of testosterone, thyroid, and DHEA. Table 15-2 shows the standard hormone blood reference ranges for men (age 60) and compares what the optimal ranges should be.

The most important blood tests for an athlete consist of a basic battery of tests that will establish a baseline reading for all pertinent systems. The recommended male panel is composed of the following tests:

- Complete blood count (CBC)/chemistry test
- Homocysteine
- Hypothalamus-pituitary-testes axis (HPTA)—total testosterone, free testosterone,
- dihydroepiandrosterone (DHEA)
- Estradiol
- Luteinizing hormone (LH)
- Follicle-stimulating hormone (FSH)
- Prostate-specific antigen (PSA)

In addition to this special male panel, the following tests are especially important for men and women over 40: fasting insulin, ferritin, cortisol, fibrinogen, thyroid-stimulating hormone (TSH), free thyroxine (T4), and free triiodothyronine (T3).

Table 15-2 Comparison of Standard Reference Range versus Optimal Range

Hormone	Standard Reference Range	Optimal Range
DHEA	42–290 mcg/dL	350–500 mcg/dL
Insulin (fasting)	6–27 mcU/mL	> 5 mcU/mL
Free testosterone	6.6–18.1 pg/mL	22–25.5 pg/mL
Estradiol	3–70 pg/mL	15–30 pg/mL
Thyroid-stimulating hormone (TSH)	0.2–5.5 mU/L	> 2.1 mU/L

For this case study, the following reference ranges are based on Labcorp test standards. Other blood testing facilities may use different reference ranges. A comprehensive hormonal panel should be performed in athletes in order to rule out any outstanding pathologies and to assess overall health status. Table 15-3 displays basic hormonal panel that can be incorporated in an athlete's training protocol:

Genetics and Blood Testing Interpretation

Blood testing provides a quantitative look at the athlete's genetic profile and allows the physician to identify any potential areas of concern: hormone/growth factor/thyroid axis; risk of diabetes, prostate cancer, metabolic syndrome, anemia, and cardiovascular

Table 15-3 Laboratory Test Results

Hormone	Actual Value	Reference Range	Optimal Range
Testosterone	520 ng/dL	300–1200 ng/dL	800–1200 ng/dL
Free testosterone	18.3 pg/mL	8.7–25 pg/mL	20–25 pg/mL
IGF-1	102 ng/mL	109–284 ng/mL	250–300 ng/mL
Estradiol	22 pg/mL	5–53 pg/mL (for adult males)	< 25 pg/mL
DHEA-s	410 µg/dL	120–520 µg/dL	400–500 µg/dL
Thyroid Panel			
T4	5.5 µg/dL	4.5–12 µg/dL	8–12 µg/dL
T3	3.1 pg/mL	2.3–4.2 pg/mL	3.5–4.5 pg/mL
TSH	2.743 µIU/mL	0.350–5.500 µIU/mL	
Lipid panel			
Total cholesterol	262 mg/dL	100–199 mg/dL	
LDL fraction	167 mg/dL	0–99 mg/dL	
HDL fraction	54 mg/dL	40–59 mg/dL	
Triglycerides	204mg/dL	0–149 mg/dL	
C-reactive protein	0.75 mg/L	(> 2 increased risk of MI and stroke)	
Other			
Homocysteine	6.3 umol/L	6.3–15 umol/L	
Alkaline phosphatase	62 IU/L	25–150 IU/L	

(continued)

Table 15-3 Laboratory Test Results (continued)

Hormone	Actual Value	Reference Range	Optimal Range
GGT	15 IU/L	0–65 IU/L	
SGOT	28 IU/L	0–40 IU/L	
SGPT	24 IU/L	0–40 IU/L	
PSA	0.6 ng/mL	0.0–4.0 ng/mL	
Creatinine	1.0 mg/dL	0.5–1.5 mg/dL	
BUN	19 mg/dL	5–26 mg/dL	
BUN/creatinine ratio	19 mg/dL	8–27 mg/dL	

Table 15-4 Amino Acid Profile

Amino Acid	Actual Value (mcmol/dL)	Reference Range (mcmol/dL)
a-Alanine	42	21–67
B-Alanine	0.9	0–1.4
a-Aminoadipic acid	0.1	0–0.3
Amino-B-guanidino-propionic acid	0	0–0.2
y-Aminobutyric acid	0	0–0.1
B-Aminoisobutyric acid	0.3	0–0.6
a-Amino-N-butyric acid	3.2	0.5–3.9
Anserine	0.9	0–1.0
Arginine	1.9	2.8–15.9
Asparagine	6.5	3.0–9.7
Aspartic acid	0.6	0–1.9
Carnosine	0.4	0–1.2
Citruline	3.3	0.7–6.5

(continued)

Table 15-4 Amino Acid Profile (continued)

Amino Acid	Actual Value (mcmol/dL)	Reference Range (mcmol/dL)
Cystathionine	3.9	0.7–6.5
Cystine	4.1	0.3–5.6
Glutamic acid	8.5	2.0–22
Glycine	23	12–46
Histidine	5.6	4.8–12.5
Homocysteine	0	0–0.2
Hydroxylysine	–	None detected
Hydroxyproline	2.1	0–4.0
Isoleucine	3.5	3.9–12.1
Leucine	6.4	6.1–20
Lysine	9.6	11.0–29
Methionine	1.6	1.4–4.7
1-Methyl-histidine	0.7	0.3–2
Ornithine	4.7	3.0–13.6
Phenylalanine	5.1	3.6–9.9
Phosphoethanolamine	0.9	0–1.8
Phosphoserine	0.9	0.3–2.1
Proline	11.6	9.8–44
Sarcosine	1.4	0–1.6
Serine	5.7	6.9–27
Taurine	2.3	3.4–14.5
Threonine	9.0	7.6–26.1
Tryptophan	4.8	2.1–9.4
Tyrosine	3.0	3.2–12.2
Valine	4.5	11.5–34

disease. Adjustments in diet, workout regimen (duration, volume, load, tempo), nutritional supplements, and herbal and pharmaceutical plans can be made to achieve optimal blood test results, which translate into optimal performance for the athlete.

Low testosterone levels can restrict musculoskeletal development and can be caused by numerous factors such as failing testes, lack of luteinizing hormone (LH, the hormone required for stimulation of testosterone production by the testes), the testes' resistance to LH, or a combination of any of these. A lack of LH usually indicates either a chemical shutdown (e.g., with exogenous testosterone) or a pituitary problem. One can have low testosterone levels with normal or high levels of LH. This indicates a failure of the testes—either they are not functioning, or they are resistant to the effects of LH. Lastly, one can have low LH and low testosterone levels. If the testes are functioning normally, then trying to increase endogenous LH is one solution (like using Clomid or Nolvadex to stimulate LH release). The other is to try using human chorionic gonadotropin (HCG, an LH analogue) to stimulate the testes to respond. In any case, it is important to try to correct these problems. If low testosterone levels cannot be corrected, then the patient may have to consider hormone replacement therapy (HRT) to maintain his baseline testosterone levels.

High estradiol levels are also a problem. High estrogen levels in men can cause gynecomastia, fat accumulation, excessive water retention, fatigue, enlarged prostate, and reduced libido. High prolactin levels can cause many of the same problems in addition to impotence and a gynecomastia of the residual lactation glands in males. It is important to keep these hormone levels in check. An aromatase inhibitor (Aromasin, Femara, Arimidex) or a selective estrogen receptor modulator (Clomid, Nolvadex) can be used for regulating high estrogen levels. Dopamine receptor agonists (Dostinex, Bromocriptine) or a progesterone receptor modulator (Winstrol) adequately control prolactin levels.

Cardiovascular function, blood chemistry, thyroid function, adrenal function, and pancreatic function are the most important systems to be monitored. If any of these systems are failing or abnormal, it makes it difficult or impossible for the athlete to benefit from any pharmaceutical enhancement.

Diagnosis

Athletes who suffer from osteitis pubis have been classified into four different stages, based on clinical presentation (Rodriguez et al., 2001). Table 15-5 describes the various classifications identified by Rodriguez and colleagues (2001).

Treatment

Until now osteitis pubis has not been understood or diagnosed, and consequently it has not been properly treated by some health practitioners. Conventionally, groin pain—and specifically osteitis pubis—has been treated by using muscle strengthening and stretching exercises, anti-inflammatory analgesics, rest, local anesthetic, and only in chronic cases, surgery (Fricker et al., 1991; Holt et al., 1995; Machlum & Bahr, 2004). In another study, conservative management included oral ibuprofen (800 mg 3 times per day for 14 days), daily application of therapeutic modalities (cryomassage, laser therapy, ultrasound, or electrical stimulation) for 14 days, and rehabilitation exercises (Rodriguez et al., 2001). This type of management demonstrated positive results in as little as three to eight weeks (Rodriguez et al., 2001).

However, a more effective treatment of the athlete at hand involved a multidisciplinary approach that focused on enhancing fascia regeneration efficiently, resulting in a fast resumption of sports activity. Table 15-6 outlines the treatment protocol used in this case study.

Abbreviations

ACS	autologous conditioned serum
BFGF	basic fibroblast growth factor (also FGF-2)
IGF-1	insulin-like growth factor-1

Table 15-5 Stages of Osteitis Pubis

Stage of Injury	Description of Injury
Stage I	Unilateral symptoms involving kicking leg and inguinal pain in the adductor muscles.
Stage II	Bilateral symptoms with inguinal pain involving the adductors; pain increases after training session.
Stage III	Bilateral inguinal pain involving adductor muscles and abdominal symptoms; pain with kicking ball, sprinting, changing positions form sitting to standing, walking long distances, and stair climbing; in this stage, the athlete cannot participate in sport.*
Stage IV	Describes pain in adductors and abdominal muscles referred to as the pelvic girdle and lumbar spine with defecation, sneezing, and walking on uneven terrain.

* For the athlete examined in this case study, the diagnosis was that of stage III osteitis pubis.

Table 15-6 Protocol Used for an Athlete Diagnosed with Stage III Osteitis Pubis

Day(s)	Treatment Protocol	Description
1	Low-level laser—635 nm	Sites treated—rectus abdominus insertion into symphysis pubis, myofascial trigger points in adductors, and rectus abdominus
		Acupuncture points—CV-5, CV-4, CV-3, SP-11 bilaterally, LR-8 bilaterally, SP-6, SP-11, SP-13 bilaterally, GB-34, LR-3, Ki-3, Ki-9 all bilaterally
1	Ice for 5 minutes	Anatomical points listed above
1	Intravenous infusion of vitamin C	High dose—50 grams per infusion daily
1	Nutritional protocol: EPA/DHA—1 gram twice daily Cetylated fatty acids—1,050 mg three times daily Proteolytic enzymes—bromelain and serrapeptidase Avoid excitatoxins—glutamate, aspartate, cysteines. Reduce intake of hydrogenated fatty	

(continued)

Table 15-6 Protocol Used for an Athlete Diagnosed with Stage III Osteitis Pubis (continued)

Day(s)	Treatment Protocol	Description
	acids and saturated fatty acids (pro-inflammatories). Consume 5–9 fruits daily.	
1	Autologous conditioned serum: sc injection of cell-free serum containing (bFGF, IGF-1, IL-1B, IL-1Ra, IL-7, NGF, PDGF-AB, TGF-β1)	
2	Low-level laser—635 nm	Sites treated—rectus abdominus insertion into symphysis pubis, myofascial trigger points in adductors and rectus abdominus Acupuncture points—CV-5, CV-4, CV-3, SP-11 bilaterally, LR-8 bilaterally, SP-6, SP-11, SP-13 bilaterally, GB-34, LR-3, Ki-3, Ki-9 all bilaterally
2	Heat—apply for 15 minutes.	Sites treated—adductors bilaterally and rectus abdominus insertion
2	Ice (cryotherapy)—apply for 5 minutes.	Sites treated—adductors bilaterally and rectus abdominus insertion
2	Alternate heat and cold—repeat thermotherapy–cryotherapy cycle twice.	
2	Static stretching	Sites stretched—adductor muscles and rectus abdominus
2	Intravenous infusion of vitamin C	High dose—50 grams per infusion daily
2	Nutritional protocol: EPA/DHA—1 gram twice daily Cetylated fatty acids—1,050 mg three times daily Proteolytic enzymes—bromelain and serrapeptidase Avoid excitatoxins—glutamate, aspartate, cysteines. Reduce intake of hydrogenated fatty acids and saturated fatty acids (pro-inflammatories). Consume 5–9 fruits daily.	

Table 15-6 Protocol Used for an Athlete Diagnosed with Stage III Osteitis Pubis (continued)

Day(s)	Treatment Protocol	Description
3	Fascial release (50–50)	Sites released—adductors and rectus abdominus
3	Chiropractic manipulation called diversified technique (CMT-D)	Joint manipulated—left sacroiliac joint
3	Low-level laser—635 nm	Sites treated—rectus abdominus insertion into symphysis pubis, myofascial trigger points in adductors and rectus abdominus
		Acupuncture points—CV-5, CV-4, CV-3, SP-11 bilaterally, LR-8 bilaterally, SP-6, SP-11, SP-13 bilaterally, GB-34, LR-3, Ki-3, Ki-9 all bilaterally
3	Nutritional protocol: Arginine—10 grams daily Carnosine—100 mg daily Copper—5 mg daily EPA/DHA—1 gram twice daily Cetylated fatty acids—1,050 mg three times daily Proteolytic enzymes—bromelain and serrapeptidase Avoid excitatoxins—glutamate, aspartate, cysteines. Reduce intake of hydrogenated fatty acids and saturated fatty acids (pro-inflammatories). Consume 5 to 9 servings of fruits and vegetables daily.	
3	Initiate functional rehabilitation program (see below for details)	
4	Low-level laser—635 nm	Sites treated—rectus abdominus insertion into symphysis pubis, myofascial trigger points in adductors and rectus abdominus
		Acupuncture points—CV-5, CV-4, CV-3, SP-11 bilaterally, LR-8 bilaterally, SP-6, SP-11, SP-13 bilaterally, GB-34, LR-3, Ki-3, Ki-9 all bilaterally

(continued)

Table 15-6 Protocol Used for an Athlete Diagnosed with Stage III Osteitis Pubis (continued)

Day(s)	Treatment Protocol	Description
4	Fascial release	Sites released—adductors and rectus abdominus
4	Active Release Technique (ART)®	Protocols 51 (adductors) and 55 (gracilis) of the lower extremity, and Protocol 50 for the left sacroiliac joint
4	Functional rehabilitation program	
4	Nutritional protocol: Arginine—10 grams daily Carnosine—100 mg daily Copper—5 mg daily EPA/DHA—1 gram twice daily Avoid excitatoxins—glutamate, aspartate, cysteines. Reduce intake of hydrogenated fatty acids and saturated fatty acids (pro-inflammatories). Consume 5–9 servings of fruits and vegetables daily.	
5	Low-level laser—635 nm	Sites treated—rectus abdominus insertion into symphysis pubis, myofascial trigger points in adductors and rectus abdominus Acupuncture points—CV-5, CV-4, CV-3, SP-11 bilaterally, LR-8 bilaterally, SP-6, SP-11, SP-13 bilaterally, GB-34, LR-3, Ki-3, Ki-9 all bilaterally
5	Static stretching	Sites stretched—adductor muscles and rectus abdominus
5	Autologous conditioned serum: sc injection of cell-free serum containing (bFGF, IGF-1, IL-1B, IL-1Ra, IL-7, NGF, PDGF-AB, TGF-β1)	
5	Functional rehabilitation program	
5	Nutritional protocol: Arginine—10 grams daily Carnosine—100 mg daily Copper—5 mg daily EPA/DHA—1 gram twice daily	

Table 15-6 Protocol Used for an Athlete Diagnosed with Stage III Osteitis Pubis (continued)

Day(s)	Treatment Protocol	Description
	Avoid excitatoxins—glutamate, aspartate, cysteines. Reduce intake of hydrogenated fatty acids and saturated fatty acids (pro-inflammatories). Consume 5–9 fruits daily.	
6	Repeat day 4.	
7	Repeat day 4.	
8	Repeat day 4.	
9	Repeat day 4.	
10	Repeat day 4 with a follow-up MRI scan.	

IL-1β	interleukin-1 beta
IL-1Ra	interleukin 1 receptor antagonist
IL-7	interleukin 7
NGF	nerve growth factor
PDGF	platelet-derived growth factor
TGF-β1	transforming growth factor beta 1

Functional Rehabilitation

The functional rehabilitation program, which involves full weight-bearing and sport-specific exercises, begins when the team doctor considers that prefunctional treatment of the player's injury has been successfully completed (Machlum & Bahr, 2004).

The functional stage of rehabilitation is comprised of 10 sequential test elements grouped into 3 phases (Fuller & Walker, 2006):

Phase 1—fitness elements, endurance, speed–endurance, speed, power and agility

Phase 2—ball and match skill elements, basic ball skills (short passing, kicking, half volleying, volleying); advanced ball skills (long passing, kicking, half volleying, volleying); basic match skills (dribbling, heading, juggling); advanced match skills (crossing, shooting, ball control, defending)

Phase 3—match pace football element. Player performance in an exercise was assessed during functional rehabilitation by the responsible therapist using a subjective six-point scale that took into account the player's normal uninjured capabilities:

- ○ 0—player unable to continue
- ○ 1—poor
- ○ 2—moderate
- ○ 3—good
- ○ 4—very good
- ○ 5—excellent (equated to the player's benchmark standard when uninjured)

In each exercise, the minimum acceptable assessment score was 3. The levels of performance rated were as follows: fitness element, skills element, and soccer element.

In the fitness elements, the requirements were (1) complete the exercise free of pain with no evidence of swelling at the injury site on the completion of the exercise, (2) experience no discomfort during motion at all speeds and in all directions, and (3) complete the exercise with a normal gait pattern.

In the skills elements, players must:

- Maintain coordination and concentration
- Achieve adequate ball control and timing
- Experience no pain during the exercise

During the match pace soccer element, players must:

- Complete all normal match activities at normal match speed
- Remain pain free throughout the assessment period (Machlum & Bahr, 2004)

In phases 1 and 2, the player is required to achieve an assessment score of 3 in two exercises available for each element. The players progressed through phases 1, 2, and 3 only when all elements of each phase were subsequently completed. "Satisfactory completion of each exercise achieved a player recovery score of 5% in phases 1 and 2 and a recovery score of 10% on completion of the single match pace element in phase 3; players were considered to be fit to return to normal team training and competition when they had achieved a 100% recovery score" (Fuller & Walker, 2006). Note that the recovery score refers to a subjective rating scale of each player's performance.

During rehabilitation, the soccer player typically received 2 hours of treatment a day for 10 days from the attending medical staff. The players progressed from the prefunctional stage to the functional stage of rehabilitation when they were pain free and when the soft tissue practitioner, in conjunction with the radiologist, confirmed that tissue healing was complete.

Return to Play Following Muscle Strains

There are no consensus guidelines or agreed-upon criteria for the safe return to sport following a muscle strain such as a fascia tear that completely eliminates the risk of recurrence and maximizes performance (Orchard, Best, & Verrall, 2005). Improved prognostic assessment of the fascia tear with injury identification (MRI) and injury assessment (isokinetic testing) can assist the practitioner to lower, but does not eliminate, recurrent injuries.

Generally the goal of determination of fitness for return to play from most injuries involves an assessment that the recurrence risk is minimal and the performance is optimal. However, with respect to muscle strains, allowing an early return to play may be a sensible strategy, albeit with a cost of an increased recurrence rate (Verrall et al., 2003). The decision regarding determination of fitness for return to play is generally based on an expert opinion level of evidence only. Despite the lack of high-quality evidence, an athlete's ability to manage return to play can be improved if the following factors are taken into consideration: strength and flexibility testing, imaging, functional field testing, and risk management strategies (Orchard et al., 2005).

Strength and Flexibility Testing

It has long been held that correcting any flexibility deficit is equally important to a strength deficit in terms of determining return to play (Garrett, 1996; Worrell & Perrin, 1992; Worrell, Smith, & Winegardner, 1994). For groin strains, a decreased range of hip abduction has been associated with a higher incidence and recurrence of groin injuries (Arnason, Sigurdsson, Gudmundsson, Ingar Holme, Lars Engebretsen, et.al, 2004; Ekstrand & Gillquist, 1983).

Imaging

In recent years, the use of MRI imaging for assessing severity of muscle strain has become more prevalent (Gibbs, Cross, Cameron, & Houang, 2004; Cross, Gibbs, Cameron, & Houang, 2004). Diagnostic ultrasound may also be used and is a reasonable alternative at a lower cost, although MRI appears to be superior for predicting prognosis (Connell, Schneider-Kolosky, Hoving, Malara, Buchbinder, Koulouris et al., 2004). The use of high-resolution imaging has allowed separation of two distinct entities of posterior thigh injury—the hamstring muscle strain (as proven by MRI scan) and the MRI-negative posterior thigh injury (Verrall, Slavotinek, Barnes, Fon, & Spriggins, 2001).

Functional Field Testing

The traditional method for determining fitness for return to play has been the following:

1. Allow training after manually assessed strength and flexibility have returned to levels comparable to the unaffected side.

2. Test functional ability (to accelerate, reach maximum speed, change direction) at training and allow return to play if all tasks can be completed without pain or obvious limitation.

It is recognized that these steps can almost certainly be passed before a player has returned to full strength (as measured by isokinetic device) or the abnormal signal on MRI scan has been resolved (Orchard & Best, 2002).

The rigor of a functional test can be theoretically increased by adding tasks beyond what is normally expected of players at training (for example, extra run-through sprints in a fatigued state). This may increase the likelihood that a player will fail the fitness test and be declared unfit to play. However, a substantial number of muscle strain injuries and reinjuries occur during training itself, so the trade-off for a more rigorous testing session is likely to be an increase in risk of recurrence at that session. With respect to the functional activity most likely to cause an injury or reinjury, full sprinting and bending forward (e.g., to catch a football) while running at high speed are thought to be the activities of greatest risk for hamstring strains, whereas taking off (acceleration) for calf strains, kicking on the run for quadriceps strains, and change of direction are the activities of greatest risk for adductor strains (Orchard, 2002).

Risk Management Strategies

Because it is recognized that many players can successfully return to competition prior to full recovery, Orchard and Best have suggested an approach of risk minimization rather than risk elimination. It has been shown in the Australian Football League that while a substantial percentage of muscle strains recur at a later stage during the season, of the recurrent injuries, only a minority are reinjured in the first return match (Orchard & Best, 2002). This observation suggests that to reduce the recurrence rate to much closer to zero, players would need to be kept out for perhaps double the recovery time rather than simply an extra week. Waiting for complete recovery of the muscle strain injury in a team sport may be an unnecessarily conservative approach, because while it would certainly decrease the recurrence rate of injury, it would increase the overall time missed through muscle strain injuries (as it would preclude many players who would have otherwise successfully returned from being able to play). While many players in team sports are able to return to play successfully without complete recovery of the muscle group, they are probably doing so with subtle biomechanical alterations that protect the injured muscle but that may also minimally sacrifice maximum performance.

Results

Using the protocol described earlier, the athlete in this case study was able to return to soccer training in just 10 days following initialization of treatment. Within one week (seven days), symptoms were reduced by 80% as indicated on visual analog scales (VAS) and pain diagrams. A MRI scan taken of the adductor region revealed a negative fascia tear at

Fukushima, K., Badlani, N., Usas, A., Riano, F., Fu, F., & Huard, J. (2001). The use of an antifibrosis agent to improve muscle recovery after laceration. *American Journal of Sports Medicine, 29*(4), 394–401.

Gallucci, R. M., Sugawara, T., Yucesoy, B., Berryann, K., Simeonova, P. P., Matheson, J. M., et al. (2001). Interleukin-6 treatment augments cutaneous wound healing in immunosuppressed mice. *Journal of Interferon & Cytokine Research, 21*(8), 603–609.

Hankenson, K. D., Watkins, B. A., Schoenlein, I. A., Allen, K. G., & Turek, J. J. (2000). Omega-3 fatty acids enhance ligament fibroblast collagen formation in association with changes in interleukin-6 production. *Proceedings of the Society for Experimental Biology and Medicine, 223*(1), 88–95.

Hendradi, E., Obata, Y., Isowa, K., Nagai, T., & Takayama, K. (2003). Effect of mixed micelle formulations including terpenes on the transdermal delivery of diclofenac. *Biological & Pharmaceutical Bulletin, 26*(12), 1739–1743.

Jaeger, B., & Skootsky, S. A. (1987). Double blind controlled study of different myofascial trigger point injection techniques. *Pain, 4*(Suppl.), 560.

Jimenez, P. A., & Rampy, M. A. (1999). Keratinocyte growth factor-2 accelerates wound healing in incisional wounds. *Journal of Surgery Research, 81*(2), 238–242.

Komarcevic, A. (2000). The modern approach to wound treatment. *Medicinski Pregled, 53*(7–8), 363–368.

Kweon, J. H., Chi, S. C., & Park, E. S. Transdermal delivery of diclofenac using microemulsions. *Archives of Pharmacal Research, 27*(3), 351–356.

Li, Y., Foster, W., Deasy, B. M., Chan, Y., Prisk, V., Tang, Y., Cummins, J., & Huard, J. (2004). Transforming growth factor-beta1 induces the differentiation of myogenic cells into fibrotic cells in injured skeletal muscle: A key event in muscle fibrogenesis. *American Journal of Pathology, 164*(3), 1007–1019.

MacGregor, J., & Parkhouse, W. S. (1996). The potential role of insulin-like growth factors in skeletal muscle regeneration. *Canadian Journal of Applied Physiology, 21*(4), 236–250.

McCourt, M., Wang, J. H., Sookhai, S., & Redmond, H. P. Pro-inflammatory mediators stimulate neutrophil directed angiogenesis. *Archives of Surgery, 134*(12), 1325–1331.

Neer, C. S. (1983). Impingement lesions. *Clinical Orthopaedics, 173,* 70–77.

Negishi, S., Li, Y., Usas, A., Fu, F. H., & Huard, J. (2005). The effect of relaxin treatment on skeletal muscle injuries. *American Journal of Sports Medicine, 33*(12), 1816 - 1824

Nelson, I., Degoul, F., Obermaier-Kusser, B., Romero, N., Borrone, C., Marsac, C., et al. (1989). Mapping of heteroplasmic mitochondrial DNA deletions in Kearns-Sayre syndrome. *Nucleic Acids Research, 17*(2), 8117–8124.

Nycomed Website. (n.d.). [Actovegin]. Retrieved October 21, 2007, from http://www.nycomed. com.cn/english/wmdcp/awz/biaoti.html

Paino, I. M., Ximenes, V. F., da Fonseca, L. M., Kanegae, M. P. P., Khalil, N. M., & Brunetti, I. L. (2005). Effect of therapeutic plasma concentrations of non-steroidal anti-inflammatory drugs on the production of reactive oxygen species by activated rat neutrophils. *Brazilian Journal of Medical & Biological Research, 38*(4), 543–551.

Raschke, M., Kolbeck, S., Bail, H., Schmidmaier, G., Flyvbjerg, A., Lindner, T., et al. (2001). Homologous growth hormone accelerates healing of segmental bone defects, *Bone, 29*(4), 368–373.

Sato, K., Li, Y., Foster, W., Fukushima K., Badlani, N., Nodachi, N., Usas, A., Fu, F. H., & Huard, J. (2003). Improvement of muscle healing through enhancement of muscle regeneration and prevention of fibrosis. *Muscle & Nerve, 28*(3), 365–372.

the os pubis, hence suggesting a better prognosis in terms of recovery time and risk of recurrence. After 10 days the player was placed off the injury reserve list of his team and returned to full playing time, thus preventing the onset of muscle imbalances and altered biomechanics that can hamper physical performance on the field.

Discussion

In addition to the "traditional" treatment protocol (rest, rehabilitation exercises, modalities) for therapy of osteitis pubis, the use of laser therapy, fascial techniques, and ART® did contribute to the quick recovery time of this patient. The mechanism of action of low-level laser therapy (such as the Erchonia® laser) is not completely understood; however, some theories have been established based on existing scientific evidence. First, low-level laser does promote the proliferation of endothelial cells, which can partially explain an increase in newly formed blood vessels (angiogenesis) following treatment (Fricker, 1997). In addition, there has also been evidence of increased mitotic activity, fibroblast numbers, and the synthesis of collagen (Mirsky, Krispel, Shoshany, Maltz, & Oron, 2002). In fact, in one study it was shown how fibroblasts proliferated faster with 665–675 nm of light, whereas 810 nm of light was inhibitory to fibroblasts (Gomez-Villamandos, Valenzuela, & Calatrava, 1995). These characteristics of laser therapy play an important role in promoting wound healing, accelerating the inflammatory process, and modulating pain.

The use of myofascial techniques is critical to further accelerating the healing process of osteitis pubis. Tension or stress on the fascial network may result from active or reflex muscular contractions producing tension upon a bone and its associated articulations. Such is the case with osteitis pubis. The case presentation involved an athlete with pain in his pubic symphysis as well as fixation of his sacroiliac joint. Since osteitis pubis involves the antagonistic tension forces placed on the pubic symphysis by the abdominal fascia and adductor fascia and muscles, it is important to work on the myofascial

system. Moreover, it is important to treat the fascia in relation to the direction of fiber orientation and attachment onto the pubic symphysis.

As described, if the fascial system is strained, the mechanical conditions under which the muscles function are also altered. The Active Release Technique Soft Tissue Management System (ART®) has proven to be clinically promising in treating soft issue injuries (Buchberger, 1993; Moore, Ridgway, Higbee, Howard, & Lucroy, 2005). Soft tissue insult will reduce circulation in the area of concern, ultimately leading to tissue hypoxia. Related research has indicated that as the partial pressure of oxygen (PO_2) begins to decrease due to hypoxic conditions, fibroblasts are stimulated by such conditions; they start to proliferate at the site of injury, causing excess collagen deposition (Fal Falanga, Zhou, & Yufit, 2002; Leahy & Mock, 1991). In addition, the injured area is also usually filled with a hematoma. Growing granulation tissue slowly replaces the hematoma, eventually resulting in the formation of scar tissue (Saed, Zhang, & Diamond, 2001). Fibrous scar tissue formation is one of the major factors that can slow down soft tissue healing (Li, Fu, & Huard, 2005).

Isokinetic strength testing and MRI assessment may be appropriate steps toward the clearance of an athlete for return to play; however, full functional recovery is probably needed to allow a good performance. In assessing the best time for an athlete to return to play, a number of factors as described in Table 15-7 may all be taken into account. Some of these factors relate to the injury itself, and others relate to the baseline risk of other circumstances.

The general treatment strategy incorporated in this case study could be equally applied to other injuries and sports if appropriate sport-specific exercises are incorporated in the program.

Summary

The case presented was that of a 17-year-old soccer player who presented with groin pain of 10 months in duration. The patient had not progressed extensively over the initial 10-month period of treatment

Table 15-7 Factors Considered in Guiding Decision Regarding Return to Play

Factors Indicating a More Conservative Approach	Factors That May Allow More Rapid Return to Play
Persisting strength deficit	Strength equal to uninjured side
Persisting flexibility deficit	Flexibility equal to uninjured side
Inability to complete full training without pain or limping	Ability to do all functional activities at training
Large area of abnormal signal on imaging	Normal ultrasound and/or MRI scan
100-m sprinter or team player in high-risk position (outfield soccer player)	Team sport player in low-risk position (goal keeper)
Older player	Younger player (but with experience of playing with injury)
Early stage of season	Playoff or must-win game with no adequate replacement player
Strain in high-risk location (biceps femoris, central tendon of rectus femoris, medial head of gastrocnemius, adductor longus or magnus)	Strain in low-risk location (semimembranosus vastus muscles, lateral head of gastrocnemius, gluteal muscles)

provided under the care of another health practitioner. This section outlined a more effective and efficient way to treat osteitis pubis that will ensure a quicker return of the athlete to activity.

Groin injuries are some of the most challenging injuries in the field of sports medicine. Symptoms can be vague and diffuse. Thus, a thorough history, proper physical examination, imaging, and a multidisciplinary approach are needed for effective treatment of these conditions.

References

Agrios, P., & Crawford, J. W. (1999). Double crush syndrome of the upper extremity. *Journal of Sports Chiropractic & Rehabilitation, 13*(3), 111–114.

Arnason, A., Sigurdsson, S., Gudmundsson, A., Gudmundsson, A., **Holme, I.**, Engebretsen, L., & Bahr, R. (2004). Risk factors for injury in football. *American Journal of Sports Medicine, 32*, 5S–16S.

Baer, J. (1999). Iliotibial band syndrome in cyclists: Evaluation and treatment; a case report. *Journal of Sports Chiropractic & Rehabilitation, 13*(2), 66–69.

Bednar, D. A., Orr, F. M., & Simon, T. (1995). Observations on the pathomorphology of the toracolumbar fascia in chronic mechanical back pain. *Spine, 20*(10), 1161–1164.

Blankenbaker, D. G., & De Smet, A. A. (2004). MR Imaging of muscle injuries. *Applied Radiology, 33*(4), 14–26.

Buchberger, D. J. (1993). Scapular dysfunctional impingement syndrome as a cause of grade two rotator cuff tear: A case study. *Chiropractic Sports Medicine, 7*, 38–45.

Buchberger, D. J. (1999). Use of active release techniques in the postoperative shoulder. *Journal of Sports Chiropractic & Rehabilitation, 13*(2), 60–66.

Buchberger, D. J., Rizzoto, H., & McAdam, B. J. (1996). Median nerve entrapment resulting in unilateral action tremor of the hand. *Journal of Sports Chiropractic & Rehabilitation, 10*(4), 176–180.

Croisier, J. L., Forthomme, B., Namurois, M. H., Vanderthommen, M., & Crielaard, J. M. (2002). Hamstring muscle strain recurrence and strength performance disorders. *American Journal of Sports Medicine, 30*(2), 199–203.

Cross, T., Gibbs, N., Cameron, M., Michael T. Houang, (2004). Acute quadriceps muscle strains: Magnetic resonance imaging features and prognosis. *American Journal of Sports Medicine, 32,* 710–719.

Connell, D., Schneider-Kolosky, M., Hoving, J., Malara, F., Buchbinder, R., Koulouris, G., Burke, F., & Bass, C. (2004). Longitudinal study comparing sonographic and MRI assessments of acute and healing hamstring injuries. *AJR American Journal of Roentgenology, 183,* 975–984.

Danto, J. B. (2003). Review of integrated neuromusculoskeletal release and the novel application of a segmental anterior/posterior approach in the thoracic, lumbar, and sacral regions. *Journal of the American Osteopathic Association, 103*(12), 583–596.

Drover, J. M., Forand, D. R., & Herzog, W. (2004). Influence of active release technique on quadriceps inhibition and strength: A pilot study. *Journal of Manipulative & Physiological Therapeutics, 27*(6), 408–414.

Ekstrand, J., & Gillquist, J. (1983). The avoidability of soccer injuries. *International Journal of Sports Medicine, 4,* 124–128.

Fal Falanga, V., Zhou, L., & Yufit, T. (2002). Low oxygen tension stimulates collagen synthesis and COL1A1 transcription through the action of TGF-beta1. *Journal of Cellular Physiology, 191*(1), 42–50.

Fricker, P. A. (1997). Osteitis pubis. *Sports Medicine & Arthroscopy Review, 5,* 305–312.

Fricker, P. A., Taunton, J. E., & Ammann, W. (1991). Osteitis pubis in athletes: Infection, inflammation, or injury? *Sports Medicine, 12,* 266–279.

Fuller, C. W., & Walker, J. (2006). Quantifying the functional rehabilitation of injured football players. *British Journal of Sports Medicine, 40,* 151–157.

Garrett, W. E. (1996). Muscle strain injuries. *American Journal of Sports Medicine, 24,* S2–S8.

Gibbs, N., Cross, T., Cameron, M., Houang M. (2004). The accuracy of MRI in predicting recovery and recurrence of acute grade one hamstring muscle strains within the same season in Australian Rules football players. *Journal of Science & Medicine in Sport, 7,* 248–258.

Gomez-Villamandos, R. J., Valenzuela, J. M. S., & Calatrava, I. R. (1995). He-Ne laser therapy by fibroendoscopy in the mucosa of the equine upper airway. *Lasers in Surgery & Medicine, 16,* 184–188.

Grzanna, R., Lindmark, L., & Frondoza, C. G. (2005). Ginger—a herbal medicinal product with broad anti-inflammatory actions. *Journal of Medicinal Food, 8*(2), 125–132.

Hammer, W. I. (1996). Muscle imbalance and post-facilitation stretch. In W. I. Hammer (Ed.), *Functional soft tissue examination and treatment by manual methods,* 2nd ed. (pp. 415–445). Baltimore, MD: Aspen.

Hennessy, L., & Watson, A.W.S. (1993). Flexibility and posture assessment in relation to hamstring injury. *British Journal of Sports Medicine, 27*(4), 243–246.

Holt, M., Keene, J., Graf, B., & Helwig, D. (1995). Treatment of osteitis pubis in athletes: Results of corticosteroid injections. *American Journal of Sports Medicine, 23*(5), 601–606.

Jonhagen, S., Nemeth, G., & Eriksson, E. (1994). Hamstring injuries in sprinters: The role of concentric and eccentric hamstring muscle strength and flexibility. *American Journal of Sports Medicine, 22*(2), 262–266.

Kaplan, P. A., Dussault, R. D., Helms, C. A., et al. (2001). Tendons and muscles. In *Musculoskeletal MRI* (pp. 55–87). Philadelphia: WB Saunders.

Kazemi, M. (2000). Adhesive capsulitis: A case report. *Journal of the Canadian Chiropractic Association, 44*(3), 169–177.

Kjaer, M. (2004). Role of extracellular matrix in adaptation of tendon and skeletal muscle to mechanical loading. *Physiological Review, 84*, 649–698.

Kruger, L. Cutaneous sensory system. (1987). In G. Adelman, (Ed.), *Encyclopedia of neuroscience* (vol. 1, pp. 293–294). Cambridge, MA: Birkhauser Boston.

Kujala, U. M., Orava, S., & Jarvinen, M. (1997). Hamstring injuries: Current trends in treatment and prevention. *Sports Medicine, 23*(6), 397–404.

Leahy, M. P. (1996). Active release techniques: Logical soft tissue treatment. In W. I. Hammer (Ed.), *Functional soft tissue examination and treatment by manual methods,* 2nd ed. (pp. 549–562). Baltimore, MD: Aspen.

Leahy, P. M., & Mock, L. E. (1991). Altered biomechanics of the shoulder and the subscapularis. *Chiropractic Sports Medicine, 5*, 62–66.

LeBlanc, K. E., & LeBlanc, K.A. (2003). Groin pain in athletes. *Hernia, 7*(2), 68–71.

Li, Y., Fu, F. H., & Huard, J. (2005, May). Cutting edge muscle recovery: Using antifibrosis agents to improve healing. *Physician and SportsMedicine,* 44–50.

Machlum, S., & Bahr, R. (2004). Treating sports injuries. In R. Bahr & S. Machlum (Eds.), *Clinical guide to sports injuries* (pp. 25–37). Champaign, IL: Human Kinetics.

McHugh, M. P., Connolly, D.A.J., Eston, R. G., Kremenic, I. J., Nicholas, S. J., & Gleim, G. W. (1999). The role of passive muscle stiffness in symptoms of exercise-induced muscle damage.

American Journal of Sports Medicine, 27(5), 594–599.

Mirsky, N., Krispel, Y., Shoshany, Y., Maltz, L., & Oron, U. (2002). Promotion of angiogenesis by low level laser. *Antioxidants & Redox Signaling,4(5),* 785–790.

Moore, K. L., & Dally, A. F. (1999). *Clinically oriented anatomy,* 4th ed. Baltimore, MD: Williams & Wilkins.

Moore, P., Ridgway, T. D., Higbee, R., Howard, E. W., & Lucroy, M. D. (2005). Effect of wavelength on low-intensity laser irradiation-stimulated cell proliferation in vitro. *Lasers in Surgery & Medicine, 36,* 8–12.

Morelli, V., & Smith, V. (2001). Groin injuries in athletes. *American Family Physician, 64*(8), 1405–1414.

Myers, T. (2001). The anatomy trains: Myofascial meridians for manual and movement therapies. London: Churchill Livingstone.

Orchard, J. (2002). Biomechanics of muscle strain injury. *New Zealand Journal of Sports Medicine, 30,* 92–98.

Orchard, J., & Best, T. (2002). The management of muscle strain injuries: An early return versus the risk of recurrence. *Clinical Journal of Sport Medicine, 12,* 3–5.

Orchard, J., Best, T. M., & Verrall, G. M. (2005). Return to play following muscle strains. *Clinical Journal of Sport Medicine, 15,* 436–441.

Pajaczkowski, J. A. (2003). Mimicking turf toe: Myofasopathy of the first dorsal interosseous muscle treated with ART®. *Journal of the American Chiropractic Association, 47*(1), 28–32.

Pool-Goudzwaard, A. L., Vleeming, R. S., Snijders, C. J., & Mens, J.M.A. (1998). Insufficient lumbopelvic stability: A clinical, anatomical and biomechanical approach to "a-specific" low back pain. *Manual Therapy, 3*(1), 12–20.

Puranen, J., & Orava, S. (1998). The hamstring syndrome: A new diagnosis of gluteal sciatic pain. *American Journal of Sports Medicine, 16*(5), 517–521.

Rodriguez, C., Miguel, A., Lima, H., & Heinrichs, K. (2001). Osteitis pubis syndrome in the professional athlete: A case report. *Journal of Athletic Training, 36*(4), 437–440.

Saed, G. M., Zhang, W., & Diamond, M. P. (2001). Molecular characterization of fibroblasts isolated from human peritoneum and adhesions. *Fertility & Sterility, 75*(4), 763–768.

Stanton, P., & Purdam, C. (1989). Hamstring injuries in sprinting–the role of eccentric exercise. *Journal of Orthopaedic & Sports Physical Therapy, 10*(9), 343–349.

Swanik, K. A. (2002). The effects of shoulder plyometric training on proprioception and selected muscle performance characteristics. *Journal of Shoulder & Elbow Surgery, 11*(6), 579–586.

Turl, S. E., & George, K. P. (1998). Adverse neural tension: A factor in repetitive hamstring strain? *Journal of Shoulder & Elbow Surgery, 27*(1), 16–21.

Turner, A. M., Owings, M., & Schwane, J. A. (2003). Improvement in running economy after 6 weeks of plyometric training. *Journal of Strength & Conditioning Research, 17*(1), 60–67.

Van Wingerden, J. P., Vleeming, A., Snijders, C. J., **Pool**-Goudzwaard, A.L., & Stoeckart, R. A. (1993). Functional-anatomical approach to the spine-pelvis mechanism: Interaction between the biceps femoris and the sacrotuberous ligament. *European Spine Journal, 2,* 140–144.

Verrall, G. M., Slavotinek, J. P., Barnes, P. G., & Fon, G. T. (2003). Diagnostic and prognostic value of clinical findings in 83 athletes with posterior thigh injury: Comparison of clinical findings with magnetic resonance imaging documentation of hamstring muscle strain.

American Journal of Sports Medicine, 31(6), 969–973.

Verrall, G., Slavotinek, J., Barnes, P., Fon, G. T., & Spriggins, A. J. (2001). Clinical risk factors for hamstring muscle strain injury: A prospective study with correlation of injury by magnetic resonance imaging. *British Journal of Sports Medicine, 35,* 435–440.

Vleeming, A., Pool-Goudzwaard, A. L., Hammudoghlu, D., Stoeckart, R., Snijders, C., & Mens, J. M. A. (1996). The function of the long dorsal sacroiliac ligament: Its implication for understanding low back pain. *Spine, 21*(5), 556–562.

Vleeming, A., Stoeckart, R., & Snijders, C. J. (1989). The sacrotuberous ligament: A conceptual approach to its dynamic role in stabilizing the sacroiliac joint. *Clinical Biomechanics, 4*(4), 201–203.

Vleeming, A., Van Wingerden, J. P., Snijders, C. J., Stoeckart, R., & Stijnen, T. (1989). Load application to the sacrotuberous ligament; influences on sacroiliac joint mechanics. *Clinical Biomechanics, 4(4),* 204–209.

Worrell, T. W. (1994). Factors associated with hamstring injuries: An approach to treatment and preventative measures. *Sports Medicine, 17*(5), 338–345.

Worrell, T., & Perrin, D. (1992). Hamstrings muscle injury: The influence of strength, flexibility, warm-up and fatigue. *Journal of Orthopaedic & Sports Physical Therapy, 16,* 12–18.

Worrell, T. W., Smith, T. L., & Winegardner, J. (1994). Effect of hamstring stretching on hamstring performance. *Journal of Orthopaedic & Sports Physical Therapy, 20,* 154–159.

Young, H. Y., Luo, Y. L., Cheng, H. Y., Hsieh, W. C., Liao, J. C., & Peng, W. H. (2005). Analgesic and anti-inflammatory activities of [6]-gingerol. *Journal of Ethnopharmacology, 96,* 207–210.

INDEX

Page numbers followed by "f" denote figures and "t" denote tables

A

Abdomen
external, 25t–26t
fascia of, 25t–27t

Achilles tendon
illustration of, 108f
repair of, case study involving, 252–253

Actin filaments, 13, 42, 63

Actin geodomes, 41–42

Actin polymerization, 42

Active release technique
adhesive capsulitis treated with, 133
applications of, 180t–181t
description of, 118–119, 179, 181, 268
hamstring injury treated with, 243–245, 247–249

Actovegin, 236

Acupuncture
connective tissue winding, 176–177
description of, 175–176
mechanical signal transduction, 177, 178f
needle grasp, 177–179
pressure points, 56, 58f

Acute inflammation, 220, 226

Acute trauma, 124–125

Adductors
imaging characteristics of, 104f
injuries to, 102

Adenosine triphosphate, 170, 206, 210, 236

Adhesions
articular pumping for treating, 118
causes of, 179, 220
characteristics of, 72, 72f, 74, 76
localization of, 235
palpation of, 174, 235

Adhesive capsulitis treatment and rehabilitation
active release technique, 133
articular pumping
of glenohumeral joint, 126t–131t
of pretracheal fascia, 131t
of scapula, 132t, 133f
D2 flexion-extension pattern, 142
dynamic joint stability, 136
functional motor patterns, 138
interval throwing program, 146, 146t–147t
isometric strengthening exercises, 138–140, 139f–141f
muscle activation technique, 133–134
muscle reactivation, 137
neuromuscular control, 135–141
overview of, 124
phase I, 124–125
phase II, 125–141
phase III, 141–144
phase IV, 144–146
preparatory activation, 137
proprioceptive and kinesthetic awareness, 135–141
proprioceptive neuromuscular facilitation, 135, 142
range of motion exercises, 134–135
returning to prior activity level, 146

rhythmic stabilization against perturbation, 137, 137f–138f
scapula
seated scapular pinches, 141
stabilization exercises, 142–143, 143f
shoulder exercises
dynamic blackburn, 139–140, 140f
external rotation, 139
plyometric, 143–144, 144f
stretch, 134
three-way stretch, 139, 139f
sound-assisted soft tissue mobilization, 133
supine cervical retractions, 141
weight-bearing shift exercises, 136–137, 137f

Adipose cells
cellulite caused by hypertrophy of, 18
description of, 3–4

Adipose tissue
brown, 3, 83
insulin resistance and, 85
subcutaneous, 85
white, 3, 83–84

Adiposity, 19

Advanced glycation end products, 85, 87, 194

Adverse neural tension, 248

Aging
advanced glycation end products and, 194
collagen fiber changes, 54f, 85, 86f
cross-linking increases secondary to, 82
free radical theory of, 183

Aging, *continued*
glycation and, 85, 87
ground substance affected by, 11

Alanine, 191t

Aloe vera, 197, 201t

Amino acids. *See also specific amino acid*
characteristics of, 190, 191t–193t
laboratory profile of, 258t–259t
supplementation of, 195

Anesthetic injections, 235–236

Anterior cruciate ligament rehabilitation
benefits of, 148
cardiovascular training, 150, 152–155
case study of, 155–162, 251–252
closed-chain exercises, 148
overview of, 146–147
phase I, 156–159
phase II, 159–161
phase III, 161–162
phase IV, 162
pool training, 149–150, 150t–151t
reconditioning, 148–149
strength endurance training, 150, 152–155

Antifibrotics, 231–232

Antioxidants, 199, 205, 208

Antithrombin, 209

Aponeurosis palmaris, 31t

Aponeurosis plantaris, 34t, 82

Arachidonic acid, 222, 225

Arachnoid mater, 58–59

Areolar tissue layer, 80

Arginine, 125t–126t, 191t, 195–196, 200t

Articular dysfunction, 95

Articular pumping
description of, 118

of glenohumeral joint, 126t–131t
of pretracheal fascia, 131t
of scapula, 132t, 133f

Ascorbic acid, 6, 198. *See also* Vitamin C

Asparagine, 191t

Aspartic acid, 191t

Attachment stage, of cellular motility, 42

Autonomic motor neurons, 60

Autonomic nervous system, 60

B

Back fascia, 29t

Biceps femoris, 101

Bike conditioning programs, 154, 155t

Biological field theory, 174

Bioluminescence theory, 172, 174

Biomedicine, 168

Bipennate muscles, 104

Blood tests, 256–257

Blood vessels
distention resistance by, 84
free radicals' effect on endothelial lining of, 207

Body temperature
brown adipose tissue's role in maintaining, 83
water's role in regulation of, 71

Boswellia, 221

Bovine colostrum, 125t–126t

Bromelain
description of, 125t–126t, 197, 201t
ischemia treated with, 212–213
platelet aggregation decreased using, 214

Brown adipose tissue, 3, 83

Buccal aponeurosis, 21t

C

Calcium, 211t

Caloric intake, 190

Camper's fascia, 25t

Carbohydrates, 12, 194

Carbon dioxide, 65

Cardiovascular training, 150, 152–155

Carnitine, 191t

Carnosine, 125t–126t, 196, 200t

Carpal tunnel syndrome, 107f

Case studies
Achilles tendon repair, 252–253
anterior cruciate ligament repair, 155–162, 251–252
groin injury, 254–266
hamstring injuries, 243–249
osteitis pubis, 254–266
supraspinatus muscle tear, 249–251

Catalase, 210

Cat's claw, 224

Celestone Soluspan injectable suspension, 236

Cell(s)
adipose, 3–4, 18
description of, 2, 69
endothelial. *See* Endothelial cells
fibroblasts. *See* Fibroblast(s)
intrafascial, 63–65
macrophages, 4
mast, 2–3, 81f, 220–221
smooth muscle. *See* Smooth muscle cells
stiffening of, 43

Cell spreading, 40

Cellular motility
actin geodomes' role in, 41–42
description of, 40–41
stages of, 42

Cellular oscillation theory, 174

Cellular tensegrity
    description of, 39–42
    somatic recall and, 46–47

Cellulite, 18

Centella, 198

Central nervous system, 56–59

Cerebrospinal fluid, 58

Cetylated monounsaturated fatty
    acid, 200, 201t, 225

Chemical mediators, 3

Chondroitin sulfate, 3, 10t

Choroid plexus, 58

Chromium GTF, 211t

Chronic inflammation, 220

Citrulline, 191t

Closed-chain exercises, 148

Clotting factors, 208

Coagulation
    activation of, 206
    pathways of, 208–210
    platelets' role in, 209

Coagulation cascade, 208–209

Collagen
    alpha chains, 4
    cross-linking, 72–73, 125
    description of, 69
    elastin and, 8
    epithelia adhesion to, 12
    food intake effects on, 190
    piezoelectrical property of, 7
    sol-to-gel transition in, 45
    stress-strain curve for, 53–54, 55f
    structure of, 4, 6
    training effects on, 82
    types of, 4t–5t, 87
    water molecules in, 71

Collagen fibers
    adaptation to changes, 81
    aging effects on, 54f, 85, 86f
    arrangement of, changes in, 81
    crimping of, 53
    dehydration of, 72–73
    density of, 54f

    description of, 4, 6, 45
    elastic fibers and, 8
    endothelial cells and, 7
    glycosylation cross-links in, 6
    half-life of, 51
    histology of, 80f–81f
    longitudinal relaxation of, 75, 75f
    microfailure of, 54–55
    properties of, 6–7
    tensile strength of, 6, 73

Collagen fibrils, 1

Collageno-elastic complex, 8

Colles' fascia, 18–19, 28t

Compartment syndrome, 88

Complement pathway, 209

Complementary medicine
    active release technique. See
        Active release technique
    acupuncture. See Acupuncture
    description of, 168–169
    earthing, 181–183
    frequency-specific microcurrent
        therapy, 169–171
    low-level laser therapy,
        171–175, 173f, 268

Complex carbohydrates, 12

Compression of injury, 116

Connective tissue
    collagen types in, 4, 4t–5t
    components of, 1
    composition of, 69
    functions of, 1
    lubrication of, 10
    microtrauma destruction of, 199
    periarticular, 53
    protein derived from, 193
    remodeled, 55
    with sliding, 81f
    stiffening of, 45
    stress-strain curve of, 56f
    subcutaneous, 81
    tension on, 8
    thixotropic properties of, 45
    "whorls" of, 176f
    winding, 176–177
    without sliding, 80f

Connective tissue fiber
    deformation, 51, 177

Continuum communication, 47,
    73, 169

Copper, 125t–126t, 196, 200t, 211t

Corticosteroids, 236

COX-2 inhibitors, 234–235

Cranial nerves, 59

Cranium, 56

C-reactive protein, 221

Creep, 55

Cross-bridges, 72

Cross-bridging, 44

Crossed extensor reflex, 60

Cross-linking
    age-related increases in, 82
    description of, 72–73
    during phase II of treatment, 125

Cross-links, 55

Cryotherapy, 116

Crystallinity, 46t, 168–169

Cumulative injury cycle, 244–245

Curcumin, 197–198, 201t,
    221–222

Cyclooxygenase enzymes. See
    COX-1; COX-2

Cysteine, 191t

Cystine, 191t

Cytokines, 198, 220, 222, 231

Cytoskeleton
    extracellular matrix, 13, 39
    intermediate filaments, 13,
        39–40, 40f
    microfilaments, 40f, 40–41
    microtubules, 40

D

D2 flexion-extension pattern, 142

Decorin, 231–232, 233f

Deep fascia
    characteristics of, 79
    composition of, 80
    description of, 18, 20
    gliding movements,
        80–81
    muscle and, 80–81, 82f

Dehydration
    blood flow affected by, 74
    chemical mediators released
        during, 72
    of collagen fibers, 72–73
    tensegrity matrix system
        affected by, 71–74

Dermatan sulfate, 10t

Di qi, 176

Diclofenac, 235

Dietary recommendations, 195

Dimethylglycine, 191t

Docosahexaenoic acid, 225

Dry needling, 235–236

Dura mater, 57–58

Dural tube, 18

Dynamic blackburn,
    139–140, 140f

E

Earthing, 181–183

Eicosanoids, 194, 234f

Eicosapentaenoic acid, 196–197,
    225

Elastic fibers
    adaptation to changes, 82
    characteristics of, 6–8
    collagen fibers and, 8
    in deep fascia, 80
    histology of, 80f–81f
    of plantar aponeurosis, 82

Elasticity
    determinants of, 70
    hydration effects on, 75

Elastin
    advanced glycation end
        product accumulation on, 85
    description of, 7–8, 84

Elastin fibers, 6, 69

ELDOA, 118, 159f, 250–251

Electrical muscle stimulation, 148

Electromagnetic healing of
    fractured bone, 168

Electromyography, 94

Elevation of injury, 116

Elliptical cross-trainer exercise, 152

Endomysium
    definition of, 96
    description of, 79, 81
    force transmission, 83
    histology of, 86f

Endosteal layer, of cranial dura
    mater, 57

Endothelial cells
    blood flow maintenance by, 207
    of capillaries, 211
    collagen fibers and, 7
    fibrin deposition, 209
    injury to, 209, 211

Energy medicine
    electromagnetism, 168, 184
    principles of, 167
    summary of, 184

Enzymes, for ischemia, 212–214

Epidermal growth factor, 230

Epimysium
    definition of, 4, 96
    description of, 79–80, 82
    transmission of tension across, 83

Estradiol, 256t, 260

Euglobulin fibrinolytic activity, 213

Exteroreceptors, 61

Extracellular matrix
    adaptation of, 81–82
    characteristics of, 168–169
    composition of, 8–9
    cytoskeleton, 13, 39

description of, 1–2, 39
    fibroblasts in, 12
    fibronectin, 11
    focal adhesion complex
        attachment to, 41
    glycoproteins, 11
    glycosaminoglycans, 9
    ground substance, 9–11
    hyaluronic acid, 9–10
    integrins, 12–13
    laminin, 11–12
    proteoglycans, 9
    water content, 11, 70

F

Fascia. *See also specific fascia*
    anatomy of, 53
    characteristics of, 20, 46t, 46–47
    contraction of, 63–64
    definition of, 18, 189
    degenerative changes to, 243
    functions of, 79
    mechanical roles of. *See*
        Mechanical roles
    neurophysiology of, 56, 57f.
        See also Nervous system
    physiological roles of. *See*
        Physiological roles
    tensegrity. *see* Tensegrity
    thixotropy, 44

Fascia abdominis profunda, 26t

Fascia abdominis superficialis, 25t

Fascia antebrachii, 30t

Fascia axillaris, 25t

Fascia brachii, 30t

Fascia buccopharyngea, 21t

Fascia capitis profunda, 20t–21t

Fascia capitis superficialis, 20t

Fascia clavipectoralis, 24t

Fascia colli profunda, 22t

Fascia colli superficialis, 21t

Fascia coracoclavicularis, 24t

Fascia coxae profunda, 32t

Fascia cruris, 54, 56f

Fascia cruris profunda, 33t–34t

Fascia dorsalis manus, 31t

Fascia dorsalis pedis, 34t

Fascia dorsi profunda, 29t

Fascia dorsi superficialis, 29t

Fascia endothoracica, 24t–25t

Fascia interossea dorsalis manus, 31t

Fascia interpterygoidea, 21t

Fascia lata, 33t

Fascia lumbodorsalis, 29t

Fascia nuchae profunda, 23t

Fascia nuchae superficialis, 23t

Fascia of hypothenar, 31t

Fascia paravertebralis, 22t–23t

Fascia parotideomasseterica, 21t

Fascia pectoralis profunda, 23t–24t

Fascia pectoralis superficialis, 23t

Fascia pedis profunda, 34t

Fascia plantaris pedis, 34t

Fascia profunda, 18, 20

Fascia profunda inferioris
    extremitatis, 32t

Fascia profunda superioris
    extremitatis, 29t

Fascia scapulae profunda, 30t

Fascia subserosa, 27t

Fascia superficialis. *See also*
    Superficial fascia
    description of, 18
    sex-based variations in, 18–19
    zones of adherence, 19t, 19–20

Fascia superficialis inferioris
    extremitatis, 32t

Fascia superficialis superioris
    extremitatis, 29t

Fascia temporalis, 21t

Fascia transversalis, 26t–27t, 85

Fascia volaris manus, 30t–31t

Fasciae pelvis parietalis, 27t

Fasciae pelvis visceralis, 28t

Fasciae perinea profunda, 28t

Fasciae perinea superficialis, 28t

Fascial planes, 20, 20t–34t

Fascial plasticity, 56

Fascial therapy. *See* Myofascial
    therapy

Fasciculus, 96

Fats, 194–195

Females, 18

Fibers
    collagen. *See* Collagen fibers
    elastic, 6–8
    reticular, 7

Fibrin
    description of, 207–208
    hypercoagulability effects
      on, 214
    nutritional products used to
      remove, 213–214

Fibrin degradation products, 213

Fibrinolytic pathways, 208–210

Fibroblast(s)
    actin filaments in, 42
    collagen precursor production
      by, 6
    description of, 2
    in dura mater, 57
    in extracellular matrix, 12

Fibroblast growth factor-10, 231

Fibromyalgia, 95

Fibronectin, 11

Fibrosis, 232, 232f

Fight-or-flight response, 64

Fish oil, 125t–126t, 225

Fixed macrophages, 4

Flavonoids
    Boswellia, 221
    cat's claw, 224
    definition of, 220

ginger, 222, 224
quercetin, 221
resveratrol, 222, 223f
turmeric, 221–222

Flexibility testing, 266

Flexor/withdrawal reflex, 60

Focal adhesion complexes,
    40–41, 41f

Foramen magnum, 58

Force transmission, 83

Forearm-strengthening
    exercises, 141

Fractured bone, 168

Free macrophages, 4

Free radicals, 182–183, 207, 209, 211

Frequency-specific microcurrent
    therapy, 169–171

Functional field testing, 266

Functional rehabilitation
    program, 265–266

G

Gamma-aminobutyric acid, 192t

Ganglion cyst, 106f

Gastrocnemius injuries
    magnetic resonance imaging
      of, 102–103
    ultrasound of, 104f

Ginger, 222, 224

Give and restriction, 114–115, 115t

Glenohumeral joint
    adhesive capsulitis of. *See*
      Adhesive capsulitis
    articular pumping of, 126t–131t

Gliding movements, 80–81

Global stabilizers, 117

Glucose, 194

Glutamic acid, 192t

Glutamine, 192t, 196

Glutathione, 192t, 210

Glycine, 192t

Glycocalyx, 12

Glycoproteins, 1, 11, 169

Glycosaminoglycans
  dehydration effects on, 73
  description of, 9, 10t, 12, 54
  glucose and, 194
  types of, 87

Glycosylation cross-links, 6

Golgi receptors, 61, 62t

Golgi tendon organ, 6, 61, 135

Gotu kola, 198, 201t

Grade I muscle strain, 97, 98f,
  104f, 104–105

Grade II muscle strain, 97–99,
  98f, 105, 105f

Grade III muscle strain, 99, 100f,
  105, 105f

Groin injuries, 253–269

Groin pain, 102

Ground substance
  description of, 9–10t
  functions of, 74
  half-life of, 51
  hyaluronic acid, 9–10, 10t, 74
  proteoglycans, 1, 9, 74
  water-binding qualities of, 74–76

Growth factors, 230–231, 237

H

Hamstring injuries
  active release technique for,
    243–245, 247–249
  anatomy of, 245
  case study of, 243–249
  cumulative injury cycle,
    244–245, 248
  description of, 101f,
    101–102, 108f
  etiologic factors, 244,
    247–248

  myofascial meridians, 245,
    247–249
  onset of, 244
  prevalence of, 244
  tension that causes, 247–248
  treatment approaches for, 244

Head fascia, 20t–21t

Healing
  copper effects on, 196
  description of, 73, 87
  immune response during, 231
  initial phase of, 198
  laser therapy for, 172
  nutritional intake effects on,
    190–195
  zinc's role in, 196

Hematoma
  elevation effects on formation
    of, 116
  with hamstring strain, 101f
  with muscle strain, 99, 100f

Hemodynamics, 84

Heparan sulfate, 10t

Heparin, 3, 10t

Hexosamine, 9

Histidine, 192t

Hormones, 256t

Human chorionic gonadotropin,
  260

Human growth hormone, 230

Humeral tubercle, 127f

Hyaluronic acid, 9–10, 10t,
  74, 81, 87

Hyaluronidase, 10

Hydration, 75, 169

Hypercoagulability, 214

Hypercoagulation, 208

Hyperventilation, 65

Hypoglycemia, 194

I

Ice, 116

Imaging. See also Magnetic
  resonance imaging; Ultrasound
  myofascial injuries, 95–96
  skeletal muscle, 96–97

Immune complexes, 213

Immune response, 231

Immunoglobulin E, 3, 220

Infections, 88

Inflammation
  acute, 220, 226
  chronic, 220
  corticosteroids for, 236
  cytokines involved in, 220, 222
  definition of, 219
  description of, 124
  earthing effects on, 182
  flavonoids for. See Flavonoids
  markers of, 221
  nutrients associated with,
    224–225
  pro-inflammatory
    compounds, 214
  signs of, 219

Inflammation cycle, 244

Inflamyar, 175

Instantaneous axis of
  rotation, 114

Insulin, 256t

Insulin resistance, 85

Insulin-like growth factor, 230

Integrins, 12–13

Inter-articular dysfunction, 115t

Interferon-gamma, 231

Interleukin-1, 220

Interleukin-6, 198, 220, 231

Intermediate filaments, 13,
  39–40, 42f

Interstitial fibers, 63, 76

Interstitial receptors, 61–62, 76

Interval throwing program, 146

Intra-articular dysfunction, 115t

Intrafascial cells, 63–64

Intrafascial pre-tension, 63

Ischemia
adenosine triphosphate
production affected
by, 206
cell injury caused by, 207
definition of, 205
energy production affected
by, 206
microcirculation changes, 210
nutritional treatment of
bromelain, 212–213
enzymes, 212–214
fibrin removal, 213–214
immune complex
removal, 213
minerals, 211t, 211–212
nattokinase, 213
oxygen-derived free radicals
in, 209–210
pro-inflammatory compounds
in, 214
vascular endothelium affected
by, 206

Isokinetic strength testing, 268

Isoleucine, 192t

Isometric exercises
description of, 119–120
shoulder strengthening,
138–140, 139f–141f

Isotonic exercise, 120

K

Keratan sulfate, 10t

Klebsiella pneumoniae, 88

L

Laboratory tests, 257t–258t

Lactoferrin, 224–225

Lamellipodia, 42

Lamina intertendinosa dorsalis
manus, 31t

Lamina media, 22t

Lamina profunda, 22t–23t

Lamina profunda fasciae
abdominis superficialis,
25t–26t

Lamina superficialis, 22t

Lamina superficialis dorsalis
manus, 31t

Lamina superficialis fasciae
abdominis superficialis, 25t

Laminin, 11–12

Laser therapy, 171–175, 173f, 268

Leucine, 192t

Ligamentum denticulatum, 59

5-Lipoxygenase, 222, 224

Loading, external, 53–54

Local anesthetic injections,
235–236

Local injection therapies, 235–236

Lower extremity
adductors, 102
fascia of, 32t–34t
gastrocnemius, 102–103,
104f
hamstrings. *See* Hamstring
injuries
myofascial injuries, 100–103
quadriceps, 102

Low-level laser therapy, 171–175,
173f, 268

Luteinizing hormone, 260

Lymphatic capillaries, 73

Lymphatic system, 84–85

Lysine, 192t

M

Macrophages, 4

Magnesium, 211t, 212

Magnetic resonance imaging
advantages of, 103

gastrocnemius injuries
evaluated using, 102–103
indications for, 108
muscle strains evaluated
using, 97–99, 98f,
100f, 267
principles of, 95

Magnetic therapy, 168

Males, 18–19

Manganese, 211t

Manual fascia therapy,
55–56

Manual resistance technique, 119

Massage therapy, 168

Mast cells, 2–3, 81f, 220–221

Mechanical properties, 70

Mechanical roles
movement, 80–81
transmission of force, 83

Mechanical signal transduction,
177, 178f

Mechanical traction
microtrauma, 254

Mechanoreceptors, 56, 61, 63t, 76,
119, 179

Mechanotransduction, 42–43,
46, 51

Medicine ball throws, 144f

Meningeal layer, of cranial dura
mater, 57–58

Meninges
arachnoid mater, 58–59
dura mater, 57–58
pia mater, 59

Metabolism, 83–84

Methionine, 192t

Microcirculation, ischemia-related
changes in, 210

Microcurrent therapy, frequency-
specific, 169–171

Microfailure, 54–55

Microfilaments, 40f, 40–41

Microtubules, 13, 40

Minerals, 211t, 211–212

Mitochondrial oxidative stress, 184

Monocytes, 87

Motor neurons, 60

Movement, gliding, 80–81

Movement dysfunction
  description of, 114–115
  rehabilitation strategy
    for, 117

Multisegmental dysfunction,
  115–116

Muscle
  amino acids derived from, 190,
    191t–193t
  anatomy of, 104, 104f
  deep fascia and, interface
    between, 80–81, 82f, 87
  imaging of, 104
  protein from, 190
  regeneration of, 197–198
  skeletal. See Skeletal muscle

Muscle activation technique,
  133–134

Muscle strains
  characteristics of, 104
  gastrocnemius, 102f
  grade I, 97, 98f, 104f, 104–105
  grade II, 97–99, 98f, 105, 105f
  grade III, 99, 100f, 105, 105f
  groin, 266
  hamstring. See Hamstring
    injuries
  magnetic resonance imaging
    of, 97–99, 98f, 100f
  muscles predisposed to, 104
  return to play after,
    266–268, 269t

Musculoskeletal system
  tensegrity in, 43
  thixotropy, 44–45, 47

Myofascia
  definition of, 245
  dysfunction of,
    242–243

Myofascial injuries
  adductors, 102
  hamstrings. See Hamstring
    injuries
  imaging of, 95–96
  lower extremity, 100–103
  pectoralis major tears, 99–100
  quadriceps, 102
  sequelae of, 242
  upper extremity, 99–100, 101f

Myofascial meridians, 245,
  247–249

Myofascial pain
  causes of, 94
  differential diagnosis, 94–95
  laboratory tests for, 95–99
  recurrent, 242
  trigger points that cause, 94

Myofascial sling, 247

Myofascial stretching
  for Achilles tendon repair, 253
  for anterior cruciate ligament
    repair, 252
  description of, 118
  for supraspinatus muscle repair
    rehabilitation, 250

Myofascial therapy
  focus of, 179
  goals of, 76
  osteitis pubis treated
    with, 268
  taking out the slack, 54
  tissue plasticity in, 64f

Myofascial trigger points, 55, 94

Myofibroblasts, 63–64

Myotendinous junction, 96,
  101, 105

N

N-acetylcysteine, 191t

NAD(P)H oxidase, 182–184

Nattokinase, 213

Neck fascia, 21t–23t

Necrotizing fasciitis, 88

Nervous system
  autonomic, 60
  central, 56–59
  description of, 56
  peripheral, 56, 59–60

Neural plasticity, 62

Neural tension, adverse, 248

Neurotransmitters, 65

Neutrophils, 87, 233

Nicotinamide-adenine
  dinucleotide, 210

Nitric oxide, 182

Nociceptors
  description of, 59–60, 62
  pain transmission by, 62
  sleeping, 63
  stability and plasticity of,
    62–63
  tissue injury reactions by, 63

No-flow phenomenon, 210

Nonsteroidal anti-inflammatory
  drugs, 233–235, 237

Nuclear factor kappa beta,
  197, 222

Nutrition
  caloric intake, 190
  carbohydrates, 194
  connective tissue healing
    affected by, 190–195
  fats, 194–195
  inflammation and, 224–225
  ischemia treated with. See
    Ischemia, nutritional
    treatment of
  protein, 190, 193–194
  recommendations for, 195

Nutritional supplements
  aloe vera, 197, 201t
  arginine, 125–126, 191t,
    195–196, 200t
  bromelain, 125–126, 197, 201t
  carnosine, 125–126, 196, 200t
  Centella, 198

cetylated monounsaturated
  fatty acid, 200, 201t
copper, 125–126, 196, 200t
curcumin, 197–198, 201t
eicosapentaenoic acid, 196–197
glutamine, 192t, 196
orthosilicic acid, 196, 200t
summary of, 200t–201t
superoxide dismutase, 198,
  201t
vitamin A, 198, 201t
vitamin B$_5$, 200, 201t
vitamin C, 198–200, 201t
zinc, 196, 200t

O

Omega-3 fatty acids, 194,
  196–197, 225
Omega-6 fatty acids, 194
Ornithine, 193t
Orthosilicic acid, 196, 200t
Oschman, James, 167
Osteitis pubis, 254–269
Oxidative stress, 184
Oxygen-derived free radicals,
  209–210

P

Pacinian corpuscle, 62t, 76
Pain
  Boswellia for, 221
  myofascial. See Myofascial pain
  nociceptive transmission of, 62
Papain, 212
Parasympathetic nervous system, 60
Pathological conditions
  compartment syndrome, 88
  infections, 88
  insulin resistance, 85
  plantar fasciitis, 88–89
  scarring, 87–88, 88f

Pectoralis major
  tears of, 99–100, 101f
Pelvis fascia, 27t–28t
Perifascial fluid, 97
Perimysial space, 85
Perimysium
  definition of, 4
  description of, 4, 79
  imaging of, 86f, 104f
Peripheral nervous system,
  56, 59–60
PH$_4$, 6
Pharmacology
  antifibrotics, 231–232
  definition of, 229
  growth factors, 230–231, 237
  nonsteroidal anti-inflammatory
    drugs, 233–235, 237
Phenylalanine, 193t
Physiological roles
  hemodynamics, 84
  lymphatics, 84–85
  metabolism, 83–84
Pia mater, 59
Piezoelectricity
  characteristics of, 46t, 168
  description of, 51
Plantar aponeurosis, 34t, 82
Plantar fasciitis, 88–89
Plasmin, 207, 213
Plasticity, 51, 56, 70
Platelet-activating factor, 209, 212
Platelets, 209, 214
Plexuses, 59
Plyometrics
  description of, 120
  shoulder exercises,
    143–144, 144f
Polymorphonuclear leukocytes, 211
Polysaccharide gel complex. See
  Ground substance

Polyunsaturated fatty acids,
  194, 196
Pompage, 118
Posterior longitudinal ligament, 58
Potassium, 211t
Pretracheal fascia, 131t
Procollagen, 4, 6
Proelastin, 7
Profilin, 42
Pro-inflammatory compounds, 214
Proline, 73
Proprioception, 119, 251
Proprioceptive neuromuscular
  facilitation, 135
Proprioceptors, 61
Prostaglandins
  COX-1–derived reduction in, 234
  description of, 225
  E2, 194, 197
Protein
  amino acids, 191t–193t
  from connective tissue, 193
  description of, 190
  from muscle, 190
Protein malnutrition, 193
Proteoglycans, 1, 9, 74
Prothrombin, 208
Protrusion stage, of cellular
  motility, 42
Pyridoxal 5'-phosphate, 224

Q

Quadriceps injuries, 102
Quercetin, 221

R

Radiculopathy, 95
Range of motion exercises, 134–135

Reactive oxygen species
  description of, 182–183, 205, 207, 221
  nonsteroidal anti-inflammatory drug inhibition of, 233

Receptors
  interstitial, 61–62, 62t, 76
  mechanoreceptors, 56, 61, 62t, 76
  sensory, 60–61

Rectus femoris, 105f

Redox signaling, 182–183

Reflex, 60

Reflex arc, 60

Regional dysfunction, 115t

Rehabilitation
  adhesive capsulitis. See Adhesive capsulitis treatment and rehabilitation
  anterior cruciate ligament. See Anterior cruciate ligament rehabilitation
  dynamic stability restoration through, 117
  functional stage of, 265–266
  principles of, 115–116
  return to play after, 266–268, 268t
  RICE therapy, 116
  risk management strategies after, 267

Relaxin, 232

Reperfusion injury, 206–207

Resistance, 70

Rest, 116

Resveratrol, 222, 223f

Reticular fibers, 7

Retromammary space, 18

RICE therapy, 116

Risk management, 267

Ruffini angle, 180t

Ruffini endings, 61, 63

Ruffini's organ, 76

S

Satellite cells, 87

Scapula
  articular pumping of, 132t, 133f
  seated scapular pinches, 141
  stabilization exercises for, 138, 142–143, 143f

Scar tissue, 87–88, 88f, 220. See also Adhesions

Scarpa's fascia, 18–19, 25t–26t

Seated scapular pinches, 141

Segmental translational motion, 114

Selenium, 211t, 212

Semiconduction, 48t, 168

Sensory receptors, 60–61

Serine, 193t

Short saphenous vein, 84, 84f

Short-range elastic component, of muscle tissue, 44

Shoulder
  adhesive capsulitis treatment and rehabilitation. See Adhesive capsulitis treatment and rehabilitation
  external rotation exercises for, 139
  isometric strengthening exercises for, 138–140, 139f–141f
  three-way stretch of, 139, 139f

Shoulder pain, 106f–107f

Shoulder stretch, 134

Signal production, 46

Signal transduction, 42, 177, 178f

Skeletal muscle
  anatomy of, 96
  description of, 83
  fibers of, 96
  imaging of, 96–97
  lymph flow in, 84

Skeletal muscle cells, 96

Sleeping nociceptors, 63

Smooth muscle cells
  carbon dioxide effects on, 65
  contraction caused by, 63, 65
  description of, 57f, 63

Snelson model, 38f

Soft tissue injuries
  active release technique for. See Active release technique
  local injection therapies for, 235–236
  manual therapy for, 118–120
  pharmacological management of. See Pharmacology
  rehabilitation of, 115–117
  RICE therapy for, 116

Soluble fibrin monomer, 209

Somatic motor neurons, 60

Somatic recall, 45–47

Somatic reflexes, 60

Sound-assisted soft tissue mobilization, 133

Spatia interaponeurotica pedis, 34t

Spinal nerves, 59

Strain. See Muscle strains

Strength endurance training, 150, 152–155

Stress fibers, 41

Stretch reflex, 60

Stretching, 118

Subarachnoid space, 58–59

Subcutaneous connective tissue, 81

Subcutaneous tissue. See also Fascia superficialis
  description of, 85
  stretch of, 2, 3f

Subscapularis, 142–143

Subtalar joint, 247

Superficial back line, 245, 247–248

Superficial fascia. See also Fascia superficialis
  characteristics of, 79

description of, 8
functions of, 79

Superficial front line, 245,
247–248

Superoxide anion, 208

Superoxide dismutase, 198, 201t,
210, 225

Supine cervical retractions, 141

Supraspinatus muscle
function of, 250
tear of, 249–251
tendon, 105f

Suramin, 231

Sympathetic nervous system, 60

T

T mast cells, 3

Taking out the slack, 54

Taurine, 193t

TC mast cells, 3

Tendinopathy, 106f

Tendon
Achilles. See Achilles tendon
cross-sectional area of, 82
supraspinatus muscle, 105f

Tennis leg, 102

Tensegrity
adhesions, 74
at cellular level, 39–42
history of, 38
in musculoskeletal system,
43
myofascia and, 43
summary of, 47

Tensegrity structures
application of force to, 43
dehydration effects on,
71–74
description of, 38–39

Testosterone, 256t–257t, 260

Thenar fascia, 31t

Thixotropy
description of, 43–45, 47
plasticity and, 51

Thorax fascia, 23t–25t

Threonine, 193t

Thrombin, 206, 208–209

Thrombin–antithrombin
complexes, 209

Thyroid-stimulating hormone, 256t

Tissue factor, 206

Tissue plasminogen activator, 207

Tissue plasticity, 51

Tissue stretching
collageno-elastic complex
response to, 8
fibroblast reaction to, 2, 3f

Traction stage, of cellular
motility, 42

Traditional Chinese medicine, 176

Transforming growth factor beta-
1, 220, 231–232, 232f

Transmission of force, 83

Traumeel, 236

Treadmill retrograde hill walk,
152–153, 154t

Treatment
adhesive capsulitis. See
Adhesive capsulitis treatment
and rehabilitation
anterior cruciate ligament. See
Anterior cruciate ligament
rehabilitation
osteitis pubis, 260, 261t–265t
pharmacologic. See
Pharmacology

Tropocollagen, 6–7, 71

Tropoelastin, 7

Tryptase, 3

Tryptophan, 193t

Tumor necrosis factor,
198, 220

Turmeric, 221–222

T1-weighted images, 97

T2-weighted images, 97

Tyrosine, 193t

U

Ultrasound
advantages of, 103
description of, 95
indications for, 108
muscle strains evaluated using,
104–105, 105f
musculoskeletal interventions
guided using, 105–106,
106f–108f
principles of, 103

Unipennate muscles, 104

Upper extremity
fascia of, 29t–31t
pectoralis major tears, 99–100,
101f

Uronic acid, 9

V

Vagal tone, 63

Valine, 193t

Vanadium, 211t

Vascular endothelial growth
factor, 231

Vascular system, 84

Vasoconstriction, 87

Vibrations, 168, 184

Visceral reflexes, 60

Viscosity, 70

Vitamin A, 198, 201t

Vitamin B$_5$, 200, 201t

Vitamin B$_6$, 224

Vitamin C, 198–200, 201t

Vitamin E, 199

W

Water
  assessments of, 75
  body percentages of, 70
  body temperature regulation
    by, 71
  in collagen, 71
  daily intake of, 76–77
  extracellular matrix content
    of, 11
  after frequency-specific
    microcurrent therapy, 171
  functions of, 76
    ground substance and, 74–76
    lubricant properties of, 70
    maintenance dose of, 76–77
    physiological purposes of, 70–71

White adipose tissue, 5, 83–84

Wound healing. *See* Healing

X

Xanthine dehydrogenase,
  210–211

Xanthine oxidase, 210

Z

Zellulisan ointment, 175

Zinc
  description of, 196, 200t
  ischemia treated with,
    211t, 212

Zones of adherence, 19t,
  19–20